**NATIONAL** *Sciences*
**ACADEMIES** *Engineering*
*Medicine*

T0295439

NATIONAL
ACADEMIES
PRESS
Washington, DC

# Evidence Review of the Adverse Effects of COVID-19 Vaccination and Intramuscular Vaccine Administration

Anne R. Bass, Kathleen Stratton,
Ogan K. Kumova, and Dara Rosenberg, *Editors*

Committee to Review Relevant Literature
Regarding Adverse Events Associated with Vaccines

Board on Population Health and
Public Health Practice

Health and Medicine Division

Consensus Study Report

**THE NATIONAL ACADEMIES PRESS 500 Fifth Street, NW Washington, DC 20001**

This activity was supported by a contract between the National Academy of Sciences and Health Resources and Services Administration, which includes funds from the Centers for Disease Control and Prevention. Any opinions, findings, conclusions, or recommendations expressed in this publication do not necessarily reflect the views of any organization or agency that provided support for the project.

International Standard Book Number-13: 978-0-309-71832-5
International Standard Book Number-10: 0-309-71832-5
Digital Object Identifier: https://doi.org/10.17226/27746
Library of Congress Control Number: 2024941529

This publication is available from the National Academies Press, 500 Fifth Street, NW, Keck 360, Washington, DC 20001; (800) 624-6242 or (202) 334-3313; http://www.nap.edu.

Suggested citation: National Academies of Sciences, Engineering, and Medicine. 2024. *Evidence review of the adverse effects of COVID-19 vaccination and intramuscular vaccine administration.* Washington, DC: The National Academies Press. https://doi.org/10.17226/27746.

The **National Academy of Sciences** was established in 1863 by an Act of Congress, signed by President Lincoln, as a private, nongovernmental institution to advise the nation on issues related to science and technology. Members are elected by their peers for outstanding contributions to research. Dr. Marcia McNutt is president.

The **National Academy of Engineering** was established in 1964 under the charter of the National Academy of Sciences to bring the practices of engineering to advising the nation. Members are elected by their peers for extraordinary contributions to engineering. Dr. John L. Anderson is president.

The **National Academy of Medicine** (formerly the Institute of Medicine) was established in 1970 under the charter of the National Academy of Sciences to advise the nation on medical and health issues. Members are elected by their peers for distinguished contributions to medicine and health. Dr. Victor J. Dzau is president.

The three Academies work together as the **National Academies of Sciences, Engineering, and Medicine** to provide independent, objective analysis and advice to the nation and conduct other activities to solve complex problems and inform public policy decisions. The National Academies also encourage education and research, recognize outstanding contributions to knowledge, and increase public understanding in matters of science, engineering, and medicine.

Learn more about the National Academies of Sciences, Engineering, and Medicine at **www.nationalacademies. org**.

# COMMITTEE TO REVIEW RELEVANT LITERATURE REGARDING ADVERSE EVENTS ASSOCIATED WITH VACCINES

**GEORGE J. ISHAM** (*Chair*), Senior Fellow, HealthPartners Institute

**ANNE R. BASS** (*Vice Chair*), Professor of Clinical Medicine, Department of Medicine, Division of Rheumatology, Hospital for Special Surgery, Weill Cornell Medicine

**ALICIA CHRISTY,** Professor of Obstetrics and Gynecology, Uniformed Services University; Adjunct Professor, Howard University School of Medicine

**DeLISA FAIRWEATHER,** Professor of Medicine, Director of Translational Research, Department of Cardiovascular Medicine; Codirector of Research for the Ehlers-Danlos Syndrome Clinic, Department of General Internal Medicine, Mayo Clinic (Jacksonville, FL)

**JAMES S. FLOYD,** Codirector of the Cardiovascular Health Research Unit, Associate Professor of Medicine, Adjunct Professor of Epidemiology, University of Washington

**ERIC J. HEGEDUS,** Professor and Chair, Department of Rehabilitation Science, Tufts University School of Medicine

**CHANDY C. JOHN,** Ryan White Professor of Pediatrics, Professor of Medicine, Professor of Microbiology and Immunology, Director of the Ryan White Center for Pediatric Infectious Diseases and Global Health, Indiana University School of Medicine

**JOHN EDWARD KUHN,** Schermerhorn Professor of Orthopaedic Surgery, Chief of Shoulder Surgery, Department of Orthopaedic Surgery, Vanderbilt University Medical Center

**EVAN MAYO-WILSON,** Associate Professor, Department of Epidemiology, University of North Carolina Gillings School of Global Public Health

**THOMAS LEE ORTEL,** Chief, Division of Hematology, Department of Medicine; Professor of Medicine and Pathology, Duke University School of Medicine

**NICHOLAS S. REED,** Assistant Professor, Department of Epidemiology, Johns Hopkins Bloomberg School of Public Health; Assistant Professor, Department of Otolaryngology, Division of Otology/Audiology, Johns Hopkins University School of Medicine

**ANDY S. STERGACHIS,** Professor and Associate Dean of Pharmacy, School of Pharmacy; Professor of Global Health, School of Public Health, University of Washington

**MICHEL TOLEDANO,** Assistant Professor of Neurology, Department of Neurology, Mayo Clinic (Rochester, MN)

**ROBERT B. WALLACE,** Irene Ensmenger Stecher Professor Emeritus of Epidemiology and Internal Medicine, University of Iowa

**OUSSENY ZERBO,** Research Scientist II, Vaccine Study Center, Division of Research, Kaiser Permanente Northern California

*National Academy of Medicine Fellow*

**INMACULADA HERNANDEZ,** Professor, San Diego Skaggs School of Pharmacy and Pharmaceutical Sciences, University of California

*Health and Medicine Division Staff*

**KATHLEEN STRATTON,** Study Director
**OGAN K. KUMOVA,** Program Officer (*since February 2023*)
**DARA ROSENBERG,** Associate Program Officer
**NERISSA HART,** Senior Program Assistant (*through May 2023*)
**OLIVIA LOIBNER,** Senior Program Assistant (*since June 2023*)
**MISRAK DABI,** Finance Business Partner

# Reviewers

This Consensus Study Report was reviewed in draft form by individuals chosen for their diverse perspectives and technical expertise. The purpose of this independent review is to provide candid and critical comments that will assist the National Academies of Sciences, Engineering, and Medicine in making each published report as sound as possible and to ensure that it meets the institutional standards for quality, objectivity, evidence, and responsiveness to the study charge. The review comments and draft manuscript remain confidential to protect the integrity of the deliberative process.

We thank the following individuals for their review of this report:

**DOUGLAS B. CINES,** Director, Coagulation Laboratory; Director, Office of Faculty Development, Pathology and Laboratory Medicine; Professor of Pathology and Laboratory Medicine (Hematology-Oncology), University of Pennsylvania School of Medicine

**BETTY DIAMOND,** Director, Institute of Molecular Medicine, The Feinstein Institutes for Medical Research North Shore-LIJ Health System, Northwell Health

**KATHRYN EDWARDS,** Professor of Pediatrics; Sarah H. Sell and Cornelius Vanderbilt Chair, Vanderbilt Vaccine Research Program, Vanderbilt University Medical Center

**MARIE GRIFFIN,** Professor Emerita, Vanderbilt University School of Medicine

**AKIKO IWASAKI,** Howard Hughes Medical Institute Investigator; Director, Center for Infection and Immunity; Sterling Professor of Immunobiology and Molecular, Cellular, and Developmental Biology, Yale University

**EMILY JUNGHEIM,** Chief of Reproductive Endocrinology and Infertility in the Department of Obstetrics and Gynecology, Northwestern University

**GRACE M. LEE,** Professor of Pediatrics, Stanford Medicine Children's Health

**TIANJING LI,** Associate Professor, University of Colorado Anschutz Medical Campus

**JENNIFER S. LIN,** Distinguished Investigator, Kaiser Permanente Center for Health Research

**CLAUDIA LUCCHINETTI,** Dean, Dell Medical School; Senior Vice President for Medical Affairs, University of Texas at Austin

**H. CODY MEISSNER,** Professor of Pediatrics and Medicine, Geisel School of Medicine at Dartmouth; Senior Vaccine and Biologics Development Analyst, Biomedical Advanced Research and Development Authority; Administration for Strategic Preparedness and Response, U.S. Department of Health and Human Services

**BRIAN OLSHANSKY,** Emeritus Professor of Internal Medicine–Cardiovascular Medicine, Carver College of Medicine, University of Iowa, University of Iowa Hospitals and Clinics

**JAMES SEGARS,** Director, Division of Reproductive Sciences and Women's Health Research, Johns Hopkins University School of Medicine

**UMASUTHAN SRIKUMARAN,** Assistant Professor, Orthopaedic Surgery, Johns Hopkins University

**GRETA C. STAMPER,** Audiology Division Chair, Audiology Externship Program Director, Consultant in Otorhinolaryngology, Mayo Clinic

Although the reviewers listed above provided many constructive comments and suggestions, they were not asked to endorse the conclusions or recommendations of this report, nor did they see the final draft before its release. The review of this report was overseen by coordinator **DAVID SAVITZ,** Professor of Epidemiology, Brown University, and monitor **WALTER FRONTERA,** Professor of Physical Medicine, Rehabilitation, and Sports Medicine, University of Puerto Rico School of Medicine. They were responsible for making certain that an independent examination of this report was carried out in accordance with the standards of the National Academies and that all review comments were carefully considered. Responsibility for the final content rests entirely with the authoring committee and the National Academies.

# Acknowledgments

The Committee to Review Relevant Literature Regarding Adverse Events Associated with Vaccines and the committee staff would like to thank many individuals for their contributions throughout all phases of the study: Misrak Dabi (Finance Business Partner), Crysti Park (Program Coordinator), Lori Brenig (Editorial Projects Coordinator), Taryn Young (Report Review Associate), Leslie Sim (Senior Report Review Officer), Benjamin Hubbert (Communications Specialist), Amber McLaughlin (Director of Communications), Tasha Bigelow (Copy Editor), Rebecca Morgan (Senior Research Librarian), and Anne Marie Houppert (Senior Research Librarian).

The committee acknowledges and thanks the members of the public who provided valuable insight to the committee via email correspondence and in public comments.

# Contents

# Boxes, Figures, and Tables

## BOXES

## FIGURES

## TABLES

# Preface

In the 4 years since the first case of COVID-19 was recognized and after a pandemic was declared by the World Health Organization 3 months later in March 2020, an estimated 3.5 million died from SARS-CoV-2 infection. Millions more became ill, and some have suffered long-term effects ("long COVID") that are not yet understood fully. Aside from its health impact, the pandemic has caused marked social, economic, and political upheaval. We doubt any have had lives unchanged by COVID-19.

The response to the pandemic has been extraordinary. By spring 2021, only 1 year after the pandemic declaration, vaccines authorized by the Food and Drug Administration for emergency use were being administered across the United States, indeed, around the world. It is estimated that more than 14 million lives were saved in the year after vaccines became available, with one death avoided for every 124 full vaccination courses. Lives were also saved by other public health interventions and often-heroic efforts of health care workers and health care systems.

In the 3 years since vaccines against SARS-CoV-2 came into use, their safety and efficacy have been established. Booster vaccinations and vaccines targeting new SARS-CoV-2 strains have been introduced and are now administered routinely alongside other vaccinations such as for influenza. While local, nonserious side effects, such as malaise or sore arm, are seen as with any vaccine, in rare instances, serious adverse events thought to be linked to SARS-CoV-2 vaccination have been noted.

The National Academies of Sciences, Engineering, and Medicine (the National Academies) have long tackled challenging questions about vaccine safety, beginning with an assessment of the oral polio vaccine in 1977. When Congress enacted the National Childhood Vaccine Injury Act in 1986, it charged the Institute of Medicine (IOM) with reviewing the literature regarding adverse events associated with vaccines covered by the program. The IOM[1] has addressed questions about the safety of routinely administered vaccines 11 times since then. Following in this tradition, the National Academies tasked this consensus committee to assess the scientific evidence dispassionately regarding a list of harms potentially associated with vaccination against SARS-CoV-2, as well as an important potential harm associated with the administration of any vaccine, shoulder injury.

Thanks to the extraordinary efforts of investigators around the world who rapidly pivoted their research efforts to focus on this new virus (including its treatment and prevention), we now have a large body of evidence to consider. However, despite that large body of evidence, our consensus committee found that in many, if not most,

---

[1]As of March 2016, the Health and Medicine Division continues the consensus studies and convening activities previously carried out by the Institute of Medicine (IOM).

cases, the evidence was insufficient to accept or reject causality for a particular potential harm from a specific COVID-19 vaccine. In other cases, however, the committee considered the evidence to be *sufficient* to "favor rejection" of, to "favor acceptance" of, or to "establish causality."

Limitations inherent in applying population-level average effects to draw conclusions about causes of specific events in individual subjects exist. For this reason, there is asymmetry in the committee's conclusions, with options to conclude that the evidence "establishes a causal relationship," "favors acceptance of causal relationship," or "favors rejection of a causal relationship," but not one to "establish rejection of a causal relationship."

For every potential harm assessed, the committee evaluated the totality of evidence and did not apply what could be seen as arbitrary rules or thresholds regarding the number or types of studies required to draw conclusions. For the evaluation of select postulated vaccine harms, some study types were simply not available or were uninformative. For some cases, there was strong mechanistic as well as epidemiologic evidence supporting a causal relationship (e.g., thrombosis with thrombocytopenia syndrome), while, in others, the evidence was drawn largely from case reports.

COVID-19 has, understandably, dominated headlines over the past 3 years, yet routine vaccinations, such as for seasonal influenza, are still given. The harms our committee was tasked to review were those for which the Health Resources and Services Administration had claims for compensation. Perhaps surprisingly, only a minority of these claims related to SARS-CoV-2 vaccination. In fact, over 60 percent of claims focused on shoulder injury associated with intramuscular vaccine administration.

The term "SIRVA" (shoulder injury related to vaccine administration) has been introduced into the literature in recent years and was included in the committee's Statement of Task. However, the term "SIRVA" encompasses many disparate shoulder conditions, and due to its lack of precision, the committee decided to dispense with this terminology. Instead, the committee addressed potential causal relationships between vaccine administration and specific shoulder-related medical diagnoses (e.g., subacromial bursitis, radial nerve injury).

This report does not address benefits of vaccination against SARS-CoV-2 or other pathogens, and readers will hopefully view causality findings in that broader context. Even when evidence of causality was established for some harms, the frequency of these harms was low. However, this report explicitly does not attempt to define point estimates for levels of risk.

Many talented, knowledgeable individuals volunteered hours of their time to analyze and report the evidence. Initially strangers, the members of this committee worked through difficult methodological questions together, at times engaging in spirited debate. In the process, we learned from one another, became a team, and became friends. Equally important, members of that team were the committee staff—Dara Rosenberg, Ogan Kumova, and Olivia Loibner, led by the incredibly wise and knowledgeable Kathleen Stratton and Rose Marie Martinez. The staff worked tirelessly every step of the way, providing indispensable support and guidance, and contributing greatly to the report itself.

This is not the first HMD/National Academies report regarding vaccine safety. Nor will it be the last. We anticipate new vaccines and expect that ongoing and future scientific research may challenge the findings reported here. This report necessarily reflects a snapshot in time, albeit a momentous one, and represents our best effort to report the truth.

George J. Isham, *Chair*
Anne R. Bass, *Vice Chair*
Committee to Review Relevant Literature Regarding
Adverse Events Associated with Vaccines

# Acronyms and Abbreviations

AAOS        American Academy of Orthopaedic Surgeons
ACE2        angiotensin-converting enzyme 2
ADE         antibody dependent enhancement
ADEM        acute disseminated encephalomyelitis
AFC         antral follicle count
AIDP        acute inflammatory demyelinating polyneuropathy
AMAN        acute motor axonal neuropathy
AMH         anti-Müllerian hormone
AV          adenovirus vector

BP          Bell's palsy
bpm         beats per minute

CAR         coxsackie and adenoviral receptor
CDC         Centers for Disease Control and Prevention
CGRP        calcitonin gene–related peptide
CI          confidence interval
CICP        Countermeasures Injury Compensation Program
CIDP        chronic inflammatory demyelinating polyneuropathy
CLS         capillary leak syndrome
CPRD        Clinical Practice Research Datalink
CRPS        complex regional pain syndrome
CSF         cerebrospinal fluid
CT          computed tomography
CVST        cerebral venous sinus thrombosis

DCM         dilated cardiomyopathy
DNA         deoxyribonucleic acid
DTaP        diphtheria, tetanus, and acellular pertussis vaccine

DVT                deep vein thrombosis

EMG                electromyogram
EMR                electronic medical record
EUA                Emergency Use Authorization
EV                 extracellular vesicle

FDA                Food and Drug Administration
FR                 fecundity rate
FSH                follicle-stimulating hormone

GBS                Guillain-Barré syndrome
GC                 germinal center

HIT                heparin-induced thrombocytopenia
HLA                human leukocyte antigen
HPV                human papillomavirus
HR                 hazard ratio
HRSA               Health Resources and Services Administration
HS                 hemorrhagic stroke
HSV                herpes simplex virus

ICD                International Classification of Diseases
ICHD               International Classification of Headache Disorders
IFN                interferon
Ig                 immunoglobulin
IL                 interleukin
IOM                Institute of Medicine
IQR                interquartile range
IR                 incidence rate
IRR                incidence rate ratio
ITP                immune thrombocytopenic purpura
IV                 intravenous

LH                 luteinizing hormone
LLPC               long-lived plasma cell
LNP                lipid nanoparticle

MI                 myocardial infarction
MRI                magnetic resonance imaging
mRNA               messenger ribonucleic acid
MS                 multiple sclerosis

NCS                nerve conduction study
NCVIA              National Childhood Vaccine Injury Act
NIH                National Institutes of Health
NR                 not reported

O:E                observed-to-expected ratio
OHCA               out-of-hospital cardiac arrest

| OPV | oral polio vaccine |
| OR | odds ratio |
| | |
| PE | pulmonary embolism |
| PF4 | platelet factor 4 |
| POTS | postural orthostatic tachycardia syndrome |
| PPV | positive predictive value |
| PTS | Parsonage-Turner syndrome |
| | |
| RBD | receptor-binding domain |
| RCT | randomized controlled trial |
| RI | relative incidence |
| RNA | ribonucleic acid |
| RR | relative risk or risk ratio |
| RSV | respiratory syncytial virus |
| | |
| SARS-CoV-2 | severe acute respiratory syndrome coronavirus-2 |
| SCCS | self-controlled case series |
| SHBG | sex hormone binding globulin |
| SIDIAP | Information System for the Development of Research in Primary Care |
| SIR | standardized incidence ratio |
| SIRVA | shoulder injury related to vaccine administration |
| SPOR | Strategy for Patient-Oriented Research |
| SSNHL | sudden sensorineural hearing loss |
| SSP | supraspinatus |
| SUD | sudden unexpected death |
| | |
| Tfh | T follicular helper |
| TLR | Toll-like receptor |
| TM | transverse myelitis |
| TNF | tumor necrosis factor |
| TTH | tension-type headache |
| TTS | thrombosis with thrombocytopenia syndrome |
| | |
| UI | uncertainty interval |
| | |
| VAED | vaccine-associated enhanced disease |
| VAERS | Vaccine Adverse Event Reporting System |
| VICP | Vaccine Injury Compensation Program |
| VITT | vaccine-induced immune thrombotic thrombocytopenia |
| VSD | Vaccine Safety Datalink |
| VTE | venous thromboembolism |
| | |
| WHO | World Health Organization |
| | |
| YLD | years lived with disability |
| YLL | years of life lost |

# Summary

Vaccines are a major public health success story, preventing or mitigating the effects of a myriad of infectious diseases. However, the threat of litigation over safety concerns related to the whole cell pertussis vaccines in particular led manufacturers to slow vaccine research and development and leave the market. In 1986, Congress addressed this looming crisis for public health by passing the National Childhood Vaccine Injury Act (P.L. 99-660) to improve federal coordination of vaccine efforts around research and development and address the concerns of those who asserted that they or their children were injured by vaccines. The Vaccine Injury Compensation Program (VICP), housed in the Health Resources and Services Administration (HRSA) in the Department of Health and Human Services and jointly administered by the Department of Justice, serves as a key policy solution developed by Congress. The program includes vaccines recommended for routine use in children or pregnant women, and anyone who receives those vaccines is eligible to apply for compensation. The VICP has long depended on the reports from the National Academies of Sciences, Engineering, and Medicine (the National Academies) as an important scientific contribution to its compensation decisions.

HRSA also administers the Countermeasures Injury Compensation Program (CICP) for those harmed by medical countermeasures, which include vaccines, medications, devices, or other preventions, diagnostics, or treatments for a public health emergency or security threat. Established by the Public Readiness and Emergency Preparedness Act of 2005 (P.L. 148, Division C), CICP differs significantly from VICP (HRSA, 2023a).

On January 31, 2020, the Secretary of Health and Human Services declared a public health emergency related to severe acute respiratory syndrome coronavirus-2 (SARS-CoV-2) under Section 319 of the Public Health Service Act. The public health emergency expired on May 11, 2023. The public health emergency was declared because SARS-CoV-2 and the disease caused by SARS-CoV-2, COVID-19, led to the greatest public health crisis to date of the 21st century. As of February 2024, it had led to an estimated 7 million deaths worldwide, including 1.2 million deaths in the United States (WHO, 2024). COVID-19 was a major cause of death and illness in both adults and children. In 2021, COVID-19 was the third most common cause of death in adults in the United States (CDC, 2021), and from 2020 to 2022, COVID-19 was among the top 10 causes of death in children in the United States (Flaxman et al., 2023).

Part of the public health emergency was the announcement of "Operation Warp Speed," a rapid response by the federal government to speed vaccine development (for detailed information, see GAO, 2021). Four vaccines were developed and used in the United States, all under Emergency Use Authorization (EUA) (see FDA, 2023), with some now fully approved by the Food and Drug Administration (FDA). However, as of June 1, 2023,

FDA revoked the EUA from Ad26.COV2.S for safety concerns (FDA, 2023). EUA allowed vaccines to be used before all phase 3 trials were completed.[1] COVID-19 vaccines, introduced in 2020, are highly effective in adults and children (CDC, 2023) and were key to control of the pandemic. COVID-19 vaccines are estimated to have prevented 14.4 million deaths worldwide in the first year of vaccination alone (Watson et al., 2022). Although in this report the committee is tasked with evaluating the causal association with select serious harm, a comparative study analyzing the prevalence and types of side effects following COVID-19 vaccination showed that the most common side effects across different vaccines were flu-like syndrome and local reactions at the injection site, which aligns with the side effect profiles of many vaccines (Yadegarynia et al., 2023).

## STATEMENT OF TASK

HRSA requested that the National Academies convene a committee to review the evidence regarding specific potential harms (see Box S-1 for the Statement of Task) related to the COVID-19 vaccines used in the United States. See Table 1-1 for a list of the vaccines and naming conventions used in this report. The list of harms includes those for which, when the project began, HRSA had claims for compensation. The committee added postural orthostatic tachycardia syndrome to its review after presentations at its second public meeting.

HRSA also requested that the committee review the evidence regarding any vaccine, not specifically COVID-19 vaccines, and shoulder injuries, to help VICP better understand whether vaccination can cause very specific types of shoulder injuries or a more general syndrome that it designated as shoulder injury related to vaccine administration (NASEM, 2023). Claims regarding shoulder injuries after routinely administered vaccines are handled by VICP; COVID-19 vaccines are currently the purview of CICP (HRSA, 2023b).

For the committee's work, it was irrelevant whether a vaccine is covered under VICP or CICP; the committee did not consider VICP or CICP processes when reviewing the evidence.

The National Academies convened an ad hoc committee comprising 15 members with expertise in epidemiology, causal inference, cardiology, rheumatology, gynecology, audiology, neurology, infectious disease, pediatrics, internal medicine, hematology, orthopedics, and immunology. The committee held two sessions open to the public. On January 30, 2023, it heard from representatives of HRSA and the Centers for Disease Control and Prevention on how they intend to use its report and why they asked for the review. On March 30, 2023, the committee held an open session during which members of the public registered to provide 3-minute statements concerning its task.

Although the committee reviewed the literature thoroughly, it did not conduct what is commonly referred to as a "systematic review," the formal steps of which were described by the Institute of Medicine (IOM) in 2011 (IOM, 2011). The processes and time frame for a systematic review were considered incompatible with this work, and, more importantly, the goals were different from those of most systematic reviews and clinical guidelines. The committee was not tasked with estimating the magnitude or strength of associations between vaccinations and outcomes. To fulfill its narrower goals, the committee did incorporate important attributes of good systematic reviews, such as searching multiple databases, using structured search terms, prespecifying a final date of searching, and using multiple reviewers to screen out irrelevant abstracts identified in the search. The committee does not address the benefits of vaccines, which have been established for COVID-19 vaccines and all vaccines covered by VICP. This review addresses evidence only about specific potential harms and vaccines available in the United States. The committee does not make conclusions regarding specific patient cases (such as reported in published case reports) or whether VICP or CICP should award compensation in individual cases or in general.

Vaccines and other medical products can cause both benefits and harms. Harms are sometimes described, including by previous IOM committees, using terms such as "adverse event," "adverse effect," "side effect," or "safety." Such terms might not convey the importance of unwanted medical events. Moreover, readers might be confused by the use of different terms with overlapping meanings or the same terms to mean different things in different contexts (Qureshi et al., 2022). For example, "adverse events" are defined in regulatory research as unwanted events not necessarily related to an intervention (e.g., a vaccine, a drug). By comparison, "adverse effects" are both unwanted and related to an intervention. On the other hand, "side effects" might be desirable or unwanted,

---

[1] The sentence was updated after the report was shared with the sponsor to clarify the EUA process.

---

**BOX S-1**
**Statement of Task**

The National Academies of Sciences, Engineering, and Medicine will convene an ad hoc committee to review the epidemiological, clinical, and biological evidence regarding the relationship between

- COVID-19 vaccines and specific adverse events i.e., Guillain-Barré Syndrome (GBS), chronic inflammatory demyelinating polyneuropathy (CIDP), transverse myelitis, Bell's palsy, hearing loss, tinnitus, chronic headaches, infertility, sudden death, myocarditis/pericarditis, thrombosis with thrombocytopenia syndrome (TTS), immune thrombocytopenic purpura (ITP), thromboembolic events (e.g., cerebrovascular accident (CVA), myocardial infarction (MI), pulmonary embolism, deep vein thrombosis (DVT)), capillary leak syndrome, and
- intramuscular administration of vaccines and shoulder injuries.

The committee will make conclusions about the causal association between vaccines and specific adverse events.

---

and they are related to an intervention. Following best practices (Junqueira et al., 2023; Zorzela et al., 2016), this report uses plain language to describe the opposite of benefits as "harms." To emphasize that an individual might or might not experience specific benefits or harms, this report sometimes describes them as "potential." Identifying a "harm" does not mean that it occurs frequently; harms associated with vaccines are rare. For example, vaccine-associated paralytic polio is an established harm of the oral polio vaccine (OPV), but it is estimated to occur at a rate of 1 in 2.7 million first doses of OPV (WHO, 2023).

The committee used different types of evidence to draw conclusions concerning possible associations between vaccination and potential harms. Some study types were not available or were considered uninformative for certain outcomes. Conclusions about causality were informed by the totality of the evidence without applying arbitrary rules or thresholds regarding the number or types of studies required to draw conclusions. For each outcome, the committee discussed the totality of the evidence and used consensus methods to draw conclusions about causality. Iterative discussions about the evidence were particularly important given the committee's decision not to use a formal grading system for each published article or for the causality conclusions. The committee used expert judgment based on clinical and research expertise and analysis, paying careful attention that all outcomes under study were evaluated similarly to ensure that a consistent approach to the causal conclusions was maintained.

The committee adopted the wording for the categories of causal conclusions used by the IOM vaccine safety committees (IOM, 1991, 1994, 2012), and approached the evaluation of evidence from a position of neutrality, presuming neither causation nor lack of causation. The conclusion categories are necessarily asymmetrical: although evidence can establish a causal relationship, the committee determined that it was unlikely that it could establish the *absence* of one for any harm. Similar to other evidence-review efforts, the committee incorporated the potential role of future research in determining the appropriate conclusion, as described below. See Box S-2 for a description of the categories.

## CONCLUSIONS

Given that this review occurred shortly after vaccines were available, the information in this report is a snapshot in time. New vaccines will be developed, and more research will be conducted. For example, the evidence does not address the real-world use of the COVID-19 vaccines in which many individuals received a "mix and match" sequence of them. Many people vaccinated for COVID-19 received other vaccines (e.g., influenza) simultaneously. Most of the evidence regarding COVID-19 vaccines was from the primary series; because children were among

---

**BOX S-2**
**Categories of Causation**

- *Evidence establishes a causal relationship*—The totality of the evidence suggests that vaccination can cause this harm. Further research is unlikely to lead to a different conclusion.
- *Evidence favors acceptance of a causal relationship*—The totality of the evidence suggests that vaccination might cause this harm, but meaningful uncertainty remains. Studies that better minimize bias and confounding, and studies that estimate effects more precisely, could lead to a different conclusion.
- *Evidence is inadequate to accept or reject a causal relationship*—The available evidence is too limited (e.g., few studies in humans, biased, imprecise) or inconsistent to draw meaningful conclusions in support of or against causality. Future research could lead to a different conclusion. This conclusion also applies to situations in which no studies were identified.
- *Evidence favors rejection of a causal relationship*—The totality of the evidence suggests that vaccination does not cause this harm, but meaningful uncertainty remains. The committee acknowledges that individual causal effects are difficult to ascertain and that limitations exist for applying population average effects to draw conclusions about the causes of specific events in individual people. For example, it is possible that both vaccination and disease cause certain harms. Thus, (1) an event could be more common in an unvaccinated than a vaccinated population, and (2) some of the events in the vaccinated population could be caused by vaccination. Research demonstrating a clear mechanism of action, or research demonstrating increased risk among vaccinated people compared with unvaccinated people, could lead to a different conclusion.

---

the last groups to be vaccinated, less evidence exists about them. The committee was not charged to evaluate the benefits of vaccines. All conclusions must be assessed in the context of the established harms of the infections against which a vaccine is directed and the well-documented benefits of vaccines in preventing those harms.

The committee makes 85 conclusions in eight chapters about the causal relationship between vaccines and possible harms. Although the committee lacked evidence to establish, accept, or reject a causal relationship for many possible harms, it identified sufficient evidence for 20 conclusions. It is not surprising that evidence is insufficient for the majority; many of the conditions had relatively few studies in the literature from which to draw conclusions. As Box S-2 indicates, the committee incorporated the notion that further research might lead to a different conclusion for all but conclusions establishing causation. See Tables S-1 and S-2 for all committee conclusions.

### Conclusions by Vaccine

Most of the evidence the committee reviewed addressed BNT162b2.[2] This is not surprising, as it was the first available in the United States and many other countries; mRNA-1273[3] followed quickly, and many studies addressed it as well. Conversely, NVX-CoV2373 was the last vaccine available in the United States, and the committee identified no published studies relevant for review. FDA revoked the authorization for Ad26.COV2.S,[4] and the small number of studies reflected that short availability.

The causality conclusions for the two messenger ribonucleic acid (mRNA) vaccines (BNT162b2 and mRNA-1273) were almost identical; the committee found convincing evidence that established a causal relationship with myocarditis. In contrast, the committee concluded that the evidence favored rejection of a causal relationship between both mRNA vaccines and thrombosis with thrombocytopenia syndrome (TTS), infertility, Guillain-Barré syndrome

---

[2] Refers to the COVID-19 vaccine manufactured by Pfizer-BioNTech under the name Comirnaty®.

[3] Refers to the COVID-19 vaccine manufactured by Moderna under the name Spikevax®.

[4] Refers to the COVID-19 vaccine manufactured by Janssen.

**TABLE S-1** Causal Conclusions Regarding COVID-19 Vaccines

| Chapter | Potential Harm | Causality Conclusions | | | |
|---|---|---|---|---|---|
| | | BNT162b2 (Pfizer-BioNTech) | mRNA-1273 (Moderna) | Ad26.COV2.S (Janssen) | NVX-CoV2373 (Novavax) |
| 3 | Guillain-Barré syndrome | Favors rejection of a causal relationship | Favors rejection of a causal relationship | Favors acceptance of a causal relationship | I |
| | Chronic inflammatory demyelinating polyneuropathy | I | I | I | I |
| | Bell's palsy | Favors rejection of a causal relationship | Favors rejection of a causal relationship | I | I |
| | Transverse myelitis | I | I | I | I |
| | Chronic headache | I | I | I | I |
| | Postural orthostatic tachycardia syndrome | I | I | I | I |
| 4 | Sensorineural hearing loss | I | I | I | I |
| | Tinnitus | I | I | I | I |
| 5 | Thrombosis with thrombocytopenia syndrome | Favors rejection of a causal relationship | Favors rejection of a causal relationship | Favors acceptance of a causal relationship | I |
| | Immune thrombocytopenic purpura | I | I | I | I |
| | Capillary leak syndrome | I | I | I | I |
| 6 | Myocardial infarction | Favors rejection of a causal relationship | Favors rejection of a causal relationship | I | I |
| | Ischemic stroke | Favors rejection of a causal relationship | I | I | I |
| | Hemorrhagic stroke | I | I | I | I |
| | Deep vein thrombosis, pulmonary embolism, venous thromboembolism | I | I | I | I |
| 7 | Myocarditis | Establishes a causal relationship | Establishes a causal relationship | I | I |
| | Pericarditis without myocarditis | I | I | I | I |
| 8 | Sudden death | I | I | I | I |
| 9 | Female infertility | Favors rejection of a causal relationship | Favors rejection of a causal relationship | I | I |

NOTE: "I" indicates that the evidence was inadequate to accept or reject a causal relationship.

**TABLE S-2** Conclusions Regarding Shoulder Injuries After Any Vaccination

| Specific Shoulder Injury (Chapter 10) | Causality Conclusion |
|---|---|
| Subacromial/subdeltoid bursitis caused by direct injection into the bursa | Establishes a causal relationship |
| Acute rotator cuff or acute biceps tendinopathy caused by direct injection into or adjacent to the tendon | Establishes a causal relationship |
| Chronic rotator cuff disease | Favors rejection of a causal relationship |
| Adhesive capsulitis | I |
| Septic arthritis | I |
| Bone injury caused by direct injection into or adjacent to the bone | Establishes a causal relationship |
| Axillary or radial nerve injury caused by direct injection into or adjacent to the nerve | Establishes a causal relationship |
| Parsonage-Turner syndrome | I |
| Complex regional pain syndrome | I |

NOTE: "I" indicates that the evidence was inadequate to accept or reject a causal relationship.

(GBS), Bell's palsy (BP), and myocardial infarction (MI). The committee identified numerous studies supporting the conclusions about GBS, BP, and MI. The evidence for TTS and infertility was more limited but still suggestive of no effect. The committee also concluded that the evidence favored rejection of a causal relationship between BNT162b2 and ischemic stroke, but the evidence was inadequate to accept or reject a causal relationship between mRNA-1273 and ischemic stroke, as the data were more limited.

Despite the limited use of Ad26.COV2.S in the United States and therefore the limited number of published studies, the committee identified sufficient evidence to conclude that it favored acceptance of a causal relationship with two specific harms, TTS and GBS. The evidence base for these two conclusions were very different. The conclusion about TTS relied on strong mechanistic evidence of binding of vaccine-generated anti–platelet factor 4 antibody to platelets in people who developed TTS who had been given ChAdOx1-S, which is a similar platform to Ad26.COV2.S. Although the mechanistic findings for ChAdOx1-S were stronger, the similar findings with Ad26.COV2.S combined with pharmacovigilance data led the committee to conclude that the evidence favors acceptance of a causal relationship. The conclusion for GBS was based on strong epidemiological studies and pharmacovigilance data. Tables S-1 and S-2 contain the causality conclusions for each potential harm.

### Conclusions by Causal Category

The committee made six conclusions that the evidence *establishes* a causal relationship with vaccination. The evidence for these conclusions fell into two broad categories. The conclusions regarding myocarditis and the mRNA platform–based vaccines, BNT162b2 and mRNA-1273, relied upon extensive data from many sources and well-supported mechanistic evidence. In patients with vaccine-associated myocarditis, elevated levels of spike protein were detected in their blood and on myocardial tissue. Studies in animal models and ex vivo human samples show a connection between myocarditis and the activation of specific immune pathways, such as Toll-like receptor 4/inflammasome/interluekin 1-beta, triggered by mRNA COVID-19 vaccines. The conclusions regarding certain shoulder injuries after intramuscular injection (independent of type of vaccine) relied heavily on numerous well-documented case reports and a good mechanistic understanding that injection directly into certain areas of the shoulder could lead to injury of the bursa, tendon, bone, or nerve.

The committee also made two conclusions that the evidence *favors acceptance* of a causal relationship between Ad26.COV2.S and GBS and TTS. The evidence for these two conclusions varied quite a bit, with mechanistic data and pharmacovigilance data providing the support for TTS and epidemiological studies for GBS.

The committee made conclusions *favoring rejection* of causality for 12 possible harms. For both GBS and TTS, the committee concluded that the evidence favored rejection with both mRNA platform vaccines but convincingly supported a causal relationship with Ad26.COV2.S. This supports the understanding that the platform distinctly influenced the adverse response. The committee also favored rejection of a causal relationship for the mRNA vaccines and several other outcomes: female infertility, BP, MI, and ischemic stroke (BNT162b2 only). The evidence varied widely for these conclusions. The committee also concluded that the evidence favors rejection of a causal relationship between vaccine injection and chronic rotator cuff disease.

## Evidence in Children

As described in Chapter 1, vaccine-associated harms may differ in children and adults. For this reason, the committee conducted an in-depth review of the literature on potential harms and COVID-19 vaccines specifically in children (individuals younger than 18). At the time of the review, data on possible harms in children were available only for BNT162b2 and mRNA-1273. EUA of COVID-19 vaccines for children occurred later than for adults, and decreased uptake in children, particularly those under 11, led to far less data on possible harms from COVID-19 vaccines in children being available in the literature.

## CONCLUDING REMARKS

The COVID-19 pandemic resulted in a voluminous increase in research for many disciplines on many topics in very little time. Many factors complicated this research. Many investigators and clinicians were treating patients under very challenging circumstances while also conducting research. Vaccines were approved or authorized for use at different times for different populations in different countries. Priority groups among the first vaccines were older people and those with comorbidities that could have put them at risk for adverse events after vaccination. The communities being vaccinated had widespread SARS-CoV-2 infection, so that few studies were able to exclude patients with an infection that occurred simultaneously with vaccination. Thus, some of the outcomes observed after vaccination might reflect harms from infection instead. Patterns of non-SARS-CoV-2 infections changed dramatically during the early days of the pandemic due in part to social distancing and other public health interventions. See the discussion on GBS in Chapter 3 as an example. This complicates the use of historical controls in some studies. Many publications report surveillance findings, which do not use control populations. Rather, comparisons are made to historical trends, which are not representative of a true contemporaneous unvaccinated population. Other methodologic limitations across many of the studies include challenges in confirming vaccine receipt and diagnostic validity. Many studies in this report were not initiated to support causal inference reviews. Thus, although a particular paper might have had limited utility to this committee, it likely has relevance and immense purpose for others.

The committee appreciates the vast amount of work of researchers and clinicians during the pandemic and the contributions of the participants involved in these studies and hopes that the information and conclusions in this report are useful to vaccine researchers and the public health community at large.

## REFERENCES

CDC (Centers for Disease Control and Prevention). 2021. *Leading causes of death*. https://www.cdc.gov/nchs/fastats/leading-causes-of-death.htm (accessed March 3, 2024).

CDC. 2023. COVID-19 vaccine effectiveness update. https://covid.cdc.gov/covid-data-tracker/#vaccine-effectiveness (accessed March 8, 2024).

FDA (Food and Drug Administration). 2023. Re: Revocation of EUA 27205 - Janssen COVID-19 vaccine. https://www.fda.gov/media/169003/download?attachment (accessed March 1, 2024).

Flaxman, S., C. Whittaker, E. Semenova, T. Rashid, R. M. Parks, A. Blenkinsop, H. J. T. Unwin, S. Mishra, S. Bhatt, D. Gurdasani, and O. Ratmann. 2023. Assessment of COVID-19 as the underlying cause of death among children and young people aged 0 to 19 years in the U.S. *JAMA Network Open* 6(1):e2253590-e2253590. https://doi.org/10.1001/jamanetworkopen.2022.53590.

GAO (Government Accountability Office). 2021. *Operation warp speed: Accelerated COVID-19 vaccine development status and efforts to address manufacturing challenges* (GAO-21-319). https://www.gao.gov/products/gao-21-319 (accessed December 7, 2023).

HRSA (Health Resources and Services Administration). 2023a. *Comparison of Countermeasures Injury Compensation Program (CICP) to the National Vaccine Injury Compensation Program (VICP).* https://www.hrsa.gov/cicp/cicp-vicp (accessed December 11, 2023).

HRSA. 2023b. *Countermeasures Injury Compensation Program: Covered countermeasures.* https://www.hrsa.gov/cicp/covered-countermeasures (accessed December 20, 2023).

IOM (Institute of Medicine). 1991. *Adverse effects of pertussis and rubella vaccines.* Edited by C. P. Howson, C. J. Howe, and H. V. Fineberg. Washington, DC: National Academy Press.

IOM. 1994. *Adverse events associated with childhood vaccines: Evidence bearing on causality.* Edited by K. R. Stratton, C. J. Howe, and R. B. Johnston, Jr. Washington, DC: National Academy Press.

IOM. 2012. *Adverse effects of vaccines: Evidence and causality.* Edited by K. Stratton, A. Ford, E. Rusch and E. W. Clayton. Washington, DC: The National Academies Press.

IOM. 2011. *Finding what works in health care: Standards for systematic reviews.* Edited by J. Eden, L. Levit, A. Berg, and S. Morton. Washington, DC: The National Academies Press.

Junqueira, D. R., L. Zorzela, S. Golder, Y. Loke, J. J. Gagnier, S. A. Julious, T. Li, E. Mayo-Wilson, B. Pham, R. Phillips, P. Santaguida, R. W. Scherer, P. C. Gøtzsche, D. Moher, J. P. A. Ioannidis, and S. Vohra. 2023. CONSORT Harms 2022 statement, explanation, and elaboration: Updated guideline for the reporting of harms in randomised trials. *British Journal of Medicine* 381:e073725. https://doi.org/10.1136/bmj-2022-073725.

NASEM. 2023. *Review of relevant literature regarding adverse events associated with vaccines.* https://www.nationalacademies.org/our-work/review-of-relevant-literature-regarding-adverse-events-associated-with-vaccines (accessed December 18, 2023).

Qureshi, R., E. Mayo-Wilson, and T. Li. 2022. Harms in systematic reviews paper 1: An introduction to research on harms. *Journal of Clinical Epidemiology* 143:186–196. https://doi.org/10.1016/j.jclinepi.2021.10.023.

Watson, O. J., G. Barnsley, J. Toor, A. B. Hogan, P. Winskill, and A. C. Ghani. 2022. Global impact of the first year of COVID-19 vaccination: A mathematical modelling study. *Lancet Infectious Diseases* 22(9):1293–1302. https://doi.org/10.1016/S1473-3099(22)00320-6.

WHO (World Health Organization). 2023. *Polio: Global eradication initiative.* https://cdn.who.int/media/docs/default-source/Documents/gpei-cvdpv-factsheet-march-2017.pdf?sfvrsn=1ceef4af_0 (accessed December 17, 2023).

WHO. 2024. *Number of COVID-19 deaths reported to WHO.* https://data.who.int/dashboards/covid19/deaths?n=c (accessed March 6, 2024).

Zorzela, L., Y. Loke, J. P. A. Ioannidis, S. Golder, P. Santaguida, D. Altman, D. Moher, S. Vohra, and PRISMA Harms Group. 2016. PRISMA harms checklist: Improving harms reporting in systematic reviews. *British Journal of Medicine* 352:i157. https://doi.org/10.1136/bmj.i157.

# 1

# Introduction

Vaccines are a major public health success story, preventing or mitigating the effects of a myriad of infectious diseases. In 1986, the United States faced a problem with vaccine development and production. The threat of litigation over safety concerns related to the whole cell pertussis vaccines in particular led manufacturers to slow research and development and leave the market. Congress addressed what many considered to be a looming crisis for public health by passing the National Childhood Vaccine Injury Act (NCVIA) (P.L. 99-660) to improve federal coordination of vaccine efforts around research and development and address the concerns of those who asserted that they or their children were injured by vaccines. The Vaccine Injury Compensation Program (VICP), housed in the Health Resources and Services Administration (HRSA) in the Department of Health and Human Services and jointly administered by the Department of Justice, serves as a key policy solution developed by Congress. The program includes vaccines recommended for routine use in children or pregnant women, and anyone who receives a covered vaccine is eligible to apply for compensation. The program is funded by a federal excise tax on covered vaccines; the taxes are held in the Vaccine Injury Trust Fund (HRSA, 2023a).

VICP has long depended on the reports from the National Academies of Sciences, Engineering, and Medicine (the National Academies) as an important scientific contribution to its compensation decisions, beginning with two studies mandated by NCVIA (Sections 312 and 313 of Public Law 99-660). The Institute of Medicine (IOM, 1991, 1994) focused on assessing the causal relationship of the Centers for Disease Control and Prevention (CDC)–recommended childhood vaccines with specific potential harms. That early work was continued by other National Academies committees reviewing the scientific literature regarding the potential for vaccines to cause harm (IOM, 2002, 2012). The committees did not recommend whether or which harms should be compensated but focused on making conclusions about the causal nature of the vaccines and potential harms after a comprehensive review of biologic, clinical, and epidemiological literature. Compensation decisions remain determined by the intricate processes established by VICP (HRSA, 2023b). See HRSA (2023b) for a description of program administration and the claims process.

HRSA also administers the Countermeasures Injury Compensation Program (CICP) to provide compensation for those harms by medical countermeasures, which are vaccines, medications, devices, or other preventions, diagnostics, or treatments for a public health emergency or security threat. Established by the Public Readiness and Emergency Preparedness Act of 2005 (P.L. 148, Division C), CICP differs significantly from VICP (HRSA, 2023c).

On January 31, 2020, the Secretary of Health and Human Services declared a public health emergency related to severe acute respiratory syndrome coronavirus-2 (SARS-CoV-2) under Section 319 of the Public Health Service Act. The public health emergency expired on May 11, 2023.

The public health emergency was declared because SARS-CoV-2 and the disease caused by SARS-CoV-2, COVID-19, were the greatest public health crisis to date of the 21st century. As of February 2024, it had led to an estimated 7 million deaths worldwide, including 1.2 million deaths in the United States (WHO, 2024). COVID-19 was a major cause of death and illness in both adults and children. Long COVID is a particular concern. In 2021, COVID-19 was the third most common cause of death in adults in the United States (CDC, 2021), and from 2020 to 2022, COVID-19 was among the top 10 causes of death in children in the United States (Flaxman et al., 2023).

Part of the public health emergency was the announcement of "Operation Warp Speed," a rapid response by the federal government to speed vaccine development (for detailed information, see GAO, 2021). Four vaccines were developed and used in the United States, all under Emergency Use Authorization (EUA) (see FDA, 2023a), with some now fully approved by the Food and Drug Administration (FDA). However, as of June 1, 2023, FDA revoked the EUA from Ad26.COV2.S for safety concerns (FDA, 2023b). EUA allowed vaccines to be used before all phase 3 trials were completed.[1] COVID-19 vaccines, introduced in 2020, are highly effective in adults and children (CDC, 2023) and were key to control of the pandemic. COVID-19 vaccines are estimated to have prevented 14.4 million deaths worldwide in the first year of vaccination alone (Watson et al., 2022). Although in this report the committee is tasked with evaluating the causal association with select serious harms, a comparative study analyzing the prevalence and types of side effects following COVID-19 vaccination showed that the most common side effects across different vaccines were flu-like syndrome and local reactions at the injection site, which aligns with the side effect profiles of many vaccines (Yadegarynia et al., 2023).

## STATEMENT OF TASK

HRSA requested that the National Academies convene a committee to review the evidence regarding specific potential harms (see Box 1-1) and the COVID-19 vaccines used in the United States. See Table 1-1 for a list of those vaccines and the naming conventions used in this report. The list of harms to be addressed requested by HRSA are those for which, when the project began, HRSA had claims for compensation. The committee added postural orthostatic tachycardia syndrome (POTS) to its review after presentations at a public meeting.

HRSA also requested that the committee review the evidence regarding any vaccine, not specifically COVID-19 vaccines, and shoulder injuries. Claims for compensation for shoulder injuries after vaccination comprise over 63 percent of claims submitted to VICP in fiscal years 2021 and 2022 (NASEM, 2023). The scientific review was requested to help VICP better understand whether vaccination can cause very specific types of shoulder injuries or a more general syndrome that it designated as shoulder injury related to vaccine administration (HRSA, 2023d). Claims regarding shoulder injuries after routinely administered vaccines are handled by VICP and COVID-19 vaccines by CICP. For the committee's work, it is irrelevant whether a vaccine is covered under VICP or CICP; National Academies committees do not consider VICP or CICP processes when reviewing the evidence.

The committee comprised 15 members with expertise in epidemiology, causal inference, cardiology, rheumatology, gynecology, audiology, neurology, infectious disease, pediatrics, internal medicine, hematology, orthopedics, and immunology. Their biosketches can be found in Appendix A. The committee held two sessions open to the public. On January 30, 2023, it heard from representatives of HRSA and CDC on how they intend to use the report and why they asked for the review. On March 30, 2023, the committee held an open session during which members of the public registered to provide 3-minute statements concerning its task. Written material submitted to the committee is in a Public Access File.[2]

---

[1] The sentence was updated after the report was shared with the sponsor to clarify the EUA process.

[2] Public Access File materials can be requested by contacting the Public Access Records Office via the link on this project's webpage: www.nationalacademies.org/our-work/review-of-relevant-literature-regarding-adverse-events-associated-with-vaccines.

---

**BOX 1-1**
**Statement of Task**

The National Academies of Sciences, Engineering, and Medicine will convene an ad hoc committee to review the epidemiological, clinical, and biological evidence regarding the relationship between

- COVID-19 vaccines and specific adverse events i.e., Guillain-Barré Syndrome (GBS), chronic inflammatory demyelinating polyneuropathy (CIDP), transverse myelitis, Bell's palsy, hearing loss, tinnitus, chronic headaches, infertility, sudden death, myocarditis/pericarditis, thrombosis with thrombocytopenia syndrome (TTS), immune thrombocytopenic purpura (ITP), thromboembolic events (e.g., cerebrovascular accident (CVA), myocardial infarction (MI), pulmonary embolism, deep vein thrombosis (DVT)), capillary leak syndrome, and
- intramuscular administration of vaccines and shoulder injuries.

The committee will make conclusions about the causal association between vaccines and specific adverse events.

---

**TABLE 1-1** COVID-19 Vaccines Used in the United States

| Non-Commercial Name | Commercial Name | Manufacturer | Platform Type | Adjuvant or Functional Adjuvant | U.S. EUA Date | U.S. Full Approval Date | Approved for Use in |
|---|---|---|---|---|---|---|---|
| BNT162b2 | Comirnaty® | Pfizer and BioNTech | mRNA | Self#- LNP and mRNA | December 11, 2020 | August 23, 2021 | Adults and children aged 6+ months |
| mRNA-1273 | Spikevax® | Moderna | mRNA | Self#- LNP and mRNA | December 18, 2020 | January 31, 2022 | Adults and children aged 6+ months |
| Ad26.COV2.S* | NA | Janssen | AV | Self#- AV | February 27, 2021 | — | Adults (18+) |
| NVX-CoV2373 | NA | Novavax | Protein Subunit | Matrix-M® | July 13, 2022 | — | Adults (18+) |

NOTES: *This vaccine is the same type of platform as ChAdOx1, manufactured by AstraZeneca, but uses a different adenovirus vector. ChAdOx1 is not used in the United States. # mRNA and previously used AV vaccines in the United States do not contain discrete adjuvants. The LNP and AV function as adjuvants to activate the innate immune system. AV: adenovirus vector; EUA: Emergency Use Authorization; LNP: lipid nanoparticle; mRNA: messenger ribonucleic acid.

The committee attempted to identify and analyze published literature about the vaccines and potential harms. Although it reviewed the literature thoroughly, it did not conduct what is commonly referred to as a "systematic review," formal steps of which were described by IOM (2011). The processes and time frame for a systematic review were considered incompatible with this work, and, more importantly, the goals of this work were different from those of most systematic reviews and clinical guidelines. The committee was not tasked with estimating the magnitude or strength of associations between vaccinations and outcomes, and the evidence was not expected to be conducive to meta-analysis in any case. To fulfill its narrower goals, the committee did incorporate important attributes of good systematic reviews. A more detailed description of the process by which the committee identified and analyzed the literature follows.

The committee does not address the benefits of vaccines. This review addresses evidence only about specific potential harms and vaccines available in the United States. The committee does not make conclusions regarding specific patient cases (such as in published case reports) or whether VICP or CICP should award compensation in individual cases or in general. The committee does aim to present evidence in a way that is useful to VICP, CICP, claimants and their legal representatives, clinicians, and the public.

Vaccines and other medical products can cause both benefits and harms. Harms are sometimes described using terms such as "adverse event," "adverse effect," "side effect," or "safety." Such terms might not convey the importance of unwanted medical events. Moreover, readers might be confused by the use of different terms with overlapping meanings or the same terms to mean different things in different contexts (Qureshi et al., 2022). For example, "adverse events" are defined in regulatory research as unwanted events not necessarily related to an intervention (e.g., a vaccine, a drug). By comparison, "adverse effects" are both unwanted and related to an intervention. On the other hand, "side effects" might be desirable or unwanted, and they are related to an intervention. Following best practices (Junqueira et al., 2023; Zorzela et al., 2016), this report describes the opposite of benefits as "harms." To emphasize that an individual patient might or might not experience specific benefits or harms, this report sometimes describes them as "potential." Identifying a "harm" does not mean that it occurs frequently; harms associated with vaccines are rare. For example, vaccine-associated paralytic polio is an established harm of the oral polio vaccine (OPV), but it is estimated to occur at a rate of 1 in 2.7 million first doses of OPV (WHO, 2023).

## LITERATURE SEARCH

The committee provided the National Academies research librarian with a comprehensive list of search terms for each potential harm. The librarian conducted separate literature searches for epidemiological and mechanistic literature based on the search terms using Embase, Medline, PubMed, Scopus, and Cochrane Central Register of Controlled Trials (Ovid).

## Epidemiological Evidence

Three comprehensive epidemiological literature searches were conducted. Each search included terms specific to each potential harm in at least one search field (i.e., title, abstract, keywords). The list of search terms is available through the project Public Access File.[3]

The first search was for literature published January 1, 2020–February 28, 2023. Follow-up searches captured literature published February 28–July 7, 2023, and July 7–October 17, 2023. Thus, publications that appeared in the databases after October 17, 2023, are not included in this report. Ad hoc searches were conducted if committee members added a search term and for literature on POTS. The committee restricted its review to U.S. vaccine platforms but included studies conducted outside of the United States.

Citations were uploaded to PICO Portal, an online platform used to screen abstracts and full text. Abstracts were reviewed to screen out citations that did not address the potential harm under the committee's purview and studies that evaluated only vaccine platforms (e.g., inactivated virus vaccine) not approved in the United States. The committee focused its review on original reports and systematic reviews, excluding narrative reviews or commentaries.

For systematic reviews, committee members screened each publication and excluded those that were considered unreliable after consideration of the following: no defined criteria for selection of studies, literature search not comprehensive for eligible studies, no assessment of risk of bias in the included studies, and inappropriate methods for meta-analyses (when meta-analyses were reported). Systematic reviews were examined to determine whether they studied the potential harms of interest and for quality of evidence.

Committee members evaluated the full text of potentially relevant epidemiological studies and eliminated those that had serious methodologic limitations and were judged unlikely to contribute to the causality assessment. Studies were excluded for reasons such as misclassification of the exposure (vaccination status) and outcomes (e.g., harms were more likely to be recorded in a certain group even if they did not occur more frequently), uncontrolled

---

[3] Public Access File materials can be requested by contacting the Public Access Records Office via the link on this project's webpage: www.nationalacademies.org/our-work/review-of-relevant-literature-regarding-adverse-events-associated-with-vaccines.

confounding, selection bias, and substantial missing data (e.g., vaccination status or outcome status is unknown for a large proportion of participants). Misclassification of the exposure means that the specific vaccine was not consistently identified. Misclassification of the outcome means that the potential harms could not be reliably identified. For instance, many studies used diagnosis codes from health care encounters to identify health outcomes—for many outcomes, the codes either are known to perform poorly (e.g., individuals with the code often do not have the outcome, or the code is absent when individuals have experienced the outcome) or have unknown accuracy for validated outcomes. Confounding can occur when an association between vaccination status and the outcome is explained by a common cause that is not completely controlled for in the design and analysis; this is one of the major problems for causal inference using results from observational studies rather than randomized controlled trials (RCTs). Many studies were unable to exclude the possibility of the harms occurring due to SARS-CoV-2 infection. Data extraction was performed on articles that were included at this stage. Pharmacovigilance studies and case reports were identified through the literature search and reviewed if the evidence from the epidemiological studies did not lead the committee to accept or reject a causal relationship. A bibliography of all citations reviewed but not included in this report are available through the project Public Access File.[4]

## Mechanistic Evidence

The committee aimed to understand immune mechanisms of the vaccine platforms potentially related to harms, as described in Chapter 2, by conducting a general search. The first search was limited to studies in humans and identified literature published January 2021–March 2023. A second search looked for information specific to the potential harms under study; it identified literature published January 2000–April 2023 and explored general mechanisms underlying vaccine–immune interactions, focusing on non-SARS-CoV-2 messenger ribonucleic acid (mRNA) and adenovirus-vector (AV) vaccines. A final literature search was conducted in September 2023. Included articles encompassed a broad spectrum of research, including human trials, murine studies, other animal models, computational modeling, and in vitro studies. Ad hoc searches conducted throughout the study were particularly informative as the committee investigated possible mechanisms. The literature search aimed to identify studies elucidating the mechanism underlying specific harms of COVID-19 vaccination and to identify studies quantifying the effect of vaccination on components of the immune system in general. In addition, ad hoc literature searches were performed to review the mechanism of specific harms outside of the vaccination context (e.g., Guillain-Barré syndrome). In the case of shoulder injury, the mechanistic evidence was largely derived from imaging (e.g., magnetic resonance imaging) provided in case reports and case series.

## EVIDENCE IN CHILDREN

Adverse effects associated with vaccines may differ in children and adults. For this reason, the committee conducted an in-depth review of the literature on potential harms from COVID-19 vaccines specifically in children (those under 18). For context, the vaccines received EUA much later in children than adults, and even later in young children (5–11 years and 6 months to 4 years) than adolescents (12–17 years) (see Table 1-2).

These much later EUA dates and a decrease in SARS-CoV-2 cases after vaccination of adults led to lower immunization rates in children; in May 2023, these were only 13 percent, 39 percent, and 68 percent in children aged 6 months to 4 years, 5–11, and 12–17, respectively, according to the CDC (AAP, 2023). For these reasons, considerably less data exist on possible harms in children, especially in those under 11, compared to adults. Ad26.COV2.S[5] was never given an EUA for individuals under 18. NVX-CoV2373, although granted an EUA for those aged 12–17 on August 19, 2022, has had very little uptake, so little data exist beyond the original clinical trial on potential harms in children.[6] The committee therefore reviewed the available data on COVID-19 vaccines in

---

[4] Public Access File materials can be requested by contacting the Public Access Records Office via the link on this project's webpage: www.nationalacademies.org/our-work/review-of-relevant-literature-regarding-adverse-events-associated-with-vaccines.
[5] Refers to the COVID-19 vaccine manufactured by Janssen.
[6] Refers to the COVID-19 vaccine manufactured by Novavax.

**TABLE 1-2** COVID-19 Vaccine Food and Drug Administration Emergency Use Authorization Dates, Adults and Children

| Vaccine | Age Group | EUA Date |
|---|---|---|
| BNT162b2 | ≥16 years | December 11, 2020 |
| | 12–15 years | May 10, 2021 |
| | 5–11 years | October 29, 2021 |
| | 6 months–4 years | June 17, 2022 |
| mRNA-1273 | ≥18 years | December 18, 2020 |
| | 6 months–17 years | June 17, 2022 |
| NVX-CoV2373 | >/= 18 years | July 13, 2022 |
| | 12-17 years | August 19. 2020 |

NOTES: BNT162b2 refers to the COVID-19 vaccine manufactured by Pfizer-BioNTech under the name Comirnaty®. mRNA-1273 refers to the COVID-19 vaccine manufactured by Moderna under the name Spikevax®. EUA: Emergency Use Authorization.

children, which consisted of data from BNT162b2[7] and mRNA-1273.[8] Although there are numerous publications on COVID-19 vaccines in children, the vast majority of these are editorial, commentary or opinion pieces, or case reports or small case series. These publications typically do not provide the quality of evidence needed for evaluation of the relationship of potential harms to vaccine administration. Published data on COVID-19 vaccines in children were reviewed in depth by the committee, and all publications that provided data that could be used to evaluate the relationship of the vaccine to adverse events were included in the analysis. For children, and particularly for children younger than 12 years of age, there was a paucity of data, due to later authorization of COVID-19 vaccines for children and lower immunization rates in children as compared to adults, resulting in less study of adverse events in children than adults.

## CAUSALITY ASSESSMENT

### Types of Evidence

The committee used different types of evidence to draw conclusions concerning possible associations between vaccination and harms. Conclusions about causality were informed by the totality of the evidence without applying arbitrary rules or thresholds regarding the number or types of studies required to draw conclusions. Some study types were not available or were considered uninformative for certain outcomes, so the following chapters do not necessarily discuss all the study types described below. The committee reviewed the literature following a well-accepted hierarchy of evidence, beginning with randomized clinical trials and controlled observational epidemiological studies. The committee proceeded to review additional evidence (uncontrolled epidemiological evidence and case reports) until the committee felt it reviewed sufficient and appropriate evidence to support a specific causal conclusion. For example, the committee did not review uncontrolled pharmacovigilance studies and case reports if it felt the observational epidemiological literature was sufficient to support a conclusion or if it felt evidence of those uncontrolled designs was unlikely to contribute to a causal conclusion. The committee notes that uncontrolled studies would likely have been excluded from consideration if it had followed strict inclusion and exclusion criteria, as is done in systematic reviews. However, given the limited information regarding some of the potential harms being reviewed, the committee felt it important to be broad in its consideration of evidence.

---

[7] Refers to the COVID-19 vaccine manufactured by Pfizer-BioNTech under the name Comirnaty®.
[8] Refers to the COVID-19 vaccine manufactured by Moderna under the name Spikevax®.

*Clinical Trials*

For each potential harm, the committee examined evidence in Phase III RCTs, including published results from clinical trials and the documents reviewed and produced by FDA in consideration of the applications by manufacturers for EUA and full approval, when available.

RCTs can produce valid causal estimates (e.g., because they minimize selection bias and confounding). Associations detected in RCTs could support causal conclusions, especially for increases in common harms or very large increases in uncommon harms. The committee was aware that RCTs were not designed to assess rare harms, and RCTs did not enroll enough participants to estimate rare events reliably. Some harms are so rare that they would not be expected to occur in RCTs even if they were caused by vaccination. Lack of evidence from RCTs would usually be considered uninformative (rather than evidence of no association).

*Nonrandomized Studies*

The committee also considered evidence from nonrandomized studies (controlled observational studies and uncontrolled screening or pharmacovigilance studies) that used appropriate methods to estimate causal effects. Although the committee determined that controlled observational studies were at greater risk of bias compared with RCTs, estimates from studies that minimized bias were considered potentially informative. Notably, positive associations between vaccination and harms could provide evidence of causality. The committee interpreted negative and null findings cautiously. Compared with RCTs, large observational studies might estimate effects with greater precision but greater bias; consequently, it would be difficult to exclude small causal effects based on evidence from nonrandomized studies alone.

The committee also considered evidence from pharmacovigilance and surveillance studies, although estimates from these studies were generally considered at greater risk of bias compared with well-designed case-control and cohort studies.

*Case Reports*

The committee determined that case reports should inform causal conclusions when temporal and biological relationships between vaccination and harm were readily observable in the reports. In particular, case reports might provide useful evidence about shoulder injuries (see Chapter 10). For harms with unclear onset and myriad potential causes, the committee determined that case reports were unlikely to be informative.

*Mechanisms*

The committee considered evidence concerning possible mechanisms of action, including findings from human and other studies. Identifying a plausible mechanism could inform the committee's interpretation of evidence concerning associations in clinical trials and observational studies but not necessarily lead to conclusions favoring causal associations. Because mechanisms might be unknown, lack of mechanistic evidence did not preclude conclusions that vaccination caused harm.

*Extrapolation*

The committee considered evidence about each specific vaccine and each harm and discussed whether evidence for some vaccines should inform conclusions about others that used the same platform (e.g., mRNA, AV). For example, mechanistic and clinical evidence establishing a causal relationship between one vaccine and a harm could inform conclusions about the effects of similar vaccines. The committee extrapolated evidence from one vaccine of a specific platform to another vaccine cautiously. In particular, the literature regarding AV ChAdOx1-S (not available in the United States) was considered in assessing thrombosis with thrombocytopenia syndrome risk from Ad26.COV2.S (see Chapter 5).

## Causal Conclusions

Working groups assigned to each outcome performed the initial screen, data abstraction, and evidence review in advance of full committee discussions. Key elements in the data abstraction included study design, sample size, comparison group, risk period, vaccine and outcome ascertainment, and methodological strengths and limitations, including risk of bias considerations. Evidence tables and narratives were presented to the full committee for extensive discussion, including in-depth re-examination of individual studies and the preliminary causality conclusion in many circumstances in order to reach a common understanding of the strengths and weaknesses of the evidence and consensus conclusions. This was particularly important when a study was used by more than one working group; a particular research paper might have serious limitations or utility to the committee for one outcome but not for every outcome studied. For each outcome, the committee discussed the totality of the evidence and used consensus methods to draw conclusions about causality. Iterative discussions are particularly important given the committee's decision not to use a formal grading system for each published article or for the causality conclusions. The committee used expert judgment based on clinical and research expertise and analysis, paying careful attention that all outcomes under study were evaluated similarly to ensure that a consistent approach to the causal conclusions was maintained.

The committee adopted the wording of the causality conclusions developed by National Academies/IOM committees and approached the evaluation of evidence from a position of neutrality, presuming neither causation nor lack of causation. The causal conclusion categories are necessarily asymmetrical: although evidence can establish a causal relationship, the committee determined it was unlikely that it could establish the *absence* of one for any harm. Similar to other evidence-review efforts, the committee incorporated the potential role of future research in determining the appropriate conclusion, as described below.

The following are the categories of causation used by the committee:

- *Evidence establishes a causal relationship*—The totality of the evidence suggests that vaccination can cause this harm. Further research is unlikely to lead to a different conclusion.
- *Evidence favors acceptance of a causal relationship*—The totality of the evidence suggests that vaccination might cause this harm, but meaningful uncertainty remains. Studies that better minimize bias and confounding, and studies that estimate effects more precisely, could lead to a different conclusion.
- *Evidence is inadequate to accept or reject a causal relationship*—The available evidence is too limited (e.g., few studies in humans, biased, imprecise) or inconsistent to draw meaningful conclusions in support of or against causality. Future research could lead to a different conclusion. This conclusion also applies to situations in which no studies were identified.
- *Evidence favors rejection of a causal relationship*—The totality of the evidence suggests that vaccination does not cause this harm, but meaningful uncertainty remains. The committee acknowledges that individual causal effects are difficult to ascertain and that limitations exist for applying population average effects to draw conclusions about the causes of specific events in individual people. For example, it is possible that both vaccination and disease cause certain harms. Thus, (1) an event could be more common in an unvaccinated population than a vaccinated population, and (2) some of the events in the vaccinated population could be caused by vaccination. Research demonstrating a clear mechanism of action, or research demonstrating increased risk among vaccinated people compared with unvaccinated people, could lead to a different conclusion.

## OUTLINE OF THE REPORT

Chapter 2 contains a brief review of the major mechanisms by which vaccines affect the immune system. Chapters 3–9 address the evidence regarding COVID-19 vaccines and the specific outcomes listed in the Statement of Task. The structure of the chapters is similar but not identical. Chapters other than Chapters 8 (Sudden Death) and 9 (Female Infertility) contain conclusions about more than one outcome. Each outcome is addressed separately. Each outcome-specific section begins with a description of the outcome under review. A brief description of pathophysiologic mechanisms and the possible role of COVID-19 vaccines follows. The epidemiologic evidence section contains the evidence the committee depended upon in reaching a causal conclusion. Evidence that did not contribute is not described. The most influential evidence is portrayed in detail in tables within each section and described briefly in the text. Each section includes a summary of the most compelling argument in support of the conclusion and ends with the causal conclusion. Chapter 10 reviews the shoulder injuries after intramuscular administration of any vaccine, not limited to COVID-19 vaccines. The report ends with crosscutting summaries of the evidence in Chapter 11.

# REFERENCES

AAP (American Academy of Pediatrics). 2023. *Summary of data publicly reported by the Centers for Disease Control and Prevention.* https://www.aap.org/en/pages/2019-novel-coronavirus-covid-19-infections/children-and-covid-19-vaccination-trends (accessed December 12, 2023).

CDC (Centers for Disease Control and Prevention). 2021. Leading causes of death. https://www.cdc.gov/nchs/fastats/leading-causes-of-death.htm (accessed March 6, 2024).

CDC. 2023. COVID-19 vaccine effectiveness update. https://covid.cdc.gov/covid-data-tracker/#vaccine-effectiveness (accessed March 8, 2024).

FDA (Food and Drug Administration). 2023a. *Emergency use authorization.* https://www.fda.gov/emergency-preparedness-and-response/mcm-legal-regulatory-and-policy-framework/emergency-use-authorization (accessed December 11, 2023).

FDA. 2023b. Re: Revocation of EUA 27205 - Janssen COVID-19 vaccine. https://www.fda.gov/media/169003/download?attachment (accessed March 1, 2024).

Flaxman, S., C. Whittaker, E. Semenova, T. Rashid, R. M. Parks, A. Blenkinsop, H. J. T. Unwin, S. Mishra, S. Bhatt, D. Gurdasani, and O. Ratmann. 2023. Assessment of COVID-19 as the underlying cause of death among children and young people aged 0 to 19 years in the US. *JAMA Network Open* 6(1):e2253590. https://doi.org/10.1001/jamanetworkopen.2022.53590.

GAO (Government Accountability Office). 2021. *Operation Warp Speed: Accelerated COVID-19 vaccine development status and efforts to address manufacturing challenges* (GAO-21-319). https://www.gao.gov/products/gao-21-319 (accessed December 7, 2023).

HRSA (Health Resources and Services Administration). 2023a. *About the National Vaccine Injury Compensation Program—what is the Vaccine Injury Compensation Trust Fund?* https://www.hrsa.gov/vaccine-compensation/about (accessed December 13, 2023).

HRSA. 2023b. *Comparison of Countermeasures Injury Compensation Program (CICP) to the National Vaccine Injury Compensation Program (VICP).* https://www.hrsa.gov/cicp/cicp-vicp (accessed December 11, 2023).

HRSA. 2023c. *National Vaccine Injury Compensation Program.* https://www.hrsa.gov/vaccine-compensation/ (accessed December 6, 2023).

HRSA. 2023d. *Vaccine injury table.* Health Resources and Services Administration.

IOM (Institute of Medicine). 1991. *Adverse effects of pertussis and rubella vaccines.* Edited by C. P. Howson, C. J. Howe, and H. V. Fineberg. Washington, DC: National Academy Press.

IOM. 1994. *Adverse events associated with childhood vaccines: Evidence bearing on causality.* Edited by K. R. Stratton, C. J. Howe and R. B. Johnston, Jr. Washington, DC: The National Academies Press.

IOM. 2002. *Immunization safety review: Hepatitis B vaccine and demyelinating neurological disorders.* Edited by K. Stratton, D. A. Almario, and M. C. McCormick. Washington, DC: The National Academies Press.

IOM. 2011. *Finding what works in health care: Standards for systematic reviews.* Edited by J. Eden, L. Levit, A. Berg, and S. Morton. Washington, DC: The National Academies Press.

IOM. 2012. *Adverse effects of vaccines: Evidence and causality.* Edited by K. Stratton, A. Ford, E. Rusch, and E. W. Clayton. Washington, DC: The National Academies Press.

Junqueira, D. R., L. Zorzela, S. Golder, Y. Loke, J. J. Gagnier, S. A. Julious, T. Li, E. Mayo-Wilson, B. Pham, R. Phillips, P. Santaguida, R. W. Scherer, P. C. Gøtzsche, D. Moher, J. P. A. Ioannidis, and S. Vohra. 2023. CONSORT Harms 2022 statement, explanation, and elaboration: Updated guideline for the reporting of harms in randomised trials. *British Journal of Medicine* 381:e073725. https://doi.org/10.1136/bmj-2022-073725.

NASEM (National Academies of Sciences, Engineering, and Medicine). 2023. Review of relevant literature regarding adverse events associated with vaccines. https://www.nationalacademies.org/our-work/review-of-relevant-literature-regarding-adverse-events-associated-with-vaccines (accessed December 18, 2023).

Qureshi, R., E. Mayo-Wilson, and T. Li. 2022. Harms in systematic reviews paper 1: An introduction to research on harms. *Journal of Clinical Epidemiology* 143:186–196. https://doi.org/10.1016/j.jclinepi.2021.10.023.

Watson, O. J., G. Barnsley, J. Toor, A. B. Hogan, P. Winskill, and A. C. Ghani. 2022. Global impact of the first year of COVID-19 vaccination: A mathematical modelling study. *Lancet Infectious Diseases* 22(9):1293–1302. https://doi.org/10.1016/S1473-3099(22)00320-6.

WHO (World Health Organization). 2023. *Polio: Global eradication initiative.* https://cdn.who.int/media/docs/default-source/Documents/gpei-cvdpv-factsheet-march-2017.pdf?sfvrsn=1ceef4af_0 (accessed December 17, 2023).

WHO. 2024. Number of COVID-19 deaths reported to WHO. https://data.who.int/dashboards/covid19/deaths?n=c (accessed March 6, 2024).

Yadegarynia, D., S. Tehrani, F. Hadavand, S. Arshi, Z. Abtahian, A. Keyvanfar, A. Darvishi, A. Zarghi, L. Gachkar, I. A. Darazam, and M. Farahbakhsh. 2023. Side effects after COVID-19 vaccination: A comparison between the most common available vaccines in Iran. *Iranian Journal of Microbiology* 15(2):189–195. https://doi.org/10.18502/ijm.v15i2.12467.

Zorzela, L., Y. Loke, J. P. A. Ioannidis, S. Golder, P. Santaguida, D. Altman, D. Moher, S. Vohra, and PRISMA Harms Group. 2016. PRISMA harms checklist: Improving harms reporting in systematic reviews. *British Journal of Medicine* 352:i157. https://doi.org/10.1136/bmj.i15.

# 2

# Immunologic Response to COVID-19 Vaccines

The global pandemic stemming from the emergence of the novel severe acute respiratory syndrome coronavirus-2 (SARS-CoV-2) virus in late 2019 made it critical to develop efficacious vaccines. This public health crisis initiated global efforts to produce vaccines to reduce viral transmission and protect individuals from life-threatening infections (Diamond and Pierson, 2020). Several COVID-19 vaccines were rapidly developed using a variety of platforms. Concomitant with the release of vaccines, concerns arose around vaccine-induced harms. To better understand how vaccine-mediated harms may arise, it is important to know how specific COVID-19 vaccines initiate an immune response.

Charged with examining biological mechanisms, the committee conducted a comprehensive review of the current literature, examining the available evidence encompassing clinical trials, epidemiology studies, case reports, preclinical and translational in vitro or in silico studies, and insights gained from animal models. The committee analyzed a diverse array of vaccine-mediated harms and a variety of vaccine platforms and compiled a list of mechanisms that were deemed most plausible in contributing to the emergence of vaccine-mediated adverse reactions following COVID-19 vaccination. Throughout these deliberations, the committee engaged in in-depth discussions regarding the pathophysiology that may be involved and the requisite evidentiary support necessary to establish the presence of a particular mechanism.

## FUNDAMENTALS OF THE IMMUNE RESPONSE

The human immune response is initiated by the innate immune system, which activates the adaptive immune system. Both the innate and adaptive arms of the immune response play a pivotal role in combating pathogens, such as SARS-CoV-2, and establishing long-term immunity. They are also both important in producing an effective immune response and long-term immunity (immunological memory) after vaccination.

The innate immune system is the "first responder" to foreign agents, such as viral infections or physical tissue damage. It comprises physical defenses, such as the skin, and cellular components, such as macrophages, mast cells, dendritic cells, neutrophils, and natural killer cells. The innate immune response is not pathogen specific at the single amino acid/protein epitope level (i.e., antigen) but recognizes categories of pathogens, such as viruses, bacteria, parasites, and tissue damage, based on molecular patterns that are specific to particular microbes (Chaplin, 2010). Important to this pathogen recognition system are pattern recognition receptors, with Toll-like receptors (TLRs) being a notable subgroup. For example, TLR3 is involved in canonically recognizing double-stranded ribonucleic acid (RNA), commonly associated with viral infections; however, evidence of TLR3 recognition of single-stranded RNA vaccines has been shown (Teijaro and Farber, 2021). TLR4, which recognizes lipopolysaccharides from Gram-negative bacteria, some viral infections, and self-like ATP from damaged mitochondria, may play a role in responses to messenger ribonucleic acid (mRNA) vaccines, which contain mRNA within lipid nanoparticles (LNPs) that augment innate immune responses. TLR7 and TLR8, recognizing single-stranded RNA, are integral to the immune response against RNA-based vaccines, such as certain COVID-19 vaccines. Meanwhile, TLR9, which detects unmethylated CpG motifs in bacterial and viral deoxyribonucleic acid (DNA), is used in some vaccines as an adjuvant (a substance in vaccines that enhances the immunological response to the antigen). The activation of these TLRs triggers signaling pathways that lead to cytokine and type I interferon production, crucial for initiating adaptive immune responses (Fitzgerald and Kagan, 2020).

After activation by the innate immune system, the adaptive immune system develops an antigen-specific immune response to a specific pathogen that is based on particular amino acids/protein sequences (antigens). Macrophages and dendritic cells are fundamental in presenting antigens to adaptive immune cells, initiating an antigen-specific response crucial for establishing long-lasting immunological memory. Because of the high specificity of the adaptive immune response, it can distinguish not only a specific virus but also a specific strain of that virus. Memory occurs primarily at the T cell and B cell levels. B cells develop into plasma cells that release antigen-specific antibodies that are critical for rapidly clearing infections when they are encountered the next time. T cells, on the other hand, play a crucial role in immune memory by recognizing and responding to previously encountered antigens, aiding in the rapid mobilization of the immune system during subsequent infections. The development of strong antigen-specific T cell and B cell-antibody memory is a primary goal of vaccine development.

All types of vaccines strongly stimulate an innate immune response to direct the adaptive immune response to make protective antigen-specific T and B cells and antibody responses against the target infection. COVID-19 vaccines (see Figure 2-1), including traditional protein-based vaccines (NVX-CoV2373[1]), mRNA vaccines (e.g., BNT162b2[2] and mRNA-1273[3]) and adenovirus-vector (AV) vaccines (e.g., Ad26.COV2.S[4] and ChAdOx1/nCoV-19[5]), are engineered to stimulate both innate and adaptive immune responses. The mRNA vaccines deliver genetic material coding for the SARS-CoV-2 spike S-protein into host cells (Martinez-Flores et al., 2021) so that an antigen-specific adaptive immune response will be generated against it. The mRNA vaccine may be able to activate resident innate immune cells at the injection site, but it primarily takes effect after the spike protein is generated within cells (Verbeke et al., 2022). The mRNA strands are structurally optimized to prevent degradation by incorporating pseudouridines (Kim et al., 2022) and mRNA into LNPs (Ndeupen et al., 2021), which both further protects the RNA transcript from degradation and facilitates cell entry (Pardi et al., 2015). Certain components within the LNP layer may also act as adjuvants by activating TLRs on antigen presenting cells and the innate immune response to induce an enhanced adaptive immune response against the spike protein (Alameh et al., 2021). Protein-based vaccines often require an adjuvant to stimulate the innate immune response; AV vaccines have an innate immune-activating ability because they are viral vectors.

Innate antigen presenting cells, particularly mast cells, macrophages, and dendritic cells, are instrumental in activating an adaptive immune response. They capture, process, and present pathogen-specific antigens to T cells, inducing a highly targeted adaptive response and immunological memory. Dendritic cells are particularly important in stimulating adaptive immune responses from the draining lymph nodes while resident mast cells and macrophages play key roles at tissue sites. In the milieu of COVID-19 vaccines, antigen presenting cells are vital for identifying and presenting the vaccine-derived spike protein to helper T cells, thereby producing spike protein–specific T and B cells.

T cells, comprising helper T cells (CD4+) and cytotoxic T cells (CD8+), play multifaceted effector roles during an infection such as SARS-CoV-2. Helper T cells facilitate B cell activation and enhance the function of cytotoxic T cells, which directly attack and destroy virally infected cells. The adaptive immune cell memory induced by

---

[1] Refers to the COVID-19 vaccine manufactured by Novavax.
[2] Refers to the COVID-19 vaccine manufactured by Pfizer-BioNTech under the name Comirnaty®.
[3] Refers to the COVID-19 vaccine manufactured by Moderna under the name Spikevax®.
[4] Refers to the COVID-19 vaccine manufactured by Janssen.
[5] Refers to the COVID-19 vaccine manufactured by Oxford-AstraZeneca.

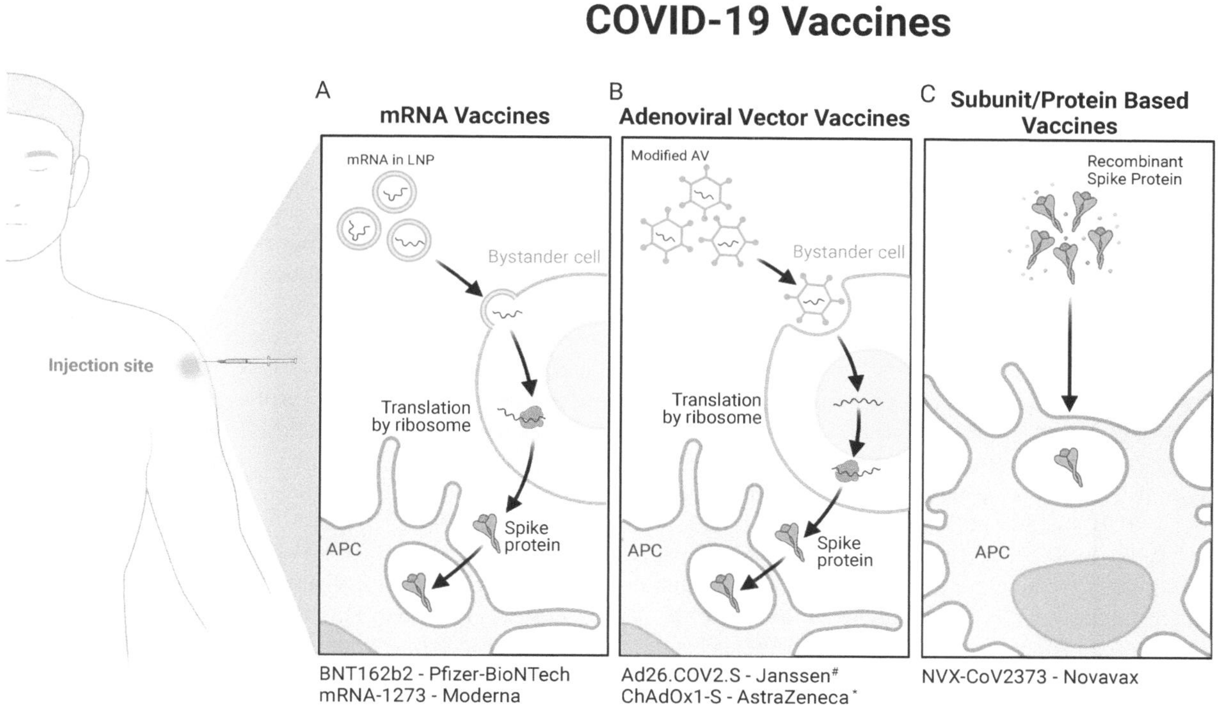

# COVID-19 Vaccines

| A mRNA Vaccines | B Adenoviral Vector Vaccines | C Subunit/Protein Based Vaccines |

**FIGURE 2-1** COVID-19 vaccines contributing to this report and their mechanism of action.
NOTES: (A) mRNA Vaccines: Upon injection, mRNA encapsulated in lipid nanoparticles (LNPs) is delivered into myocytes or bystander cells. The mRNA is released from LNPs and translated by ribosomes to produce the viral antigen, such as the spike protein (S), which is secreted. Antigen-presenting cells (APCs) such as dendritic cells (DCs) uptake the secreted antigen, initiating an immune response. (B) Adenoviral Vector Vaccines: Adenoviral vectors containing viral DNA enter myocytes or bystander cells, where they uncoat. The DNA, containing a nuclear localization signal, is transported to the nucleus and transcribed into mRNA. The extrachromosomal DNA does not integrate into the host genome. The mRNA is translated into protein, which is secreted and uptaken by APCs, initiating an immune response. (C) Subunit Vaccines: Pre-formed viral protein, such as the spike protein (S), is delivered. Antigen-presenting cells, particularly resident dendritic cells (DCs), uptake the protein to initiate an immune response. Additionally, M-matrix adjuvants enhance this response. #Ad26.COV2.S is no longer authorized under EUA in the United States as of June 1, 2023. *ChAdOx1-S is not used in the United States. Created with BioRender.com.

COVID-19 vaccines ensures a rapid antigen-specific T and B cell/antibody response when the vaccinee encounters SARS-CoV-2 in the future.

## SARS-COV-2 AND VACCINE TARGET OF THE SPIKE PROTEIN

SARS-CoV-2 is characterized by several structural proteins; the spike (S) glycoprotein and the nucleocapsid (N) protein are primary targets for the immune response (Krammer, 2020). The spike protein is a major virus surface protein crucial for viral entry into host cells; it binds to the angiotensin-converting enzyme 2 (ACE2) receptor on host cells (Walls et al., 2020). Structurally, the spike protein is a class I viral fusion glycoprotein comprising of two subunits: the S1 subunit, responsible for receptor binding, and the S2 subunit, involved in fusion. These subunits are connected by a furin cleavage site, unique to SARS-CoV-2 (rather than all SARS viruses), and the protein is cleaved posttranslationally at this furin cleavage site. The receptor-binding domain (RBD) within the

S1 subunit is particularly critical for viral entry to cells, as it directly interacts with the ACE2 receptor, initiating conformational changes leading to membrane fusion and viral entry (Kirchdoerfer et al., 2016; Wrapp et al., 2020). In addition, the spike protein is the only SARS-CoV-2 antigen recognized to stimulate neutralizing antibodies (Xiaojie et al., 2020). Several other receptors are important in viral entry but not described in this report.

The spike protein has been the primary focus in vaccine developments due to its essential role in viral entry to host cells. Vaccines contain (subunit vaccines, such as NVX-CoV2373) or generate production of (mRNA and AV vaccines) the spike protein to elicit an immune response in the absence of infection. Typically, adjuvants are also needed to induce a strong immune response because the antigen itself (without an active infection) does not do so in individuals who have not encountered SARS-CoV-2. The goal of all vaccine platforms is to contain or produce a stable form of the S protein that will not degrade or be cleared from the body without activating the immune response.

Two main mRNA vaccine strategies have been employed to stabilize the spike protein in its prefusion conformation, which is essential for preserving epitopes that are sensitive to degradation. One method, used in both mRNA-1273 and BNT162b2 vaccines, introduces mutations in the mRNA transcript (proline substitutions at positions 986 and 987), which maintain the spike glycoprotein in the prefusion state (Pallesen et al., 2017; Wrapp et al., 2020). Another strategy, not employed by the current vaccines, involves designing an mRNA construct where the full-length spike protein lacks the furin cleavage site (Δfurin), preventing posttranslational cleavage (Laczko et al., 2020; Lederer et al., 2020).

As an alternative to targeting the full-length spike protein, some vaccines focus solely on RBD (Bettini and Locci, 2021), which contains multiple epitopes that can be effective targets for virus neutralization, making it a potent target for vaccine strategies (Robbiani et al., 2020; Zost et al., 2020). For instance, the BNT162b1 vaccine candidate developed by BioNTech/Pfizer encodes a secreted trimerized version of RBD. The choice of the full-length spike protein or smaller RBD of the spike protein in vaccine design balances the benefits of eliciting a broader immune response with the full-length protein versus focusing on the highly neutralizing epitopes in the RBD. However, due to its favorable immunogenicity to reactogenicity profiles, BNT162b2, encoding full-length spike protein, was chosen as the leading vaccine candidate (Khehra et al., 2021).

## TYPES OF COVID-19 VACCINES

Several COVID-19 vaccines have been developed and authorized for use in the United States, using several different vaccine platforms (see Figure 2-1). The mRNA vaccines, such as BNT162b2 and mRNA-1273, use LNP-encapsulated mRNA to encode the SARS-CoV-2 spike protein. This technology prompts host cells to produce the spike protein, subsequently eliciting innate and adaptive immune responses and, most importantly, immunological memory. Adenovirus vector vaccines, such as Ad26.COV2.S (Emergency Use Authorization was revoked by the Food and Drug Administration [FDA] on June 1, 2023) and AZD1222 (not used in the United States), employ modified adenoviruses to deliver DNA encoding the spike protein. Protein subunit vaccines, such as NVX-CoV2373, consist of recombinantly produced viral proteins (such as the spike protein or its epitopes) combined with the Matrix-M® adjuvant, which enhances the immunogenicity of the protein antigen, leading to a more robust immune response. Each platform has distinct immunogenic profiles and mechanisms for eliciting an immune response.

## mRNA Vaccines

The advent of mRNA vaccines has marked a revolutionary leap in the field of immunology and vaccine development, particularly underscored by their critical role in combating the COVID-19 pandemic. These vaccines represent a significant departure from traditional vaccine platforms, providing a number of new advantages, including rapid development, high efficacy and safety, and rapid adaptation to new viral strains (Welsh, 2021). This technology holds promise for preventing serious outcomes and/or spread from viral infections. Developing mRNA vaccines, although conceptually straightforward, involves a complex design process. These vaccines function by delivering mRNA encoding a target antigen, such as the SARS-CoV-2 spike protein, into host cells. Once in the cytoplasm, the cells use their own machinery to translate the mRNA into the target protein, which is released from the host cell, usually in an extracellular vesicle (Trougakos et al., 2022), activating an innate immune response that also prompts the adaptive immune system to mount a memory response against the spike (S) protein. The next time the individual sees the spike protein during an active infection or vaccine boost, the immune system rapidly mounts a highly protective T and B cell/antibody response. For a detailed depiction of the sequence through which SARS-CoV-2 mRNA vaccines elicit immune responses, from their administration to the priming of T cells and initiation of germinal center (GC) reactions, refer to Figure 2-2.

One of the initial challenges of mRNA vaccines was the inherent nature of unmodified mRNA, which is extremely labile and highly immunogenic, making it unsuitable for direct use in vaccines (Pardi et al., 2018). Karikó et al. (2008) tested various modifications to nucleosides in mRNA molecules. They tested modifications, such as pseudouridine, 5-methylcytidine, N6-methyladenosine, 5-methyluridine, and 2-thiouridine. The substitution

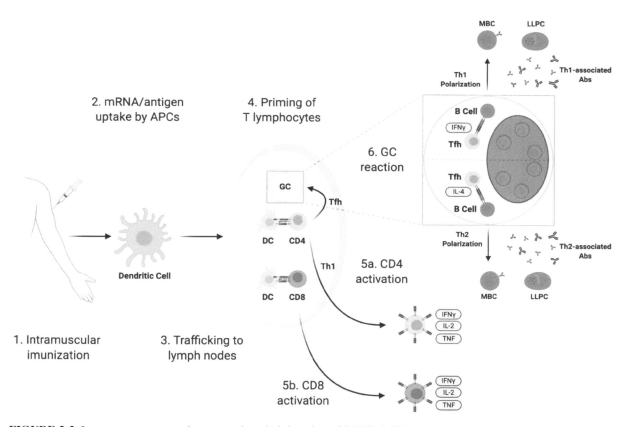

**FIGURE 2-2** Immune responses to intramuscular administration of SARS-CoV-2 mRNA vaccines.
NOTES: Immune responses triggered by SARS-CoV-2 mRNA vaccines involve a sequence of events starting with their intramuscular administration. These vaccines, which include mRNA encapsulated in lipid nanoparticles (mRNA-LNPs) or the antigen they produce, are first taken up by antigen-presenting cells (APCs) such as dendritic cells. After uptake, these APCs migrate to the lymph nodes, where they activate both CD4 and CD8 T lymphocytes. This process of T cell priming and its subsequent steps are discussed comprehensively in scientific literature. Following priming, CD8 T cells may differentiate into cytotoxic T lymphocytes capable of destroying virus-infected cells, while CD4 T cells may evolve into either Th1 cells or T follicular helper (Tfh) cells. Tfh cells are pivotal in initiating the germinal center reaction, a critical process for the development of high-affinity memory B cells and long-lived plasma cells that secrete antibodies. The direction of Tfh cell differentiation toward a Th1 or Th2 phenotype influences the isotype of antibodies produced by these plasma cells, affecting the body's immune response to the vaccine.
SOURCE: Bettini and Locci, 2021 CC BY.

of uridine with N1-methyl-pseudouridine (m1$\Psi$) led to a 10-fold increase in translation efficiency compared to unmodified mRNA (Karikó et al., 2008). Moreover, mRNA with this modification was not recognized by the pathogen-associated molecular pattern (PAMP) sensing mechanisms, such as TLRs or retinoic acid-inducible gene I (RIG-I), thus avoiding excessive inflammation, RNA degradation, and potential harms (Karikó et al., 2008; Pardi et al., 2018). This m1$\Psi$ modification has been adopted in the design of several mRNA vaccine candidates, including the widely used mRNA-1273 and BNT162b2 (Corbett et al., 2020; Walsh et al., 2020).

Although it is possible to inject naked mRNA directly for immunization, this approach is generally inefficient (Cao and Gao, 2021). For the mRNA to be translated into proteins in the host cell, it must penetrate the cell's lipid membrane to reach the cellular ribosomes. To facilitate efficient protein translation, delivery methods that ensure the cytosolic localization of mRNA are essential. Although standard laboratory lipid encapsulation methods, such as lipofectamine, were effective in vitro, they were cytotoxic and less efficient in vivo (Cao and Gao, 2021; Karikó et al., 2008). The encapsulation of mRNA into LNPs significantly contributes to its stability and uptake by the cells; LNPs effectively transport mRNA within the body and, upon intramuscular injection, can be taken up by antigen-presenting cells at the injection site and in nearby lymph nodes, facilitating both innate and adaptive immune responses. Furthermore, LNPs provide protection against nuclease-mediated degradation of the mRNA. The composition of LNPs is often proprietary, but they are known to contain a mixture of ionizable cationic lipids, cholesterol, phospholipids, and polyethylene glycols (PEGs), which self-assemble into nanoparticles of approximately 100 nanometers in diameter to encapsulate the mRNA (Cullis and Hope, 2017; Maier et al., 2013). Many of these components are known to be immunogenic and can act as adjuvants to stimulate the innate immune response to the spike protein. In fact, the composition of the LNP can be tailored to enhance the immune system's response to the vaccine by inducing robust T follicular helper (Tfh) cell and humoral responses, making LNPs not only a delivery vehicle but also an adjuvant-like component of mRNA vaccines (Alameh et al., 2021).

## Adenovirus-Vector Vaccines

AV vaccines have emerged as key players in COVID-19 vaccine development, leveraging the unique properties of adenoviruses. These linear double-stranded DNA viruses, typically responsible for respiratory infections in children and adults, possess stable genes and efficient transduction capabilities (ability to transfer genetic materials), making them ideal vaccine vectors (Lukashev and Zamyatnin, 2016). Adenoviruses do not integrate into the host genome but remain in a non-genome episomal state, meaning the injected genetic material translocates into the nucleus but does not integrate into the host DNA (Coughlan, 2020; Walsh et al., 2020). This aspect is significant because it mitigates concerns about potential long-term genetic changes in the host's cells. In some other types of viral vectors, the viral DNA could integrate into the host's genome, which could lead to unintended genetic alterations (Bulcha et al., 2021). However, with AV vaccines, this risk is greatly reduced because the adenovirus DNA remains separate from the host's DNA.

The adenovirus's nucleocapsid is composed of fiber, penton, and hexon proteins, contributing to its robustness and versatility as a vector. Over 150 primate adenoviruses have been identified, with many being developed for vaccines due to their cost-effectiveness, thermostability, and ability to induce strong immune responses (Chavda et al., 2023). A significant challenge is pre-existing immunity to common adenovirus serotypes in humans. To circumvent this, rare adenoviruses are employed, such as Ad26 or chimpanzee adenoviruses, which are less likely to be neutralized by pre-existing human antibodies. These vectors have demonstrated effectiveness in both animal models and human studies, despite the varying levels of pre-existing immunity across populations (Ewer et al., 2017; Geisbert et al., 2011).

In the context of COVID-19 vaccines, AZD1222, also known as "Covishield" by the Serum Institute of India, uses the ChAdOx1 AV. It carries the gene for the SARS-CoV-2 spike protein (ChAdOx1-S), which is expressed in its trimeric prefusion conformation (Watanabe et al., 2021).

Janssen Pharmaceuticals developed Ad26.COV2.S, using an Ad26 vector that encodes the spike protein with specific modifications (K986P and V987P) to enhance immunogenicity by locking the spike in its prefusion conformation (Bos et al., 2020). This vaccine is distinguished by its single-dose regimen.

## Protein Subunit Vaccines

Protein-based vaccines, a well-established class of vaccines, use specific proteins (or protein fragments) from a pathogen to elicit an immune response without introducing the complete pathogen. These vaccines are known for their safety, as they do not contain live components of the pathogen, reducing the risk of vaccine-induced disease, but they are also less immunogenic and require adjuvants or other interventions (Pollard and Bijker, 2021). These vaccines fall into two main categories: subunit vaccines, which include only the parts of the virus that best stimulate the immune system, and toxoid vaccines, which use a toxin produced by the pathogen that has been made harmless but still triggers immunity. Toxoid vaccines include diphtheria and tetanus vaccines, which use inactivated forms of the toxins produced by these bacteria. Subunit vaccines include hepatitis B, which uses a surface protein from the virus, the pertussis toxin component of the DtaP (diphtheria, tetanus, and acellular pertussis) vaccine, and NVX-CoV2373.

NVX-CoV2373 comprises recombinantly produced spike proteins combined with Novavax's proprietary Matrix-M® adjuvant (Keech et al., 2020). The spike protein used in the vaccine is produced by baculovirus expression in *Spodoptera frugiperda* insect cells, a method known for its ability to yield complex, properly folded proteins (Jarvis, 2003). This strategy ensures that the spike protein maintains its prefusion conformation, which is known to expose critical neutralizing epitopes more effectively than the post-fusion conformation (Bowen et al., 2021; Keech et al., 2020). The adjuvant is a critical component that significantly boosts the innate immune response to the spike protein. It is based on saponin, derived from the *Quillaja saponaria* tree, and combined with cholesterol and phospholipid to form nanoparticles. These nanoparticles enhance the immune response by stimulating the entry of the antigen into antigen-presenting cells and activating these innate cells. This adjuvant has been shown to boost both the quantity and quality of the immune response, leading to higher levels of neutralizing antibodies and a more robust T cell response (Stertman et al., 2023) to infection. In addition, adjuvants enable the use of smaller amounts of antigen. Producing neutralizing antibodies is the goal for most vaccines, as they bind to a pathogen and block its ability to infect cells, effectively neutralizing its disease-causing capabilities. In addition to antibody production, the orchestration of a robust T cell response is paramount, as these cells not only assist in the maturation of antibody-producing B cells but also identify and eliminate infected host cells, thereby mitigating the pathogen's proliferation and ensuring a comprehensive immunological defense.

This vaccine's storage and handling requirements are less stringent than those of mRNA vaccines, making it a valuable asset in global vaccination efforts, especially in regions with limited cold chain infrastructure.

## VACCINE IMMUNE RESPONSE ELICITATION

For non-single-dose COVID-19 vaccines, the first and second doses play distinct and complementary roles in eliciting an effective immune response. The initial vaccine dose largely primes the immune system, providing the antigen in a way that stimulates initial antibody production and activates specific immune cells that lead to antigen-specific memory T and B cells. Because the vaccine is not an actual infection, it may not provide the needed cues to mount an optimal immune response. Thus, the second dose, or the booster, is crucial for amplifying and broadening this response. It significantly enhances the quantity and quality of neutralizing antibodies, solidifies memory B cell and T cell responses, and induces a more robust, durable immunity. The booster dose thus ensures a more sustained and effective immune response, including against virus variants (Chu et al., 2022). Table 2-1 presents a summary of antibody responses and T cell responses in humans for each U.S. COVID-19 vaccine.

The immunogenicity of COVID-19 vaccines largely hinges on the adaptive immune system recognizing the specific spike protein fragments. B cell receptors on B cells and T cell receptors on T cells are key to this recognition when they interact with innate immune antigen-presenting cells. B cell receptors directly bind to epitopes on the spike protein, initiating B cell activation (Pettini et al., 2022). T cell receptors, however, recognize these epitopes when presented on Major Histocompatibility Complex (MHC) molecules by antigen-presenting cells (Yang et al., 2023). This dual recognition mechanism is essential for the coordinated activation of both humoral and cellular arms of the adaptive immune response (Teijaro and Farber, 2021) for viral proteins that are not superantigens.

Following vaccination, B cell activation predominantly occurs in GCs within secondary lymphoid organs (see Figure 2-2), such as lymph nodes and the spleen. In general, antigen-activated B cells undergo somatic

**TABLE 2-1** Immune Responses to U.S. COVID-19 Vaccines

| Vaccine | Platform | Dosing Regimen | Antibody Responses in Humans | T Cell Responses in Humans |
|---|---|---|---|---|
| BNT162b2 | mRNA | 30 µg mRNA 2 doses 21 days apart[a] | S1-binding antibody present after first dose, responses increased following the second dose; significant NAB was only present after second dose[b] | Increases in antigen-specific IFNγ+ CD4+ and CD8+ T cells after second dose; predominance of IFNγ and IL-2 secretion, compared with IL-4, suggesting TH1 cell polarization[c] |
| mRNA-1273 | mRNA | 100 µg mRNA 2 doses 28 days apart | S-binding antibody detected 14 days after first dose, levels increased slightly by 28 days, with marked increase after second dose[d]; minimal NAB present after first dose, peak at 14 days after second dose[e] | Significant increases in CD4+ T cells secreting TH1 type cytokines (TNF > IL-2 > IFNγ) after second dose, small increases in TNF-secreting and IL-2-secreting cells after first dose; minimal change in TH2 cell responses; low levels of CD8+ responses[d] |
| Ad26.COV2.S | Viral vector | 5 × 10^10 viral particles 1 dose[f] | S-binding and neutralizing antibody present by 28 days after vaccination in 99% of individuals and antibody levels sustained until at least 84 days post vaccination[g] | CD4+ and CD8+ T cell responses present at 14 and 28 days post-vaccination, based on presence of CD4+ and CD8+ T cells secreting IFNγ and/or IL-2 and not IL-4 or IL-3, suggesting TH1 cell polarization of the CD4+ T cell response[g] |
| NVX-CoV2373 | Protein subunit | 5 µg protein 2 doses 21 days apart[h] | S-binding antibody detected 21 days after first dose, with a marked increase after the second dose; some NAB present after the first dose, with a significant increase by 7 days after second dose[h] | CD4+ T cell responses present by 7 days after second dose, based on IFNγ, IL-2 and TNF production in response to S protein stimulation, with a strong bias toward a TH1 cell phenotype; minimal TH2 cell responses (as measured by IL-5 and IL-13)[h] |

NOTES: BNT162b2 refers to the COVID-19 vaccine manufactured by Pfizer-BioNTech under the name Comirnaty®. mRNA-1273 refers to the COVID-19 vaccine manufactured by Moderna under the name Spikevax®. Ad26.COV2.S refers to the COVID-19 vaccine manufactured by Janssen. NVX-CoV2373 refers to the COVID-19 vaccine manufactured by Novavax. CD: Cluster of Differentiation; IFN: Interferon; IL: Interleukin; mRNA: Messenger Ribonucleic Acid; NAB: Neutralizing Antibody; TH: T-helper cells; TNF: Tumor Necrosis Factor

[a] Pollard and Bijker, 2021.
[b] Walsh et al., 2020.
[c] FDA, 2021; Sadarangani et al., 2021.
[d] FDA, 2022; Jackson et al., 2020.
[e] Widge et al., 2021.
[f] Marfe et al., 2021.
[g] Sadoff et al., 2021.
[h] Keech et al., 2020.
SOURCE: Adapted from Sadarangani et al., 2021.

hypermutation, which introduces random mutations into their immunoglobulin (Ig) genes (Laidlaw and Ellebedy, 2022; Turner et al., 2021) and leads to B cells with high-affinity antibodies for the spike protein. B cells with the highest affinity are selected and differentiated into long-lived plasma cells (LLPCs) and memory B cells. LLPCs secrete neutralizing antibodies, some of which are capable of mediating sterilizing immunity, which prevents infection in the host including mucous membranes, and can potentially persist for years, continuously producing antibodies. Memory B cells quickly activate and give rise to a new wave of high-affinity antibody-secreting cells, providing rapid protection upon re-exposure to the virus (Sadarangani et al., 2021; Tam et al., 2016). For COVID-19 vaccines, in time, mutations in the spike protein may result in lower-affinity interaction between the antibodies induced by one strain and a mutated spike protein.

The role of T cells, particularly CD4+ T cells, is multifaceted. Tfh cells, a subset of CD4+ T cells, are critical for the development of GC reactions and consequently for the maturation of B cell responses. Tfh cells assist B cells in the GCs by providing necessary costimulatory signals and cytokines, facilitating the selection of high-affinity

B cells. These interactions are crucial for developing both LLPCs and memory B cells, and mRNA vaccines have been demonstrated to effectively induce Tfh cell responses, which are key to generating robust and long-lasting neutralizing immunity (Bettini and Locci, 2021; Pardi et al., 2018; Sadarangani et al., 2021). Clinically, however, immunity from COVID-19 vaccines is observed to wane over time (Menegale et al., 2023), necessitating booster doses to counteract this decline and to address the emergence of new, circulating common strains, thereby ensuring sustained protection against the virus.

Cytotoxic CD8+ T cells, which directly eliminate virus-infected cells, are another crucial component. These cells are characterized by the release of cytotoxic molecules, such as granzyme B and perforin. Upon vaccination, polyfunctional antigen-specific CD8+ T cells increase; these produce inflammatory cytokines, which are critical signaling molecules in the immune system. These include IFNγ (interferon gamma), IL-2 (interleukin-2), and TNF (tumor necrosis factor). IFNγ plays a crucial role in activating and directing other immune cells, enhancing the overall immune response to the vaccine and the virus. IL-2 is vital for the growth, proliferation, and differentiation of T cells, ensuring a robust and sustained immune response. TNF is involved in systemic inflammation and capable of inducing apoptosis or cell death in virus-infected cells. These cells exhibit markers of cytotoxic activity and contribute to the overall defense against viral infection. The ability to activate CD8+ T cell responses varies among vaccine candidates, with some inducing strong responses in both small and large animal models, while others show more variable results (Bettini and Locci, 2021; Creech et al., 2021).

Immunological memory is a hallmark of the adaptive immune response and a key goal of vaccination. Most licensed vaccines, including those for COVID-19, confer protection by eliciting long-lasting antibody responses.

The rapid and effective response to a pathogen upon re-exposure is primarily mediated by memory B and T cells. Memory B cells, upon re-exposure to the antigen, differentiate into antibody-secreting cells more quickly than naïve B cells, leading to a fast increase in antibody titers. Similarly, memory T cells, both CD4+ and CD8+, are primed to respond more rapidly and effectively than naïve T cells. Tfh cells are especially important in supporting memory B cell responses in GCs. They facilitate the selection of high-affinity memory B cells and their differentiation into LLPCs or memory B cells (Pollard and Bijker, 2021). These interactions are critical for maintaining long-lasting immunity and providing rapid protection upon subsequent exposures to the virus. Upon activation in a future infection, memory B cells rapidly produce large amounts of antigen-specific antibody, which can neutralize viral infection/entry into host cells—reducing the severity of the infection.

The duration of immunity conferred by COVID-19 vaccines and the potential need for booster doses are areas of ongoing research. Studies have shown that mRNA vaccines can induce robust CD8+ T cell responses characterized by key cytokines and cytotoxic markers upon rechallenge (Sadarangani et al., 2021; Teijaro and Farber, 2021). However, the longevity of these responses and persistence of memory T cells after vaccination is still under investigation. Some evidence suggests that the immune response elicited by these vaccines, particularly the generation of memory B and T cells, may be long lasting, but further studies are required to confirm the duration of this protection. Additionally, the need for booster doses may depend on factors such as the emergence of new viral variants/strains and the longevity of the vaccine-induced immune response (Teijaro and Farber, 2021).

## POSSIBLE MECHANISMS OF VACCINE-MEDIATED REACTIONS

Although rare, vaccine-mediated harms can range from mild, transient reactions to more serious conditions, underscoring the importance of ongoing safety monitoring and research. Certain of the most common vaccine-associated harms can arise from a few different immunological mechanisms, some of which are briefly discussed next (see Table 2-2).

Immediate-type hypersensitivity reactions are rapid immunological responses observed in certain individuals following vaccination. Mast cells and basophils play a crucial role; they become activated by IgE when individuals are re-exposed to the same antigen during vaccination (Stone et al., 2019), which triggers degranulation and the release of various mediators, such as histamine, leukotrienes, prostaglandins, and cytokines, including IL-4 and IL-5. The clinical manifestation ranges from urticaria (hives) to the more severe and potentially life-threatening anaphylaxis (McLeod et al., 2015).

**TABLE 2-2** Vaccine-Mediated Reactions and Their Mechanisms

| Type of Reaction | Immune Cells Involved | Plausible Mechanisms | Clinical Manifestation | Time of Onset |
|---|---|---|---|---|
| Immediate hypersensitivity | Mast cells, basophils | IgE-mediated mast cell/basophil activation induced by previous exposure to antigens in the vaccine, leading to degranulation and release of histamine, leukotrienes, prostaglandins, cytokines (IL-4, IL-5) | Urticaria (hives) to anaphylaxis | Rapid, post-vaccination |
| Delayed hypersensitivity | CD4+ helper T cells | Secretion of cytokines (IFN-γ, IL-2, TNF-α) upon activation | Rash, fever, joint pain | Days to weeks |
| Autoimmune reactions | Various | Molecular mimicry, bystander activation, epitope spreading, polyclonal activation, adjuvant-induced autoimmunity, and others | Varies | Varies |
| Vaccine-induced immune thrombotic thrombocytopenia (VITT) | Platelets, immune cells producing anti-PF4 antibodies | Formation of antibodies against platelet factor 4 (PF4), complement activation | Thrombosis, thrombocytopenia | Post-vaccination (variable) |
| Vaccine-associated enhanced disease (VAED) | B cells, Th2 skewed immunity | Non-neutralizing or suboptimal antibodies, generated in response to a vaccine, facilitate viral entry into host cells through Fc receptors or complement receptors | Worsening of diseases/symptoms | Upon exposure to natural virus after vaccination |
| Other | APCs, B cells, T cells | Activation of immune cells and release of cytokines (IL-1, IL-6, IL-12, TNF-α) | Varies | Post-vaccination |

NOTES: APCs: Antigen-Presenting Cells; IFN: Interferon, IL: interleukin, PF4: platelet factor 4, TNF: Tumor Necrosis Factor.
SOURCES: Chen et al., 2022b; Dabbiru et al., 2023; Lamprinou et al., 2023; Segal and Shoenfeld, 2018.

In contrast, delayed-type hypersensitivity reactions involve a different immune pathway. T cells, particularly CD4+ helper T cells, are central to these reactions. Upon exposure to an antigen that the immune system has seen before, T cells secrete cytokines, such as IFNγ, IL-2, and tumor necrosis factor-alpha (TNF-α). The symptoms associated with this reaction, such as rash, fever, and joint pain, typically develop days to weeks after vaccination, distinguishing them from the immediate-type reactions (Biedermann et al., 2000).

Autoimmune reactions in the context of vaccination encompass a variety of plausible mechanisms (Chen et al., 2022a; Lamprinou et al., 2023):

- Molecular mimicry, where vaccine antigens closely resemble the body's own proteins, potentially leading to the production of autoantibodies or autoreactive T cells that target self-tissues (Segal and Shoenfeld, 2018).
- Bystander activation, when localized inflammation exposes self-antigens, leading to the activation of previously dormant self-reactive lymphocytes.
- Epitope spreading, particularly with repeat vaccinations, where the initial immune response to vaccine antigens broadens to include self-antigens.
- Polyclonal activation and adjuvant-induced autoimmunity, where intense immune stimulation, potentially exacerbated by adjuvants, overcomes the tolerance to self-antigens, resulting in autoimmunity.

A current and significant concern is vaccine-induced immune thrombotic thrombocytopenia (VITT), an extremely rare condition characterized by forming antibodies against platelet factor 4 (PF4). This activates platelets and immune cells producing anti-PF4 antibodies (Dabbiru et al., 2023). The role of complement activation in promoting a prothrombotic state is also being explored (see Chapter 5).

Vaccine-associated enhanced disease (VAED) and antibody-dependent enhancement (ADE) are critical considerations in vaccine development, particularly highlighted by historical challenges with the formalin-inactivated respiratory syncytial virus (RSV) vaccine (Acosta et al., 2015). VAED encompasses a spectrum of phenomena where vaccination paradoxically exacerbates the disease upon exposure to the natural pathogen, mediated through mechanisms such as ADE. In ADE, non-neutralizing or suboptimal antibodies generated by the vaccine facilitate the pathogen's entry into host cells via Fc receptors, leading to increased viral replication and severe disease manifestations (Gartlan et al., 2022). The formalin-inactivated RSV vaccine is a notable example where immunization-induced antibodies not only failed to confer protection but also potentiated respiratory disease upon subsequent natural RSV infection. This outcome was partly attributed to the vaccine eliciting a skewed Th2-type immune response, promoting eosinophilic infiltration and severe lung pathology, rather than a protective Th1-type response (Gartlan et al., 2022). Additionally, immune complexes formed by the vaccine-induced antibodies could activate complement pathways, contributing to tissue damage.

Furthermore, general vaccine reactions encompass a wide array of immune responses. These involve the activation of antigen-presenting cells, B cells, and T cells. Cytokines, such as IL-1, IL-6, IL-12, and TNF-$\alpha$, play a significant role in the initial immune response to vaccines, contributing to both their protective effects and potential harms.

## ADJUVANTS

Adjuvants in vaccines serve to enhance the body's immune response to an antigen, ensuring a stronger and longer-lasting immunity by activating TLRs on antigen-presenting cells to stimulate a strong innate immune response that produces a strong adaptive immune response. For example, aluminum salts create a depot effect for sustained antigen release, and oil-in-water emulsions, such as MF59, increase cytokine release and antigen uptake (Wilkins et al., 2017). Adjuvants such as AS01, AS02, AS03, and saponins stimulate antigen-presenting cells, such as dendritic cells, to activate T cells, and CpG oligodeoxynucleotides activate TLR9 (Facciola et al., 2022). These mechanisms, although crucial for vaccine efficacy, can sometimes lead to adverse reactions, primarily localized ones, such as inflammation and soreness, due to heightened immune activation at the site of injection. Table 2-3 lists some of the most commonly used adjuvants and their mechanisms of action.

**TABLE 2-3** Most Commonly Used Adjuvants in Vaccines

| Adjuvant | Mechanism of Action |
|---|---|
| Aluminum salts (alum) | Creates a depot effect, slowly releasing antigen and enhancing antigen uptake by antigen-presenting cells. |
| MF59 (oil-in-water emulsion) | Increases cytokine release and antigen uptake, stimulating a stronger immune response. |
| AS04 (aluminum salt + monophosphoryl lipid [MPL] A) | Combines alum's depot effect with MPL to enhance the immune response. MPL activates TLR4. |
| CpG oligodeoxynucleotides | Activates TLR9, enhancing the immune response to specific pathogens. |
| AS01 (liposome based) | Stimulates dendritic cells and T cell responses, enhancing both innate and adaptive immunity. |
| Virosomes | Mimics viral infection, enhancing the immune system's recognition and response to the antigen. |
| QS-21 (saponin based) | Enhances antigen presentation and stimulates both humoral and cellular immune responses. |
| Lipopolysaccharide (LPS) | Activates TLR4, which leads to strong antibody responses by activating Th2 cells. |
| Poly-ICLC (polyinosinic-polycytidylic acid) | Mimics viral RNA, stimulating a strong immune response. |
| Matrix-M® (saponin based) | Activates antigen-presenting cells and boosts cytokine production, enhancing T cell and antibody responses. |
| Adjuvant system 03 (AS03, oil-in-water emulsion) | Contains squalene, DL-$\alpha$-tocopherol, and polysorbate 80, enhancing immune response via cytokine modulation. |

SOURCES: Stertman et al., 2023; Wilkins et al., 2017.

Matrix-M® is a saponin-based adjuvant in NVX-CoV2373, which is the only specifically adjuvanted COVID-19 vaccine. It consists of *Quillaja Saponaria Molina* extracts, known for their ability to stimulate both the innate and adaptive arms of the immune system. It enhances immune responses by activating antigen-presenting cells and boosting cytokine production, which facilitates a stronger T cell and antibody response to the vaccine antigen (Stertman et al., 2023). Its mechanism of action increases the vaccine's efficacy, but like other adjuvants, it can also contribute to or cause reactions. In the United States, FDA approves adjuvants only as components of vaccines, not as stand-alone products, because their properties can vary based on their concentration and interaction with other ingredients in the vaccine formulation.

Potential harms of vaccination necessitate a thorough investigation of mechanisms. Examining their immune response will help investigators gain insights into possible mechanisms of vaccine-related harms.

Through an examination of clinical trials, epidemiology studies, case reports, preclinical in vivo and in silico work, and insights from animal models, the committee has delved into possible mechanisms that may contribute to adverse events. Understanding these mechanisms is paramount in ensuring the safety and well-being of individuals receiving COVID-19 vaccines.

## REFERENCES

Acosta, P. L., M. T. Caballero, and F. P. Polack. 2015. Brief history and characterization of enhanced respiratory syncytial virus disease. *Clinical and Vaccine Immunology* 23(3):189–195. https://doi.org/10.1128/cvi.00609-15.

Alameh, M. G., I. Tombacz, E. Bettini, K. Lederer, C. Sittplangkoon, J. R. Wilmore, B. T. Gaudette, O. Y. Soliman, M. Pine, P. Hicks, T. B. Manzoni, J. J. Knox, J. L. Johnson, D. Laczko, H. Muramatsu, B. Davis, W. Meng, A. M. Rosenfeld, S. Strohmeier, P. J. C. Lin, B. L. Mui, Y. K. Tam, K. Karikó, A. Jacquet, F. Krammer, P. Bates, M. P. Cancro, D. Weissman, E. T. Luning Prak, D. Allman, M. Locci, and N. Pardi. 2021. Lipid nanoparticles enhance the efficacy of mRNA and protein subunit vaccines by inducing robust T follicular helper cell and humoral responses. *Immunity* 54(12):2877–2892. https://doi.org/10.1016/j.immuni.2021.11.001.

Bettini, E., and M. Locci. 2021. SARS-CoV-2 mRNA vaccines: Immunological mechanism and beyond. *Vaccines* 9(2). https://doi.org/10.3390/vaccines9020147.

Biedermann, T., M. Kneilling, R. Mailhammer, K. Maier, C. A. Sander, G. Kollias, S. L. Kunkel, L. Hultner, and M. Rocken. 2000. Mast cells control neutrophil recruitment during T cell-mediated delayed-type hypersensitivity reactions through tumor necrosis factor and macrophage inflammatory protein 2. *Journal of Experimental Medicine* 192(10):1441–1452. https://doi.org/10.1084/jem.192.10.1441.

Bos, R., L. Rutten, J. E. M. van der Lubbe, M. J. G. Bakkers, G. Hardenberg, F. Wegmann, D. Zuijdgeest, A. H. de Wilde, A. Koornneef, A. Verwilligen, D. van Manen, T. Kwaks, R. Vogels, T. J. Dalebout, S. K. Myeni, M. Kikkert, E. J. Snijder, Z. Li, D. H. Barouch, J. Vellinga, J. P. M. Langedijk, R. C. Zahn, J. Custers, and H. Schuitemaker. 2020. Ad26 vector–based COVID-19 vaccine encoding a prefusion-stabilized SARS-CoV-2 spike immunogen induces potent humoral and cellular immune responses. *NPJ Vaccines* 5:91. https://doi.org/10.1038/s41541-020-00243-x.

Bowen, J. E., A. C. Walls, A. Joshi, K. R. Sprouse, C. Stewart, M. A. Tortorici, N. M. Franko, J. K. Logue, I. G. Mazzitelli, S. W. Tiles, K. Ahmed, A. Shariq, G. Snell, N. T. Iqbal, J. Geffner, A. Bandera, A. Gori, R. Grifantini, H. Y. Chu, W. C. Van Voorhis, D. Corti, and D. Veesler. 2021. SARS-CoV-2 spike conformation determines plasma neutralizing activity. bioRxiv. https://doi.org/10.1101/2021.12.19.473391.

Bulcha, J. T., Y. Wang, H. Ma, P. W. L. Tai, and G. Gao. 2021. Viral vector platforms within the gene therapy landscape. *Signal Transduction and Targeted Therapy* 6(1):53. https://doi.org/10.1038/s41392-021-00487-6.

Cao, Y., and G. F. Gao. 2021. mRNA vaccines: A matter of delivery. *EClinicalMedicine* 32:100746. https://doi.org/10.1016/j.eclinm.2021.100746.

Chaplin, D. D. 2010. Overview of the immune response. *Journal of Allergy and Clinical Immunology* 125(2 Suppl 2):S3–S23. https://doi.org/10.1016/j.jaci.2009.12.980.

Chavda, V. P., R. Bezbaruah, D. Valu, B. Patel, A. Kumar, S. Prasad, B. B. Kakoti, A. Kaushik, and M. Jesawadawala. 2023. Adenoviral vector–based vaccine platform for COVID-19: Current status. *Vaccines* 11(2). https://doi.org/10.3390/vaccines11020432.

Chen, D. P., Y. H. Wen, W. T. Lin, and F. P. Hsu. 2022a. Association between the side effect induced by COVID-19 vaccines and the immune regulatory gene polymorphism. *Frontiers in Immunology* 13:941497. https://doi.org/10.3389/fimmu.2022.941497.

Chen, Y., Z. Xu, P. Wang, X. M. Li, Z. W. Shuai, D. Q. Ye, and H. F. Pan. 2022b. New-onset autoimmune phenomena post-COVID-19 vaccination. *Immunology* 165(4):386–401. https://doi.org/10.1111/imm.13443.

Chu, L., K. Vrbicky, D. Montefiori, W. Huang, B. Nestorova, Y. Chang, A. Carfi, D. K. Edwards, J. Oestreicher, H. Legault, F. J. Dutko, B. Girard, R. Pajon, J. M. Miller, R. Das, B. Leav, and R. McPhee. 2022. Immune response to SARS-CoV-2 after a booster of mRNA-1273: An open-label Phase 2 trial. *Nature Medicine* 28(5):1042–1049. https://doi.org/10.1038/s41591-022-01739-w.

Corbett, K. S., B. Flynn, K. E. Foulds, J. R. Francica, S. Boyoglu-Barnum, A. P. Werner, B. Flach, S. O'Connell, K. W. Bock, M. Minai, B. M. Nagata, H. Andersen, D. R. Martinez, A. T. Noe, N. Douek, M. M. Donaldson, N. N. Nji, G. S. Alvarado, D. K. Edwards, D. R. Flebbe, E. Lamb, N. A. Doria-Rose, B. C. Lin, M. K. Louder, S. O'Dell, S. D. Schmidt, E. Phung, L. A. Chang, C. Yap, J. M. Todd, L. Pessaint, A. Van Ry, S. Browne, J. Greenhouse, T. Putman-Taylor, A. Strasbaugh, T. A. Campbell, A. Cook, A. Dodson, K. Steingrebe, W. Shi, Y. Zhang, O. M. Abiona, L. Wang, A. Pegu, E. S. Yang, K. Leung, T. Zhou, I. T. Teng, A. Widge, I. Gordon, L. Novik, R. A. Gillespie, R. J. Loomis, J. I. Moliva, G. Stewart-Jones, S. Himansu, W. P. Kong, M. C. Nason, K. M. Morabito, T. J. Ruckwardt, J. E. Ledgerwood, M. R. Gaudinski, P. D. Kwong, J. R. Mascola, A. Carfi, M. G. Lewis, R. S. Baric, A. McDermott, I. N. Moore, N. J. Sullivan, M. Roederer, R. A. Seder, and B. S. Graham. 2020. Evaluation of the mRNA-1273 vaccine against SARS-CoV-2 in nonhuman primates. *New England Journal of Medicine* 383(16):1544–1555. https://doi.org/10.1056/NEJMoa2024671.

Coughlan, L. 2020. Factors which contribute to the immunogenicity of non-replicating adenoviral vectored vaccines. *Frontiers in Immunology* 11:909. https://doi.org/10.3389/fimmu.2020.00909.

Creech, C. B., S. C. Walker, and R. J. Samuels. 2021. SARS-CoV-2 vaccines. *JAMA* 325(13):1318–1320. https://doi.org/10.1001/jama.2021.3199.

Cullis, P. R., and M. J. Hope. 2017. Lipid nanoparticle systems for enabling gene therapies. *Molecular Therapy* 25(7):1467–1475. https://doi.org/10.1016/j.ymthe.2017.03.013.

Dabbiru, V. A. S., L. Muller, L. Schonborn, and A. Greinacher. 2023. Vaccine-induced immune thrombocytopenia and thrombosis (VITT)—insights from clinical cases, in vitro studies and murine models. *Journal of Clinical Medicine* 12(19). https://doi.org/10.3390/jcm12196126.

Diamond, M. S., and T. C. Pierson. 2020. The challenges of vaccine development against a new virus during a pandemic. *Cell Host & Microbe* 27(5):699–703. https://doi.org/10.1016/j.chom.2020.04.021.

Ewer, K., S. Sebastian, A. J. Spencer, S. Gilbert, A. V. S. Hill, and T. Lambe. 2017. Chimpanzee adenoviral vectors as vaccines for outbreak pathogens. *Human Vaccines & Immunotherapeutics* 13(12):3020–3032. https://doi.org/10.1080/21645515.2017.1383575.

Facciola, A., G. Visalli, A. Lagana, and A. Di Pietro. 2022. An overview of vaccine adjuvants: Current evidence and future perspectives. *Vaccines* 10(5). https://doi.org/10.3390/vaccines10050819.

FDA (Food and Drug Administration). 2021. *BLA clinical review memorandum—COMIRNATY.* https://www.fda.gov/media/152256/download (accessed December 12, 2023).

FDA. 2022. *BLA clinical review memorandum—SPIKEVAX.* https://www.fda.gov/media/156342/download (accessed December 12, 2023).

Fitzgerald, K. A., and J. C. Kagan. 2020. Toll-like receptors and the control of immunity. *Cell* 180(6):1044–1066. https://doi.org/10.1016/j.cell.2020.02.041.

Gartlan, C., T. Tipton, F. J. Salguero, Q. Sattentau, A. Gorringe, and M. W. Carroll. 2022. Vaccine-associated enhanced disease and pathogenic human coronaviruses. *Frontiers in Immunology* 13:882972. https://doi.org/10.3389/fimmu.2022.882972.

Geisbert, T. W., M. Bailey, L. Hensley, C. Asiedu, J. Geisbert, D. Stanley, A. Honko, J. Johnson, S. Mulangu, M. G. Pau, J. Custers, J. Vellinga, J. Hendriks, P. Jahrling, M. Roederer, J. Goudsmit, R. Koup, and N. J. Sullivan. 2011. Recombinant adenovirus serotype 26 (Ad26) and Ad35 vaccine vectors bypass immunity to ad5 and protect nonhuman primates against ebolavirus challenge. *Journal of Virology* 85(9):4222–4233. https://doi.org/10.1128/jvi.02407-10.

Jackson, L. A., E. J. Anderson, N. G. Rouphael, P. C. Roberts, M. Makhene, R. N. Coler, M. P. McCullough, J. D. Chappell, M. R. Denison, L. J. Stevens, A. J. Pruijssers, A. McDermott, B. Flach, N. A. Doria-Rose, K. S. Corbett, K. M. Morabito, S. O'Dell, S. D. Schmidt, P. A. Swanson, II, M. Padilla, J. R. Mascola, K. M. Neuzil, H. Bennett, W. Sun, E. Peters, M. Makowski, J. Albert, K. Cross, W. Buchanan, R. Pikaart-Tautges, J. E. Ledgerwood, B. S. Graham, J. H. Beigel, and mRNA-1273 Study Group. 2020. An mRNA vaccine against SARS-CoV-2—preliminary report. *New England Journal of Medicine* 383(20):1920–1931. https://doi.org/10.1056/NEJMoa2022483.

Jarvis, D. L. 2003. Developing baculovirus-insect cell expression systems for humanized recombinant glycoprotein production. *Virology* 310(1):1–7. https://doi.org/10.1016/s0042-6822(03)00120-x.

Karikó, K., H. Muramatsu, F. A. Welsh, J. Ludwig, H. Kato, S. Akira, and D. Weissman. 2008. Incorporation of pseudouridine into mRNA yields superior nonimmunogenic vector with increased translational capacity and biological stability. *Molecular Therapy* 16(11):1833–1840. https://doi.org/10.1038/mt.2008.200.

Keech, C., G. Albert, I. Cho, A. Robertson, P. Reed, S. Neal, J. S. Plested, M. Zhu, S. Cloney-Clark, H. Zhou, G. Smith, N. Patel, M. B. Frieman, R. E. Haupt, J. Logue, M. McGrath, S. Weston, P. A. Piedra, C. Desai, K. Callahan, M. Lewis, P. Price-Abbott, N. Formica, V. Shinde, L. Fries, J. D. Lickliter, P. Griffin, B. Wilkinson, and G. M. Glenn. 2020. Phase 1–2 trial of a SARS-CoV-2 recombinant spike protein nanoparticle vaccine. *New England Journal of Medicine* 383(24):2320–2332. https://doi.org/10.1056/NEJMoa2026920.

Khehra, N., I. Padda, U. Jaferi, H. Atwal, S. Narain, and M. S. Parmar. 2021. Tozinameran (BNT162b2) vaccine: The journey from preclinical research to clinical trials and authorization. *AAPS PharmSciTech* 22(5):172. https://doi.org/10.1208/s12249-021-02058-y.

Kim, S. C., S. S. Sekhon, W. R. Shin, G. Ahn, B. K. Cho, J. Y. Ahn, and Y. H. Kim. 2022. Modifications of mRNA vaccine structural elements for improving mRNA stability and translation efficiency. *Molecular & Cellular Toxicology* 18(1):1–8. https://doi.org/10.1007/s13273-021-00171-4.

Kirchdoerfer, R. N., C. A. Cottrell, N. Wang, J. Pallesen, H. M. Yassine, H. L. Turner, K. S. Corbett, B. S. Graham, J. S. McLellan, and A. B. Ward. 2016. Pre-fusion structure of a human coronavirus spike protein. *Nature* 531(7592):118–121. https://doi.org/10.1038/nature17200.

Krammer, F. 2020. SARS-CoV-2 vaccines in development. *Nature* 586(7830):516–527. https://doi.org/10.1038/s41586-020-2798-3.

Laczko, D., M. J. Hogan, S. A. Toulmin, P. Hicks, K. Lederer, B. T. Gaudette, D. Castano, F. Amanat, H. Muramatsu, T. H. Oguin, III, A. Ojha, L. Zhang, Z. Mu, R. Parks, T. B. Manzoni, B. Roper, S. Strohmeier, I. Tombacz, L. Arwood, R. Nachbagauer, K. Karikó, J. Greenhouse, L. Pessaint, M. Porto, T. Putman-Taylor, A. Strasbaugh, T. A. Campbell, P. J. C. Lin, Y. K. Tam, G. D. Sempowski, M. Farzan, H. Choe, K. O. Saunders, B. F. Haynes, H. Andersen, L. C. Eisenlohr, D. Weissman, F. Krammer, P. Bates, D. Allman, M. Locci, and N. Pardi. 2020. A single immunization with nucleoside-modified mRNA vaccines elicits strong cellular and humoral immune responses against SARS-CoV-2 in mice. *Immunity* 53(4):724–732. https://doi.org/10.1016/j.immuni.2020.07.019.

Laidlaw, B. J., and A. H. Ellebedy. 2022. The germinal centre B cell response to SARS-CoV-2. *Nature Reviews: Immunology* 22(1):7–18. https://doi.org/10.1038/s41577-021-00657-1.

Lamprinou, M., A. Sachinidis, E. Stamoula, T. Vavilis, and G. Papazisis. 2023. COVID-19 vaccines adverse events: Potential molecular mechanisms. *Immunologic Research* 71(3):356–372. https://doi.org/10.1007/s12026-023-09357-5.

Lederer, K., D. Castano, D. Gomez Atria, T. H. Oguin, III, S. Wang, T. B. Manzoni, H. Muramatsu, M. J. Hogan, F. Amanat, P. Cherubin, K. A. Lundgreen, Y. K. Tam, S. H. Y. Fan, L. C. Eisenlohr, I. Maillard, D. Weissman, P. Bates, F. Krammer, G. D. Sempowski, N. Pardi, and M. Locci. 2020. SARS-CoV-2 mRNA vaccines foster potent antigen-specific germinal center responses associated with neutralizing antibody generation. *Immunity* 53(6):1281–1295. https://doi.org/10.1016/j.immuni.2020.11.009.

Lukashev, A. N., and A. A. Zamyatnin, Jr. 2016. Viral vectors for gene therapy: Current state and clinical perspectives. *Biochemistry* 81(7):700–708. https://doi.org/10.1134/S0006297916070063.

Maier, M. A., M. Jayaraman, S. Matsuda, J. Liu, S. Barros, W. Querbes, Y. K. Tam, S. M. Ansell, V. Kumar, J. Qin, X. Zhang, Q. Wang, S. Panesar, R. Hutabarat, M. Carioto, J. Hettinger, P. Kandasamy, D. Butler, K. G. Rajeev, B. Pang, K. Charisse, K. Fitzgerald, B. L. Mui, X. Du, P. Cullis, T. D. Madden, M. J. Hope, M. Manoharan, and A. Akinc. 2013. Biodegradable lipids enabling rapidly eliminated lipid nanoparticles for systemic delivery of RNAI therapeutics. *Molecular Therapy* 21(8):1570–1578. https://doi.org/10.1038/mt.2013.124.

Marfe, G., S. Perna, and A. K. Shukla. 2021. Effectiveness of COVID-19 vaccines and their challenges (review). *Experimental and Therapeutic Medicine* 22(6):1407. https://doi.org/10.3892/etm.2021.10843.

Martinez-Flores, D., J. Zepeda-Cervantes, A. Cruz-Resendiz, S. Aguirre-Sampieri, A. Sampieri, and L. Vaca. 2021. SARS-CoV-2 vaccines based on the spike glycoprotein and implications of new viral variants. *Frontiers in Immunology* 12:701501. https://doi.org/10.3389/fimmu.2021.701501.

McLeod, J. J., B. Baker, and J. J. Ryan. 2015. Mast cell production and response to IL-4 and IL-13. *Cytokine* 75(1):57–61. https://doi.org/10.1016/j.cyto.2015.05.019.

Menegale, F., M. Manica, A. Zardini, G. Guzzetta, V. Marziano, V. d'Andrea, F. Trentini, M. Ajelli, P. Poletti, and S. Merler. 2023. Evaluation of waning of SARS-CoV-2 vaccine-induced immunity: A systematic review and meta-analysis. *JAMA Network Open* 6(5):e2310650. https://doi.org/10.1001/jamanetworkopen.2023.10650.

Ndeupen, S., Z. Qin, S. Jacobsen, A. Bouteau, H. Estanbouli, and B. Z. Igyarto. 2021. The mRNA-LNP platform's lipid nanoparticle component used in preclinical vaccine studies is highly inflammatory. *iScience* 24(12):103479. https://doi.org/10.1016/j.isci.2021.103479.

Pallesen, J., N. Wang, K. S. Corbett, D. Wrapp, R. N. Kirchdoerfer, H. L. Turner, C. A. Cottrell, M. M. Becker, L. Wang, W. Shi, W. P. Kong, E. L. Andres, A. N. Kettenbach, M. R. Denison, J. D. Chappell, B. S. Graham, A. B. Ward, and J. S. McLellan. 2017. Immunogenicity and structures of a rationally designed prefusion MERS-COV spike antigen. *Proceedings of the National Academy of Sciences of the United States of America* 114(35):E7348–E7357. https://doi. org/10.1073/pnas.1707304114.

Pardi, N., S. Tuyishime, H. Muramatsu, K. Karikó, B. L. Mui, Y. K. Tam, T. D. Madden, M. J. Hope, and D. Weissman. 2015. Expression kinetics of nucleoside-modified mRNA delivered in lipid nanoparticles to mice by various routes. *Journal of Controlled Release* 217:345–351. https://doi.org/10.1016/j.jconrel.2015.08.007.

Pardi, N., M. J. Hogan, F. W. Porter, and D. Weissman. 2018. mRNA vaccines—a new era in vaccinology. *Nature Reviews Drug Discovery* 17(4):261–279. https://doi.org/10.1038/nrd.2017.243.

Pettini, E., D. Medaglini, and A. Ciabattini. 2022. Profiling the B cell immune response elicited by vaccination against the respiratory virus SARS-CoV-2. *Frontiers in Immunology* 13:1058748. https://doi.org/10.3389/fimmu.2022.1058748.

Pollard, A. J., and E. M. Bijker. 2021. A guide to vaccinology: From basic principles to new developments. *Nature Reviews: Immunology* 21(2):83–100. https://doi.org/10.1038/s41577-020-00479-7.

Robbiani, D. F., C. Gaebler, F. Muecksch, J. C. C. Lorenzi, Z. Wang, A. Cho, M. Agudelo, C. O. Barnes, A. Gazumyan, S. Finkin, T. Hagglof, T. Y. Oliveira, C. Viant, A. Hurley, H. H. Hoffmann, K. G. Millard, R. G. Kost, M. Cipolla, K. Gordon, F. Bianchini, S. T. Chen, V. Ramos, R. Patel, J. Dizon, I. Shimeliovich, P. Mendoza, H. Hartweger, L. Nogueira, M. Pack, J. Horowitz, F. Schmidt, Y. Weisblum, E. Michailidis, A. W. Ashbrook, E. Waltari, J. E. Pak, K. E. Huey-Tubman, N. Koranda, P. R. Hoffman, A. P. West, Jr., C. M. Rice, T. Hatziioannou, P. J. Bjorkman, P. D. Bieniasz, M. Caskey, and M. C. Nussenzweig. 2020. Convergent antibody responses to SARS-CoV-2 in convalescent individuals. *Nature* 584(7821):437–442. https://doi.org/10.1038/s41586-020-2456-9.

Sadarangani, M., A. Marchant, and T. R. Kollmann. 2021. Immunological mechanisms of vaccine-induced protection against COVID-19 in humans. *Nature Reviews: Immunology* 21(8):475–484. https://doi.org/10.1038/s41577-021-00578-z.

Sadoff, J., G. Gray, A. Vandebosch, V. Cárdenas, G. Shukarev, B. Grinsztejn, P. A. Goepfert, C. Truyers, H. Fennema, B. Spiessens, K. Offergeld, G. Scheper, K. L. Taylor, M. L. Robb, J. Treanor, D. H. Barouch, J. Stoddard, M. F. Ryser, M. A. Marovich, K. M. Neuzil, L. Corey, N. Cauwenberghs, T. Tanner, K. Hardt, J. Ruiz-Guiñazú, M. Le Gars, H. Schuitemaker, J. Van Hoof, F. Struyf, and M. Douoguih. 2021. Safety and efficacy of single-dose Ad26.COV2.S vaccine against COVID-19. *New England Journal of Medicine* 384(23):2187–2201. https://doi.org/10.1056/NEJMoa2101544.

Segal, Y., and Y. Shoenfeld. 2018. Vaccine-induced autoimmunity: The role of molecular mimicry and immune crossreaction. *Cellular & Molecular Immunology* 15(6):586–594. https://doi.org/10.1038/cmi.2017.151.

Stertman, L., A. E. Palm, B. Zarnegar, B. Carow, C. Lunderius Andersson, S. E. Magnusson, C. Carnrot, V. Shinde, G. Smith, G. Glenn, L. Fries, and K. Lovgren Bengtsson. 2023. The matrix-M adjuvant: A critical component of vaccines for the 21st century. *Human Vaccines & Immunotherapeutics* 19(1):2189885. https://doi.org/10.1080/21645515.2023.2189885.

Stone, C. A., Jr., C. R. F. Rukasin, T. M. Beachkofsky, and E. J. Phillips. 2019. Immune-mediated adverse reactions to vaccines. *British Journal of Clinical Pharmacology* 85(12):2694–2706. https://doi.org/10.1111/bcp.14112.

Tam, H. H., M. B. Melo, M. Kang, J. M. Pelet, V. M. Ruda, M. H. Foley, J. K. Hu, S. Kumari, J. Crampton, A. D. Baldeon, R. W. Sanders, J. P. Moore, S. Crotty, R. Langer, D. G. Anderson, A. K. Chakraborty, and D. J. Irvine. 2016. Sustained antigen availability during germinal center initiation enhances antibody responses to vaccination. *Proceedings of the National Academy of Sciences of the United States of America* 113(43):E6639–E6648. https://doi.org/10.1073/pnas.1606050113.

Teijaro, J. R., and D. L. Farber. 2021. COVID-19 vaccines: Modes of immune activation and future challenges. *Nature Reviews: Immunology* 21(4):195–197. https://doi.org/10.1038/s41577-021-00526-x.

Trougakos, I. P., E. Terpos, H. Alexopoulos, M. Politou, D. Paraskevis, A. Scorilas, E. Kastritis, E. Andreakos, and M. A. Dimopoulos. 2022. Adverse effects of COVID-19 mRNA vaccines: The spike hypothesis. *Trends in Molecular Medicine* 28(7):542–554. https://doi.org/10.1016/j.molmed.2022.04.007.

Turner, J. S., J. A. O'Halloran, E. Kalaidina, W. Kim, A. J. Schmitz, J. Q. Zhou, T. Lei, M. Thapa, R. E. Chen, J. B. Case, F. Amanat, A. M. Rauseo, A. Haile, X. Xie, M. K. Klebert, T. Suessen, W. D. Middleton, P. Y. Shi, F. Krammer, S. A. Teefey, M. S. Diamond, R. M. Presti, and A. H. Ellebedy. 2021. SARS-CoV-2 mRNA vaccines induce persistent human germinal centre responses. *Nature* 596(7870):109–113. https://doi.org/10.1038/s41586-021-03738-2.

Verbeke, R., M. J. Hogan, K. Lore, and N. Pardi. 2022. Innate immune mechanisms of mRNA vaccines. *Immunity* 55(11):1993–2005. https://doi.org/10.1016/j.immuni.2022.10.014.

Walls, A. C., Y. J. Park, M. A. Tortorici, A. Wall, A. T. McGuire, and D. Veesler. 2020. Structure, function, and antigenicity of the SARS-CoV-2 spike glycoprotein. *Cell* 183(6):1735. https://doi.org/10.1016/j.cell.2020.11.032.

Walsh, E. E., R. W. Frenck, Jr., A. R. Falsey, N. Kitchin, J. Absalon, A. Gurtman, S. Lockhart, K. Neuzil, M. J. Mulligan, R. Bailey, K. A. Swanson, P. Li, K. Koury, W. Kalina, D. Cooper, C. Fontes-Garfias, P. Y. Shi, O. Tureci, K. R. Tompkins, K. E. Lyke, V. Raabe, P. R. Dormitzer, K. U. Jansen, U. Sahin, and W. C. Gruber. 2020. Safety and immunogenicity of two RNA-based COVID-19 vaccine candidates. *New England Journal of Medicine* 383(25):2439–2450. https://doi.org/10.1056/NEJMoa2027906.

Watanabe, Y., L. Mendonca, E. R. Allen, A. Howe, M. Lee, J. D. Allen, H. Chawla, D. Pulido, F. Donnellan, H. Davies, M. Ulaszewska, S. Belij-Rammerstorfer, S. Morris, A. S. Krebs, W. Dejnirattisai, J. Mongkolsapaya, P. Supasa, G. R. Screaton, C. M. Green, T. Lambe, P. Zhang, S. C. Gilbert, and M. Crispin. 2021. Native-like SARS-CoV-2 spike glycoprotein expressed by ChAdOx1 nCoV-19/AZD1222 vaccine. *ACS Central Science* 7(4):594–602. https://doi.org/10.1021/acscentsci.1c00080.

Welsh, J. 2021. Coronavirus variants—will new mRNA vaccines meet the challenge? *Engineering* 7(6):712–714. https://doi.org/10.1016/j.eng.2021.04.005.

Widge, A. T., N. G. Rouphael, L. A. Jackson, E. J. Anderson, P. C. Roberts, M. Makhene, J. D. Chappell, M. R. Denison, L. J. Stevens, A. J. Pruijssers, A. B. McDermott, B. Flach, B. C. Lin, N. A. Doria-Rose, S. O'Dell, S. D. Schmidt, K. M. Neuzil, H. Bennett, B. Leav, M. Makowski, J. Albert, K. Cross, V. V. Edara, K. Floyd, M. S. Suthar, W. Buchanan, C. J. Luke, J. E. Ledgerwood, J. R. Mascola, B. S. Graham, J. H. Beigel, and mRNA-1273 Study Group. 2021. Durability of responses after SARS-CoV-2 mRNA-1273 vaccination. *New England Journal of Medicine* 384(1):80–82. https://doi.org/10.1056/NEJMc2032195.

Wilkins, A. L., D. Kazmin, G. Napolitani, E. A. Clutterbuck, B. Pulendran, C. A. Siegrist, and A. J. Pollard. 2017. AS03- and Mf59-adjuvanted influenza vaccines in children. *Frontiers in Immunology* 8:1760. https://doi.org/10.3389/fimmu.2017.01760.

Wrapp, D., N. Wang, K. S. Corbett, J. A. Goldsmith, C. L. Hsieh, O. Abiona, B. S. Graham, and J. S. McLellan. 2020. Cryo-em structure of the 2019-nCoV spike in the prefusion conformation. *bioRxiv*. https://doi.org/10.1101/2020.02.11.944462.

Xiaojie, S., L. Yu, Y. Lei, Y. Guang, and Q. Min. 2020. Neutralizing antibodies targeting SARS-CoV-2 spike protein. *Stem Cell Research* 50:102125. https://doi.org/10.1016/j.scr.2020.102125.

Yang, G., J. Wang, P. Sun, J. Qin, X. Yang, D. Chen, Y. Zhang, N. Zhong, and Z. Wang. 2023. SARS-CoV-2 epitope-specific T cells: Immunity response feature, TCR repertoire characteristics and cross-reactivity. *Frontiers in Immunology* 14:1146196. https://doi.org/10.3389/fimmu.2023.1146196.

Zost, S. J., P. Gilchuk, R. E. Chen, J. B. Case, J. X. Reidy, A. Trivette, R. S. Nargi, R. E. Sutton, N. Suryadevara, E. C. Chen, E. Binshtein, S. Shrihari, M. Ostrowski, H. Y. Chu, J. E. Didier, K. W. MacRenaris, T. Jones, S. Day, L. Myers, F. Eun-Hyung Lee, D. C. Nguyen, I. Sanz, D. R. Martinez, P. W. Rothlauf, L. M. Bloyet, S. P. J. Whelan, R. S. Baric, L. B. Thackray, M. S. Diamond, R. H. Carnahan, and J. E. Crowe, Jr. 2020. Rapid isolation and profiling of a diverse panel of human monoclonal antibodies targeting the SARS-CoV-2 spike protein. *Nature Medicine* 26(9):1422–1427. https://doi.org/10.1038/s41591-020-0998-x.

# 3

# Neurologic Conditions and COVID-19 Vaccines

This chapter describes the potential relationship between COVID-19 vaccines and potential neurological harms Guillain-Barré syndrome (GBS), chronic inflammatory demyelinating polyneuropathy (CIDP), Bell's palsy (BP), transverse myelitis (TM), chronic headache, and postural orthostatic tachycardia syndrome (POTS) (see Boxes 3-1 through 3-6 for all conclusions in this chapter).

## GUILLAIN-BARRÉ SYNDROME

---

**BOX 3-1**
**Conclusions for Guillain-Barré Syndrome**

**Conclusion 3-1: The evidence favors rejection of a causal relationship between the BNT162b2 vaccine and Guillain-Barré syndrome.**

**Conclusion 3-2: The evidence favors rejection of a causal relationship between the mRNA-1273 vaccine and Guillain-Barré syndrome.**

**Conclusion 3-3: The evidence favors acceptance of a causal relationship between the Ad26.COV2.S vaccine and Guillain-Barré syndrome.**

**Conclusion 3-4: The evidence is inadequate to accept or reject a causal relationship between the NVX-CoV2373 vaccine and Guillain-Barré syndrome.**

---

**Background**

GBS is an acute, monophasic, immune-mediated disorder, or group of disorders, that primarily affects the peripheral nerves and roots. The typical clinical features include progressive symmetric muscle weakness and absent or depressed deep tendon reflexes. Patients may also experience tingling or prickling sensations (paresthesia) along with autonomic dysfunction, including fluctuations in blood pressure, heart rate, and respiratory distress. Cranial nerve involvement can result in facial weakness, difficulty swallowing, and speech problems, and some individuals experience significant pain, particularly in the back or legs. Symptoms usually progress over 1–2 weeks and generally plateau before 4 weeks (Fokke et al., 2014).

Diagnosing GBS is a multifaceted process that involves a comprehensive clinical evaluation, cerebrospinal fluid (CSF) analysis, and electrodiagnostic studies. A thorough clinical history and neurological examination are critical to assess the pattern of weakness and reflex abnormalities. Analysis of CSF often reveals elevated protein levels without a significant increase in white blood cells. Electrophysiological tests can confirm the diagnosis by revealing evidence of nerve demyelination in demyelinating variants of GBS and identifying pathological changes affecting both the roots and nerves.

GBS is a relatively rare disease, with a global incidence of 0.81–1.91 cases per 100,000 person-years (Shahrizaila et al., 2021). The U.S. incidence of GBS is generally in line with the global average, with an estimated 1–2 cases per 100,000 individuals each year (Bragazzi et al., 2021). Although all age groups are affected, the incidence increases by approximately 20 percent with every 10-year increase beyond the first decade of life, with a peak incidence reported between 50–69 years and a slight male predominance (Leonhard et al., 2022).

The pathophysiology of GBS remains incompletely understood and is likely heterogeneous, reflecting phenotypic variability among what is likely a group of related disorders rather than a single nosological entity. Despite this heterogeneity, more than two-thirds of patients report a history of upper respiratory tract or gastrointestinal infection weeks before the onset of neurologic symptoms, suggesting infection plays an important pathogenic role in all GBS variants (Leonhard et al., 2022). Although GBS is a global disease, regional differences occur in the distribution of variants. Demyelinating forms dominate in Europe and North America, but acute inflammatory demyelinating polyradiculoneuropathy (AIDP) accounts for 80–90 percent of cases and is characterized by ascending limb weakness. Other demyelinating variants with prominent and early cranial nerve involvement affecting eye movements and facial muscles, including the Miller-Fisher and facial diplegia with limb paresthesia variant, are rare. Axonal subtypes, such as acute motor axonal neuropathy (AMAN), dominate in Asia, particularly Bangladesh and north China (Leonhard et al., 2022). Seasonal variation of incidence tracks with infections. The risk is higher during the winter, particularly in Europe and North America, where it is associated primarily with upper respiratory infections. A summer peak occurs in Northern China, India, Bangladesh, and Latin America, where diarrheal illnesses can be more common. Incidence can also rise during outbreaks of infection, such as with Zika virus in South America or other arthropod infections, such as dengue and chikungunya (Shahrizaila et al., 2021). Globally, commonly implicated pathogens include *Campylobacter jejuni*, cytomegalovirus, Epstein-Barr virus, *Mycoplasma pneumoniae*, *Haemophilus influenzae*, influenza A virus, and Zika virus (Shahrizaila et al., 2021). *C. Jejuni* is the most commonly and extensively reported, and robust evidence suggests that molecular mimicry between microbial antigens and nerves is implicated in developing GBS.

In addition to infection, GBS cases after vaccination have also been reported, especially with the 1976 swine-influenza and seasonal 2009 H1N1 monovalent influenza vaccines. However, the overall risk of influenza vaccines if present at all appears to be small, approximately 1–2 excess cases of GBS per million people vaccinated (Vellozzi et al., 2014). While some have reported an increased risk of GBS after severe acute respiratory syndrome coronavirus-2 (SARS-CoV-2) infection, the actual incidence of GBS decreased during the pandemic, possibly due to an overall reduction in other communicable diseases (Keddie et al., 2021).

The latency period between exposure to a triggering event (infection or vaccination) and GBS can vary, but it typically occurs within a few days to a few weeks. It is crucial to understand that not everyone exposed to these risk factors will develop GBS, and the exact mechanisms continue to be the subject of ongoing research. The epidemiology of GBS can be influenced by various factors, including changes in diagnostic techniques, vaccination practices, and evolving patterns of infectious diseases, so ongoing surveillance and research are crucial to continually monitor and understand it.

## Mechanisms

GBS is heterogeneous because it is likely a group of related disorders. Demyelinating variants, such AIDP, differ from axonal variants, such as AMAN, in both the range and extent of pathological changes. Nevertheless, nerve injury appears to be immune mediated, with antecedent infection being a common potential trigger. Autopsy studies demonstrate infiltrates of lymphocytes and macrophages involved in macrophage-mediated demyelination (Asbury et al., 1969; Wanschitz et al., 2003). Complement deposition can be demonstrated within the endoneurium, on the surface of myelinated fibers, and on mononuclear cells at sites of myelin breakdown, particularly in acute cases of less than 4 weeks duration, suggesting a role for antibody-mediated injury, whereas granzyme-expressing CD8+ T cells (i.e., cytotoxic T cells) are described in cases of longer duration (Wanschitz et al., 2003). By contrast, patients with AMAN demonstrate primary axonal injury with a paucity of inflammatory infiltrates or demyelination. IgG and complement-mediated humoral immune response are directed against epitopes in the axonal membrane. Animal models of GBS have been generated by immunizing rats with myelin proteins, galactocerebroside, adoptive transfer of myelin-specific T cells (AIDP), or immunization with GM1 ganglioside, resulting in circulating anti-GM1 antibodies (AMAN) (Shahrizaila et al., 2021) (see Figure 3-1). These animal models implicate T cells and macrophages in AIDP but suggest that autoantibodies may play a greater role in AMAN (Shahrizaila et al., 2021). The mechanism of antibody-mediated damage may include interference with ion channel function, complement-dependent cytotoxicity, and/or interference with nerve regeneration; different clinical subtypes of GBS are associated with different anti-ganglioside antibodies (Shahrizaila et al., 2021).

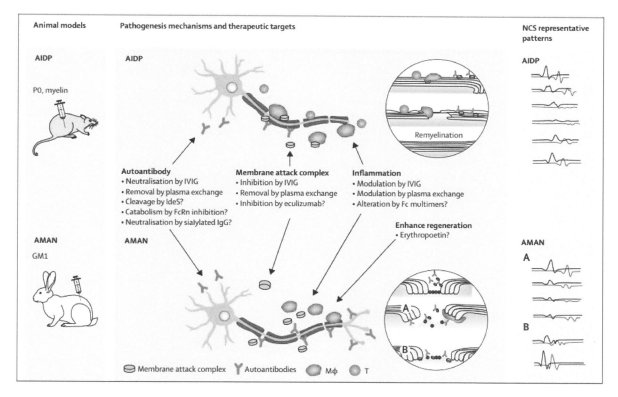

**FIGURE 3-1** Overview of the pathogenesis and therapeutic targets of the two major Guillain-Barré syndrome subtypes.
NOTE: AMAN: Acute Motor Axonal Neuropathy; AIDP: Acute Inflammatory Demyelinating Polyneuropathy; IVIG: Intravenous Immunoglobulin; Ig: Immunoglobulin; GM1: Ganglioside M1; Fc: Fragment crystallizable.
SOURCE: Shahrizaila et al., 2021. Reprinted from *The Lancet*, Vol. 397(10280), Shahrizaila, N., H. C., Lehmann, and S. Kuwabara. Guillain-Barré syndrome. 1214-1228, Copyright (2021), with permission from Elsevier.

Evidence for molecular mimicry is best supported for *C. jejuni*-associated AMAN, where the reasoning is as follows (Yuki et al., 2004):

- Patients with GBS after *C. jejuni*, but not patients with *C. jejuni* enteritis, have antibodies to GM1 ganglioside in their serum (Sheikh et al., 1998).
- The specific serotype of *C. jejuni* most commonly isolated from patients with GBS (PEN19) is rare in patients with *C. jejuni* enteritis.
- The GM1 ganglioside has an antigenic similarity with the lipopolysaccharide of *C. jejuni* serotype PEN19 (Yuki et al., 1993).
- Rabbits sensitized to *C. jejuni* lipopolysaccharide (LPS) develop AMAN and flaccid limb weakness with pathological findings similar to GBS.
- Anti-GM1 IgG from patients with GBS can block muscle action potentials in muscle-spinal cord coculture, although they do not induce weakness when injected into mice (Yuki et al., 2004).

*C. jejuni* infection can also generate antibodies against GQ1b gangliosides, which are associated with the Miller-Fisher GBS variant (Jacobs et al., 1997). Anti-ganglioside antibodies, however, are not found in association with all GBS variants. In addition, as mentioned in the background section, GBS is associated with a variety of pathogens, including potentially SARS-CoV-2, arguing against molecular mimicry as the single unifying mechanism in all forms of it.

A few in silico studies have sought peptide antigens in SARS-CoV-2 with the potential to induce antibodies that cross-react with proteins in the peripheral or central nervous system, thereby activating complement and mediating neuronal damage (Chen et al., 2022b; Kadkhoda, 2022). One such study demonstrated similarity between a peptide in SARS-CoV-2 and the NCAM L1–like protein in the myelin sheath and argued that cross-reactive antibodies might explain GBS after infection (Kadkhoda, 2022; Morsy, 2020). However, the shared peptide was in the SARS-CoV-2 envelope protein, not the spike protein, and would not provide mechanistic evidence for GBS occurring after COVID-19 vaccination.

Epidemiological evidence suggests a possible association between adenovirus-vector (AV) COVID-19 vaccines and GBS but not for the messenger ribonucleic acid (mRNA) vaccines (Hanson et al., 2022; Keh et al., 2023). This suggests the possibility of a platform-specific mechanism or immune response as opposed to one related to immune responses to the spike protein itself (such as molecular mimicry) (Rzymski, 2023). One study found high levels of complement-fixing antibodies to cytomegalovirus in a cohort of patients with GBS but no comparable antibodies to adenovirus in the same patients (Dowling et al., 1977), and adenovirus has not been historically linked with GBS in epidemiological studies. This suggests that natural adenoviral infection may not be associated with GBS.

ChAdOx1-S[1] has high affinity for the coxsackie and adenoviral receptor (CAR), whereas HAdV26 has much lower CAR affinity (Baker et al., 2021; Hemsath et al., 2022; Rzymski, 2023). CAR is widely expressed in the body, including the central nervous system (Zussy et al., 2016); however, whether it is expressed in the peripheral nervous system has not been established. Therefore, it is unknown whether ChAdOx1-S could target peripheral nerves directly.

## Epidemiological Evidence

Clinical trial results submitted to the Food and Drug Administration (FDA) for Emergency Use Authorization and full approval do not indicate a signal regarding GBS and any of the vaccines under study (FDA, 2021, 2023a,b,c). Table 3-1 presents nine studies that contributed to the causality assessment.

Keh et al. (2023) retrospectively analyzed data from the National Immunoglobulin Database linked to the National Immunisation Management System, which records all intravenous immunoglobulin (IVIG) prescriptions for GBS patients in England (IVIG is given to an estimated 86 percent of UK patients with GBS). IVIG approval requires adjudication by an independent physician panel (Keh et al., 2023). The study included 11.5 million doses

---

[1] Refers to the COVID-19 vaccine manufactured by Oxford-AstraZeneca.

**TABLE 3-1** Epidemiological Studies in the Guillain-Barré Syndrome Evidence Review

| Author | Study Design and Control Group | Location | Data Source | Vaccine(s) | Age Range | N | Number of Events | Results (95% CI) |
|---|---|---|---|---|---|---|---|---|
| Hanson et al. (2022) | Cohort/ vaccinated concurrent comparators and historical controls | US | VSD/EMR (physician adjudicated) | BNT162b2 | ≥12 years | 8.8 million doses | 9 cases meeting Brighton Collaboration criteria 1–3 during 1–21-day risk period | RR 20.56 (6.94–64.66) 15.5 excess cases in risk interval per million doses of Ad26. COV2.S compared to mRNA vaccines |
| | | | | mRNA-1273 | | 5.8 million doses | 9 cases meeting Brighton Collaboration criteria 1–3 during 1–21-day risk period | |
| | | | | Ad26. COV2.S | | 483,053 doses | 8 cases meeting Brighton Collaboration criteria 1–3 during 1–21-day risk period | |
| Keh et al. (2023) | Cohort/ vaccinated GBS cases | UK | National Immunization Database/ National Immuno-globulin Database | BNT162b2 | ≥18 years | 11.5 million doses | 21 cases in 0–42 days | No excess risk of GBS observed 0–42 days following BNT162b2 vaccine compared to vaccinated cases in control period |
| | | | | mRNA-1273 | | 300,000 doses | 1 | |
| | | | | ChAdOx1-S | | 20.3 million doses | 176 | |
| Klein et al. (2021) | Cohort/ vaccinated concurrent comparators | US | VSD/ EMR | BNT162b2 | ≥16 years | 6.8 million doses | BNT162b2 and mRNA-1273 combined: 10 | BNT162b2 and mRNA-1273 combined: RR 0.70 (0.22–2.31) |
| | | | | mRNA-1273 | | 5.1 million doses | | |

*continued*

**TABLE 3-1** Continued

| Author | Study Design and Control Group | Location | Data Source | Vaccine(s) | Age Range | N | Number of Events | Results (95% CI) |
|---|---|---|---|---|---|---|---|---|
| Li et al. (2022) | Cohort/ historical background | UK and Spain | Primary care databases linked to hospital data/ EMR | BNT162b2 (UK and Spain) | ≥18 years | UK Dose 1: 1.7 million vaccinees Dose 2: 1.2 million vaccinees | UK Dose 1: <5 Dose 2: <5 | UK N/A |
| | | | | | | Spain Dose 1: 1.9 million vaccinees Dose 2: 1.3 million vaccinees | Spain Dose 1: 5 Dose 2: <5 | Spain Dose 1: SIR 0.79 (0.33–1.91) |
| | | | | mRNA-1273 (Spain only) | | Dose 1: 244,913 vaccinees Dose 2: 160,213 vaccinees | Dose 1: 0 Dose 2: <5 cases | N/A |
| | | | | Ad26. COV2.S (Spain only) | | Dose 1: 120,731 vaccinees | Dose 1: 0 | N/A |
| | | | | ChAdOx1-S (UK and Spain) | | UK Dose 1: 3.8 million vaccinees Dose 2: 1.1 million vaccinees | UK Dose 1: 11 Dose 2: <5 | UK SIR 0.74 (0.41–1.33) |
| | | | | | | Spain Dose 1: 592,860 vaccinees Dose 2: 1.3 million vaccinees | Spain Dose 1: <5 Dose 2: 0 | Spain N/A |
| Loo et al. (2022) | Case-control study/ historical background | UK | EMR (physician adjudicated) | BNT162b2 | ≥16 years | 24 patients admitted with acute onset polyradiculo-neuropathy between January–June 2021 | 1 | 2.6-fold (1.98–3.51) increase in admissions compared with the average for the same period in the previous 3 years |
| | | | | mRNA-1273 | | | 1 | |
| | | | | ChAdOx1-S | | | 14 | |

**TABLE 3-1** Continued

| Author | Study Design and Control Group | Location | Data Source | Vaccine(s) | Age Range | N | Number of Events | Results (95% CI) |
|---|---|---|---|---|---|---|---|---|
| Morciano et al. (2023) | Cohort/self-controlled | Italy | Multi-regional databases/EMR | BNT162b2 | ≥12 years | 10.8 million vaccinees | Dose 1: 19 Dose 2: 30 | Dose 1: RI 0.85 (0.49–1.48)  Dose 2: RI 1.30 (0.80–2.10) |
| | | | | mRNA-1273 | | 1.7 million vaccinees | Dose 1: 7 Dose 2: 5 | Dose 1: RI 6.83 (2.14–21.85)  Dose 2: RI 7.41 (2.35–23.38) |
| | | | | Ad26.COV2.S | | 581,796 vaccinees | Dose 1: 7 | Dose 1: RI 1.94 (0.32–11.69) |
| | | | | ChAdOx1-S | | 2.9 million vaccinees | Dose 1: 34 Dose 2: 6 | Dose 1: RI 6.52 (2.88–14.77)  Dose 2: RI 3.56 (0.31–40.29) |
| Patone et al. (2021) | Cohort/self-controlled | England | English immunization records/EMR | BNT162b2 | ≥16 years | 12.1 million vaccinees | 34 cases during 1–28 days risk interval | IRR 0.86 (0.54–1.36) |
| | | | | ChAdOx1-S | | 20.4 million vaccinees | 153 1–28 days | IRR 2.04 (1.60–2.60) |
| Sturkenboom et al. (2022) | Cohort/background rate | European countries | Primary and secondary care databases/EMR | BNT162b2 | Varied | 6.5 million doses | 16 | IRR 1.10 (0.56–2.15) |
| | | | | mRNA-1273 | | 727,047 doses | No cases | N/A |
| | | | | Ad26.COV2.S | | 242,349 doses | 2 | IRR 5.65 (1.4–22.83) |
| | | | | ChAdOx1-S | | 4.6 million doses | 15 | IRR 1.43 (0.85–2.40) |

*continued*

**TABLE 3-1** Continued

| Author | Study Design and Control Group | Location | Data Source | Vaccine(s) | Age Range | N | Number of Events | Results (95% CI) |
|---|---|---|---|---|---|---|---|---|
| Walker et al. (2022) | Self-controlled cohort | UK | EMR | BNT162b2 | ≥18 years | 5.7 million vaccinees | 283 | IRR 1.00 (0.61–1.64) |
| | | | | mRNA-1273 | | 255,446 vaccinees | No cases | N/A |
| | | | | ChAdOx1-S | | 7.8 million vaccinees | 517 | IRR 2.85 (2.33–3.47) |

NOTES: BNT162b2 refers to the COVID-19 vaccine manufactured by Pfizer-BioNTech under the name Comirnaty®. mRNA-1273 refers to the COVID-19 vaccine manufactured by Moderna under the name Spikevax®. Ad26.COV2.S refers to the COVID-19 vaccine manufactured by Janssen. The primary series for Ad26.COV2.S is one dose. ChAdOx1-S refers to the COVID-19 vaccine manufactured by Oxford-AstraZeneca. ChAdOx1-S appears in this table because it provides support for Conclusion 3-3. The primary series for Ad26.COV2.S is one dose. Keh et al. (2023) refers to BNT162b2 as Tozinameran (Pfizer). Number of events refers to events in vaccinees only. EMR: electronic medical record; IRR: incidence rate ratio; N/A: not applicable; RI: relative incidence; RR: risk ratio; SIR: standardized incidence ratio; VSD: Vaccine Safety Datalink.
SOURCES: Hanson et al., 2022; Keh et al., 2023; Klein et al., 2021; Li et al., 2022; Loo et al., 2022; Morciano et al., 2023; Patone et al., 2021; Sturkenboom et al., 2022; Walker et al., 2022.

of BNT162b2[2] and 300,000 doses of mRNA-1273.[3] Of 196 postvaccinal cases, 21 occurred with BNT162b2 and one with mRNA-1273. Using case numbers from days 43–84 after first-dose vaccination as a comparison group, the first 42 days post-vaccination with BNT162b2 had no excess risk of GBS (Keh et al., 2023).

Patone et al. (2021) investigated the association between BNT162b2 and GBS among 32.6 million vaccinees, 12.1 million of whom received BNT162b2. This retrospective self-controlled cohort study compared the incidence rate of GBS in England at several intervals (1–7, 8–14, 15–21, 22–28, and 1–28 days after vaccination) with the rate of GBS during periods outside of this interval. GBS was defined using International Classification of Diseases 10 (ICD-10) codes and identified as the first hospital admission or as a cause of death recorded on the death certificate. Vaccination status was identified in the English National Immunisation (NIMS) Database of COVID-19 vaccination. Only 34 cases of GBS were observed for BNT162b2 during the risk interval. The study found no association between BNT162b2 and GBS at any interval, including the 1–28-day period—incidence rate ratio (IRR) 0.86 (95% confidence interval [CI]: 0.54–1.36) (Patone et al., 2021). The results do not suggest increased incidence, but the estimate is imprecise; the results are consistent with no association but could also be consistent with a small increased risk (Patone et al., 2021).

Klein et al. (2021) conducted a surveillance study within the Vaccine Safety Datalink (VSD), which includes data from eight U.S. integrated health care organizations with electronic health records. They compared incidence of GBS among vaccine recipients 1–21 days after either dose 1 or 2 of an mRNA vaccine with that of concurrent comparators who, on the same calendar day, had received their most recent dose 22–42 days earlier. After 11.8 million doses (57 percent BNT162b2), 10 GBS cases were identified in the risk interval compared with six in the controlled interval, risk ratio (RR) 0.70 (95% CI: 0.22–2.31) (Klein et al., 2021). Few events were observed, so the authors were unable to precisely estimate the measure of association. The results would be consistent with no association but could also be consistent with a small increase in risk.

Hanson et al. (2022) also analyzed data from VSD. In their primary analysis, they compared the incidence of GBS cases among vaccine recipients at two time intervals, 1–21 and 1–42 days, with that of vaccinated concurrent comparators, who, on the same calendar day, had received their most recent dose 22–42 and 43–84 days

---

[2] Refers to the COVID-19 vaccine manufactured by Pfizer-BioNTech under the name Comirnaty®.
[3] Refers to the COVID-19 vaccine manufactured by Moderna under the name Spikevax®.

earlier, respectively. In addition, incidence of GBS for individual vaccines was compared to prepandemic historical background rate (Hanson et al., 2022). GBS cases were physician adjudicated according to Brighton Collaboration criteria (Sejvar et al., 2011), and the analysis included Brighton Collaboration criteria 1–4. Level 1 has the highest level of diagnostic certainty; Level 4 includes suspected cases. The study included 14.6 million doses of mRNA vaccines (BNT162b2 or mRNA-1273) and 483,053 doses of Ad26.COV2.S.[4] During the 1–84 days following mRNA vaccines, 36 cases of GBS were confirmed, with nine cases meeting Brighton Collaboration criteria 1–3 in the 1–21 days risk period. Eleven cases of GBS were confirmed 1–84 days after Ad26.COV2.S, with eight cases meeting Brighton Collaboration criteria 1–3 in the 1–21 days period. Scan statistics identified days 1–14 after vaccination as a statistically significant cluster ($p = .003$). In a comparison of Ad26.COV2.S and mRNA vaccines, the adjusted rate ratio in the 1–21 days risk period was 20.56 (95% CI: 6.94–64.66) (Hanson et al., 2022). No association appeared between GBS and any of the vaccines based on the comparison with unvaccinated comparators (Hanson et al., 2022). However, the unadjusted incidence rate at 1–21 and 1–42 days after Ad26.COV2.S was higher than the historical background rate ($p < .001$). Excluding Brighton Level 4 cases did not significantly alter results.

Sturkenboom et al. (2022) conducted a cross-national multi-database retrospective dynamic cohort study using primary and/or secondary health care data from four European countries: Italy, the Netherlands, the United Kingdom, and Spain. They compared the incidence of GBS in vaccine recipients with nonvaccinated persons in 2020 within 28 days after each dose. Of 25.7 million people, 16 GBS cases were identified after BNT162b2, two after Ad26.COV2.S, and none after mRNA-1273. They found an increased risk of GBS 28 days after Ad26. COV2.S (IRR 5.65, 95% CI: 1.40–22.83) but no increased risk after BNT162b2 (IRR 1.10, 95% CI: 0.56–2.15). Results for BNT162b2 suggest no association, but the authors were unable to precisely estimate risk, and results could also be consistent with a small increase in risk (Sturkenboom et al., 2022).

Walker et al. (2022) analyzed primary care data from over 17 million patients in England linked to emergency care, hospital admission, and mortality records in OpenSAFELY, which is a secure analytics platform for the National Health Service electronic health records. They used a self-controlled case-series (SCCS) analytical approach where the risk interval was 4–28 days after vaccination. Among 5.7 million recipients of BNT162b2, 283 GBS cases were identified during the risk and controlled intervals; none were identified among 255,446 recipients of mRNA-1273. The results from the study suggested no association between the first dose of BNT162b2 and GBS, although the measure was imprecise and could suggest a small increase in risk (IRR 1.09, 95% CI: 0.75–1.57). Adjusting for calendar time and history of COVID-19 infection did not significantly change the measure of association (IRR 1.00, 95% CI: 0.61–1.64).

Li et al. (2022) compared rates of GBS identified through medical records among vaccinees with historical background rates. They used the Clinical Practice Research Datalink (CPRD) Aurum, which contains routinely collected data from UK primary care practices, and Spain's Information System for the Development of Research in Primary Care (SIDIAP), a primary care database that covers 80 percent of the population in Catalonia. The study included 3.6 million people who received BNT162b2, 244,913 who received mRNA-1273, 120,731 who received Ad26.COV2.S, and 14.3 million people from the general population (Li et al., 2022). Of the BNT162b2 vaccinees, <5 cases occurred within 1–21 days after a first and second dose in CPRD Aurum, compared with 10.4 and 9 expected. SIDIAP showed five cases after the first dose of BNT162b2 and <5 cases after the second dose, compared with 6.3 and 5.3 expected, respectively. For mRNA-1273, <5 cases were diagnosed after the second dose compared with 0.7 expected. No cases were observed with the first dose of mRNA-1273 or after Ad26.COV2.S (Li et al., 2022).

Morciano et al. (2023) investigated the association between COVID-19 vaccines and GBS in the population older than 12 years using an SCCS design with data from several regional health care databases in Italy. They evaluated relative incidence (RI) of GBS during a risk interval of 0–42 days after vaccination and an unexposed interval defined as any time of observation before, between, or after the risk intervals. Of 1.7 million individuals who received mRNA-1273, 25 developed GBS during the study period, with seven and five cases observed with the first and second doses, respectively, during the risk interval (RI 6.83, 95% CI: 2.14–21.85 for dose 1 and RI 7.41, 95% CI: 2.35–23.38 for dose 2) (Morciano et al., 2023). This corresponded with an estimated 0.4 and 0.3

---

[4] Refers to the COVID-19 vaccine manufactured by Janssen.

excess number of cases per 100,000 vaccinated for doses 1 and 2, respectively. The RI of GBS was not significantly increased in the 10.8 million and 581,796 individuals who received BNT162b2 and Ad26.COV2.S, respectively (Morciano et al., 2023).

Loo et al. (2022) conducted a retrospective case-control study of all patients admitted for acute polyradiculo-neuropathy to two UK neuroscience centers between January 1 and June 30, 2021. They compared vaccinees from the preceding 4 weeks to all GBS patients admitted to their centers between 2005 and 2019. A 2.6-fold (95% CI: 1.98–3.51) increase in admissions for GBS was noted during the time frame, compared to the same period in the preceding 3 years. Of 24 GBS patients, 16 were postvaccine, and all but two (one BNT162b2, one mRNA-1273) occurred after ChAdOx1-S (Loo et al., 2022).

Although some studies relied on physician adjudication for case ascertainment (Hanson et al., 2022; Keh et al., 2023; Loo et al., 2022), others relied on ICD codes from electronic data without chart confirmation. Some GBS cases identified by the ICD codes might not be true cases, which could have biased the measure of association. In addition, some studies used historical cohorts as a comparator group. Several studies have shown that annual GBS incidence decreased during the pandemic, which could have biased the measure of association.

*Pharmacovigilance and Surveillance*

Table 3-2 presents five pharmacovigilance studies that contributed to the committee's assessment based on their size, design, analytic approach, and region surveilled.

Abara et al. (2023) analyzed data from the Vaccine Adverse Event Reporting System, which is comanaged by the Centers for Disease Control and Prevention and FDA. Of 487.7 million COVID-19 vaccine doses, 209 and 253 reports of GBS occurred within 21 and 42 days, respectively. Observed-to-expected ratios were 3.79 (95% CI: 2.88–4.88) for days 1–21 and 2.34 (95% CI: 1.83–2.94) for days 1–42 after Ad26.COV2.S and less than 1 (not significantly increased) after BNT162b2 and mRNA-1273 for both post-vaccination periods (Abara et al., 2023).

Pegat et al. (2022) analyzed data from VigiBase, the World Health Organization pharmacovigilance database, and the French pharmacovigilance database to compare the frequency of facial paralysis in GBS cases after AV vaccines to that after mRNA vaccines and found that 142 of 1,256 GBS patients in VigiBase had associated facial paralysis (11.3 percent). This included 26 of 488 who received mRNA vaccines (12/328 BNT162b2, 14/160 mRNA-1273), 114 of 744 who received AV vaccines (28/114 Ad26.COV2.S, 86/630 ChAdOx1-S), and 2 of 24 who received other vaccines. Facial paralysis was significantly more frequent after AV vaccines ($\chi^2$: $p = 6.44 \times 10^{-8}$) (Pegat et al., 2022).

García-Grimshaw et al. (2022) conducted a retrospective analysis of a nationwide passive registry of GBS among recipients of 81.8 million doses of seven COVID-19 vaccines in Mexico. The overall observed incidence was 1.19 per 1 million doses (95% CI: 0.97–1.45), which was higher for Ad26.COV2.S (3.86 per 1 million doses, 95% CI: 1.50–9.93) and BNT162b2 (1.92 per 1 million doses, 95% CI: 1.36–2.71) (García-Grimshaw et al., 2022).

Ha et al. (2023) conducted a prospective regional surveillance study for GBS in the Gyeonggi Province, South Korea. Out of 38.8 million vaccine doses, 55 cases of physician adjudicated GBS were identified. The incidence rate of GBS after AV vaccines (Ad26.COV2.S, ChAdOx1-S) was 4.49 per million doses (95% CI: 2.85–6.12), compared to 0.80 per million doses after mRNA vaccines (BNT162b2, mRNA-1273) (95% CI: 0.49–1.11) (Ha et al., 2023).

Takuva et al. (2022) evaluated the incidence rate of GBS in all health care workers in South Africa registered in the national Electronic Vaccination Data System after receiving Ad26.COV2.S. Four cases of GBS were recorded, with an observed-to-expected ratio of 5.09 (95% CI: 1.39–13.02) (Takuva et al., 2022).

**TABLE 3-2** Pharmacovigilance Studies in the Guillain-Barré Syndrome Evidence Review

| Author | Study Design and Control Group | Location | Data Source | Vaccine(s) | Age Range | N | Number of Events | Results (95% CI) |
|---|---|---|---|---|---|---|---|---|
| Abara et al. (2023) | Cohort/ historical background | US | VAERS (physician adjudicated) | BNT162b2 | ≥18 years | 266.9 million doses | 21 days: 209 42 days: 253 | O:E <1 |
| | | | | mRNA-1273 | | 202.8 million doses | | O:E <1 |
| | | | | Ad26.COV2.S | | 17.9 million doses | | 1–21 days O:E 3.79 (2.88–4.88)  1–42 days O:E 2.34 (1.83–2.94) |
| García-Grimshaw et al. (2022) | Cohort/ historical background | Mexico | Mexican Epidemiological Surveillance System/ EMR (physician adjudicated) | BNT162b2 | ≥18 years | 16.6 million doses | 32 | Unadjusted Incidence 1.92 (1.36– 2.71) |
| | | | | mRNA-1273 | | 2.3 million doses | 3 | Unadjusted Incidence 1.29 (0.44–3.81) |
| | | | | Ad26.COV2.S | | 1.0 million doses | 4 | Unadjusted Incidence 3.86 (1.50–9.93) |
| | | | | ChAdOx1-S | | 38.5 million doses | 37 | Unadjusted incidence 0.96 (0.70–1.32) |
| Ha et al. (2023) | Cohort | South Korea | Gyeonggi Infectious Disease Control Center/EMR (physician adjudicated) | BNT162b2, mRNA-1273, Ad26.COV2.S | ≥12 years | 38.8 million doses | mRNA vaccines: 26 cases  Adenovirus-vectored vaccines: 29 cases | mRNA vaccines IR 0.80 per million doses (0.49–1.11) Adenovirus-vectored IR 4.49 per million doses (2.85–6.12) |
| Pegat et al. (2022) | Cohort/mRNA vaccines to Adenovirus-vectored vaccines | US, UK, Europe | VigiBase (physician adjudicated) | BNT162b2, mRNA-1273, Ad26.COV2.S, ChAdOx1 | Not stated | 488 mRNA vaccine vaccinees  788 Adenovirus-vectored vaccine vaccinees | 142/1,256 of GBS cases with facial paresis (26 mRNA vaccines, 28 adenovirus-vectored) | Facial paresis more frequent with adenovirus-vectored vaccines |
| Takuva et al. (2022) | Open-label phase 3b implementation study/ historical background | South Africa | National Electronic Vaccination Data System/ EMR (physician adjudicated) | Ad26.COV2.S | ≥18 years | 477,234 vaccinees | 4 cases | O:E 5.09 (1.39–13.02) |

NOTES: BNT162b2 refers to the COVID-19 vaccine manufactured by Pfizer-BioNTech under the name Comirnaty®. mRNA-1273 refers to the COVID-19 vaccine manufactured by Moderna under the name Spikevax®. Ad26.COV2.S refers to the COVID-19 vaccine manufactured by Janssen. ChAdOx1-S refers to the COVID-19 vaccine manufactured by Oxford-AstraZeneca. ChAdOx1-S appears in this table because it provides support for Conclusion 3-3. Ha et al. (2023) combined the number of events from adenovirus-vector vaccines (Ad26.COV2.S and ChAdOx1-S). CI: confidence interval; EMR: electronic medical record; IR: incidence rate; O:E: observed-to-expected ratio; VAERS: Vaccine Adverse Event Reporting System.
SOURCES: Abara et al., 2023; García-Grimshaw et al., 2022; Ha et al., 2023; Pegat et al., 2022; Takuva et al., 2022.

**From Evidence to Conclusions**

The totality of the evidence included several large studies that minimized confounding bias by using self-controlled or concurrent cohort design or by relying on chart review for case ascertainment; none of the epidemiological studies reported a significant risk of GBS after BNT162b2. This is reinforced by the pharma-covigilance data; although they were more prone to confounding bias, multiple large studies surveilling different population cohorts worldwide consistently identified an increased risk with AV but not mRNA vaccines despite potential differing coding trends, seasonality, co-infections, and co-administration of other vaccines.

> **Conclusion 3-1: The evidence favors rejection of a causal relationship between the BNT162b2 vaccine and Guillain-Barré syndrome.**

In general, relatively few mRNA-1273 doses were included in the studies. Only one study reported an increased risk of GBS after the first and second doses, although the CIs for the measure of association were very wide (Morciano et al., 2023). The study also reported that the excess number of cases was very small (<1 case per 100,000 doses). Morciano et al. (2023) was the only study to utilize the relatively longer risk period of 0–42 days without relying on chart review for case ascertainment. Although the study used a self-controlled strategy to minimize bias, its reliance on ICD codes combined with the prolonged risk interval may have led to inclusion of some historical cases rather than true incident cases. Two other studies included a larger number of vaccines and used a vaccinated concurrent cohort design (Hanson et al., 2022; Klein et al., 2021). As noted, the pharmacovigilance data also favored lack of an association between GBS and the mRNA vaccines, and the platforms used in mRNA-1273 and BNT162b2 are similar. Additionally, strong mechanistic evidence linking mRNA vaccines to GBS is lacking.

> **Conclusion 3-2: The evidence favors rejection of a causal relationship between the mRNA-1273 vaccine and Guillain-Barré syndrome.**

Four epidemiology studies included patients who received Ad26.COV2.S. One study found an increased risk of GBS compared to a historical cohort, even though it did not find an association in its primary analysis, which used a vaccinated concurrent cohort design (Hanson et al., 2022). Unlike other studies reviewed, cases were physician adjudicated according to Brighton Collaboration criteria, and the increased risk was still observed when Level 4 cases (suspected GBS) were excluded. Although the analysis included two risk periods, 1–21 and 1–42 days, the vast majority of cases occurred in the first period, which is in keeping with expected latency based on historical precedent and presumed mechanism. Sturkenboom et al. (2022) also found an increased risk when comparing Ad26.COV2.S recipients with a 2020 cohort of unvaccinated individuals, although the total number of events was small and the CI wide. No association was observed in the other two studies (Li et al., 2022; Morciano et al., 2023). Li et al. (2022) had a comparatively low number of vaccinees.

Although ChAdOx1-S was not formally within the purview of the committee, five of the studies observed an increased risk of GBS (Keh et al., 2023; Loo et al., 2022; Morciano et al., 2023; Patone et al., 2021; Walker et al., 2022). These included studies with a large number of participants and designs that minimize confounding bias. Additionally, two studies reported a higher rate of the facial paresis variant in patients who received either AV vaccine compared to historical cohorts (Hanson et al., 2022; Loo et al., 2022). This trend was not observed in Keh et al. (2023) despite reporting an increased risk of GBS after ChAdOx1-S. Evidence from pharmacovigilance databases spanning different regions worldwide also documented an increased risk with the AV vaccines, and one study (Pegat et al., 2022) observed an increased rate of facial paresis associated with AV but not mRNA vaccines.

The epidemiological association between GBS and ChAdOx1-S but not mRNA vaccines suggests that the mechanism is unlikely to relate to immune responses to the spike protein itself. In addition, the reported increased rates of a rare variant (facial paresis) after vaccination with both related, albeit not identical, AV vaccines suggest a potential shared mechanism, although no definitive one was identified by the committee in the mechanistic literature, and this pattern was not observed in all studies. Differences in the AV platforms and their respective receptor, however, should give pause when extrapolating from one such vaccine to another.

The totality of evidence for Ad26.COV2.S includes two well-designed, positive epidemiological studies and pharmacovigilance data, strong supporting epidemiological evidence from ChAdOx1-S, and the potential for a platform-specific mechanism in both AV vaccines. No epidemiological literature evaluated the relationship between NVX-CoV2373[5] and GBS.

**Conclusion 3-3: The evidence favors acceptance of a causal relationship between the Ad26.COV2.S vaccine and Guillain-Barré syndrome.**

**Conclusion 3-4: The evidence is inadequate to accept or reject a causal relationship between the NVX-CoV2373 vaccine and Guillain-Barré syndrome.**

## CHRONIC INFLAMMATORY DEMYELINATING POLYNEUROPATHY

---

**BOX 3-2**
**Conclusions for Chronic Inflammatory Demyelinating Polyneuropathy**

**Conclusion 3-5: The evidence is inadequate to accept or reject a causal relationship between the BNT162b2 vaccine and chronic inflammatory demyelinating polyneuropathy.**

**Conclusion 3-6: The evidence is inadequate to accept or reject a causal relationship between the mRNA-1273 vaccine and chronic inflammatory demyelinating polyneuropathy.**

**Conclusion 3-7: The evidence is inadequate to accept or reject a causal relationship between the Ad26.COV2.S vaccine and chronic inflammatory demyelinating polyneuropathy.**

**Conclusion 3-8: The evidence is inadequate to accept or reject a causal relationship between the NVX-CoV2373 vaccine and chronic inflammatory demyelinating polyneuropathy.**

---

### Background

CIDP, also known as "chronic inflammatory demyelinating polyradiculoneuropathy," is an acquired, immune-mediated disorder affecting the peripheral nerve and roots. As with GBS, CIDP is now considered a group of disorders all sharing clinical and electrodiagnostic features but with probable heterogenous underlying mechanisms. Typical CIDP, the most prevalent CIDP variant, accounts for 50–60 percent of cases and presents as relapsing-remitting or gradually progressive symmetric limb weakness over a period of months. Sensory loss is common, and deep tendon reflexes are absent or reduced. Cranial nerve involvement occurs in 10–20 percent of cases. Acute onset resembling GBS can occur in 5–16 percent of cases, but unlike GBS, where symptom progression ends within 4 weeks, symptoms continue to progress beyond 8 weeks (McCombe et al., 1987; Thomas et al., 1987) (a minimum of 2 months of symptoms is required to make the diagnosis per CIDP diagnostic criteria; Van den Bergh et al., 2010).

The reported incidence of CIDP is 0.3–1.6 cases per 100,000 person-years (Laughlin et al., 2009), with a male predominance and incidence rising with advancing age and some studies reporting a mean age at presentation of 60 years (Hafsteinsdottir and Olafsson, 2016). Electrodiagnostic evidence of nerve demyelination and elevated CSF protein with a normal leukocyte count supports the diagnosis. A nerve biopsy demonstrating segmental demyelination with or without inflammation can be diagnostic but is rarely needed. CIDP variants are recognized, and their distinctive clinical characteristics are included in European Academy of Neurology/Peripheral Nerve Society diagnostic criteria (Van den Bergh et al., 2021). These include typical, distal (or distal acquired demyelinating distal neuropathy),

---

[5] Refers to the COVID-19 vaccine manufactured by Novavax.

multifocal (or multifocal acquired demyelinating sensory and motor neuropathy), focal, motor, and sensory CIDP (Van den Bergh et al., 2021). Definitions of what constitute CIDP continue to evolve, and certain conditions classed as CIDP variants in the past, including chronic immune sensory polyradiculopathy and the autoimmune paranodopathies, were excluded from the most recent criteria because the underlying nerve injury is not definitively demyelinating.

## Mechanisms

Although the pathophysiology of CIDP and its variants is not known, evidence supports an immune-mediated mechanism as the main cause. Characteristic features include segmental demyelination and remyelination and varying degrees of endoneurial macrophage infiltration (Dalakas, 2011). Levels of T helper 17 cells are increased in the peripheral blood and CSF, as are levels of soluble adhesion molecules, chemokines, and metalloproteinases (Dalakas, 2011). The apparent effectiveness of plasmapheresis, which purportedly removes pathogenic antibodies along with other inflammatory mediators, suggests that circulating humoral factors and autoantibodies may be involved. Complement fixation on the myelin sheath of nerves of some with CIDP also suggests a potential anti-body-mediated mechanism (Dalakas and Engel, 1980). Antibodies directed against nodal and paranodal proteins, such as contactin-1 and neurofascin isoforms, are found in a subset of patients with clinical features suggestive of CIDP. However, nerve biopsies in these patients do not show the distinctive features of CIDP, and this is now considered a separate entity (autoimmune paranodopathies) (Van den Bergh et al., 2021).

One study identified potentially cross-reactive epitopes shared between the SARS-CoV-2 spike protein and neuronal structures using a bioinformatics approach (Felipe Cuspoca et al., 2022), suggesting that molecular mimicry as a cause of potential neurological harms of COVID-19 vaccines is plausible, but evidence supporting this hypothesis is lacking.

## Epidemiological Evidence

Clinical trial results submitted to FDA for Emergency Use Authorization and/or full approval do not indicate a signal regarding CIDP and any of the vaccines under study (FDA, 2021, 2023a,b,c). Table 3-3 summarizes one study that contributed to the causality assessment.

Loo et al. (2022) conducted a retrospective case-control study of all patients admitted with acute-onset polyradiculoneuropathy to two UK neuroscience centers, January 1–June 30, 2021. Of 24 GBS patients, 16 were post-vaccination and all but two (one BNT162b2, one mRNA-1273) were after ChAdOx1-S. Four cases initially classified as GBS were eventually reclassified as acute-onset CIDP due to progression or relapse past 8 weeks from onset; all four had received ChAdOx1-S.

**TABLE 3-3** Epidemiological Study in the Chronic Inflammatory Demyelinating Polyneuropathy Evidence Review

| Author | Study Design and Control Group | Location | Data Source | Vaccine(s) | Age Range | N | Number of Events | Results |
|---|---|---|---|---|---|---|---|---|
| Loo et al. (2022) | Case-control study/historical background | UK | EMR (physician adjudicated) | BNT162b2 | ≥16 years | 24 patients admitted with acute onset polyradiculo-neuropathy between January–June 2021 | 1 | 4 cases reclassified as acute onset CIDP; No cases followed mRNA vaccines |
| | | | | mRNA-1273 | | | 1 | |

NOTES: BNT162b2 refers to the COVID-19 vaccine manufactured by Pfizer-BioNTech under the name Comirnaty®. mRNA-1273 refers to the COVID-19 vaccine manufactured by Moderna under the name Spikevax®. Number of events refers to events in vaccinees only. EMR: electronic medical record.
SOURCE: Loo et al., 2022.

## From Evidence to Conclusions

Epidemiological and mechanistic evidence are absent. Only one small case-control study evaluated the association between COVID-19 vaccines and CIDP; four cases initially classified as GBS were later reclassified as acute-onset CIDP, and no historical background rate was offered for comparison.

**Conclusion 3-5: The evidence is inadequate to accept or reject a causal relationship between the BNT162b2 vaccine and chronic inflammatory demyelinating polyneuropathy.**

**Conclusion 3-6: The evidence is inadequate to accept or reject a causal relationship between the mRNA-1273 vaccine and chronic inflammatory demyelinating polyneuropathy.**

**Conclusion 3-7: The evidence is inadequate to accept or reject a causal relationship between the Ad26.COV2.S vaccine and chronic inflammatory demyelinating polyneuropathy.**

**Conclusion 3-8: The evidence is inadequate to accept or reject a causal relationship between the NVX-CoV2373 vaccine and chronic inflammatory demyelinating polyneuropathy.**

## BELL'S PALSY

---

**BOX 3-3**
**Conclusions for Bell's Palsy**

**Conclusion 3-9: The evidence favors rejection of a causal relationship between the BNT162b2 vaccine and Bell's Palsy.**

**Conclusion 3-10: The evidence favors rejection of a causal relationship between the mRNA-1273 vaccine and Bell's Palsy.**

**Conclusion 3-11: The evidence is inadequate to accept or reject a causal relationship between the Ad26.COV2.S vaccine and Bell's Palsy.**

**Conclusion 3-12: The evidence is inadequate to accept or reject a causal relationship between the NVX-CoV2373 vaccine and Bell's Palsy.**

---

## Background

BP is an idiopathic, unilateral, self-limited, acute facial nerve paresis or paralysis. It occurs with equal frequency on either side of the face and usually resolves within weeks or months. It can lead to severe temporary oral insufficiency and an incapability to close the eyelids, resulting in potentially permanent eye injury. In approximately 25 percent of patients, moderate-to-severe facial asymmetry may persist and affect quality of life (Zhang et al., 2020).

BP is the most common acute mononeuropathy (Zhang et al., 2020), with an incidence of 11.5–53.3 per 100,000 person-years (Baugh et al., 2013). It is estimated that every year, about 40,000 U.S. people are affected (NORD, 2022). The risk factors are poorly understood. Risk may increase with age, but no indication exists that one sex or geographical area is more at risk (Kim and Park, 2021). BP symptoms typically develop quickly, with maximum symptoms occurring within 72 hours (Zhang et al., 2020).

## Mechanisms

The etiology of BP is unknown, but theories fall into five categories: anatomical, viral, ischemic, inflammatory, and due to cold exposure (based on season or local climate) (Zhang et al., 2020). When considering the possibility of a vaccine trigger of BP, it is unlikely that anatomy, ischemia, or cold stimulation would play a role.

Evidence supporting inflammation includes demonstrated gadolinium enhancement of the facial nerve on magnetic resonance imaging (MRI) of the brain and CSF pleocytosis in many patients with BP (Steiner and Mattan, 1999). Histopathology from one autopsy study demonstrated a lymphohistiocytic infiltrate within all layers of the nerve and inflammation that extended to the geniculate ganglion but spared most ganglion cells (Liston and Kleid, 1989).

Infection may be a cause of BP. Infectious facial palsy has been most clearly linked to *Borrelia burgdorferi* (the bacteria that causes Lyme disease) and varicella zoster virus reactivation (Ramsay Hunt syndrome). Many have argued for a link between herpes simplex virus type 1 (HSV-1) reactivation and BP (Zhang et al., 2020), and acyclovir is routinely prescribed to patients with BP. Arguments against a pathophysiological role for HSV-1 include that it resides in the peripheral sensory ganglia, and reactivation is not associated with motor weakness; that it tends to recur, whereas BP tends to be monophasic; and that HSV-1 outbreaks are common, whereas BP is rare (Steiner and Mattan, 1999). Finally, in a randomized controlled trial with a factorial design in which patients received 10 days of prednisolone, acyclovir, both, and placebo, prednisolone significantly improved outcomes, whereas acyclovir did not (Sullivan et al., 2007).

Infection may also cause BP via a post-infectious immune-mediated mechanism rather than by direct invasion of the nerve. Such mechanisms could include bystander activation, epitope spreading, or polyclonal activation of previously dormant self-reactive lymphocytes (see Chapter 2). Arguments favoring an infectious trigger of BP include that it can occur in epidemic clusters (Leibowitz, 1969) and displays seasonal variation (Kim and Park, 2021). Potential triggers include cytomegalovirus, Epstein-Barr virus, mumps, rubella, and HIV (Steiner and Mattan, 1999). An intranasal influenza vaccine that has since been removed from the market was associated with BP (Wratten et al., 1977). In this case-control study, BP most often occurred within 31–60 days following vaccination, arguing against a direct toxic effect and in favor of an immune-mediated mechanism. Recent evidence has suggested a possible association between COVID-19 infection and BP (Rafati et al., 2023). The fact that there are multiple putative viral triggers argues against molecular mimicry as a mechanism.

Patients with BP have been shown to have elevated levels of the cytokines IL-6 (interleukin-6), IL-8, and TNF-alpha compared to controls (Yılmaz et al., 2002). Some have argued that cytokine-mediated neuronal damage, in particular by type 1 interferon (type 1 IFN), might mediate neurological adverse events after COVID-19 vaccination (Chen et al., 2022a; Shemer et al., 2021). Because BP has been seen as a complication of type 1 IFN treatment for hepatitis C (Hwang et al., 2004), some have postulated that an elevation of type 1 IFN after COVID-19 vaccination could be associated with it (Shemer et al., 2021). Single-cell transcriptomics demonstrate a strong interferon signature after booster mRNA vaccination (Arunachalam et al., 2021), but this has not been correlated with neurological harms. Adenoviral vaccines have also been shown to induce an interferon signature, at least in mice (Sheerin et al., 2021). However, no studies link cytokine responses after vaccination to neurological events.

## Epidemiological Evidence

Clinical trial results submitted to FDA for Emergency Use Authorization and/or full approval do not indicate a signal regarding BP and any of the vaccines under study (FDA, 2021, 2023a,b,c). Table 3-4 presents 11 studies that contributed to the causality assessment.

Patone et al. (2021) investigated the association between BNT162b2 and BP among 12.1 million vaccinees in England using an SCCS study. They compared the incidence rate of BP in the interval of 1–28 days after vaccination with that during periods outside of this interval. BP was defined using ICD-10 codes and identified as the first hospital admission or as a cause of death recorded on the death certificate (Patone et al., 2021). Vaccination status was identified in the English National Immunisation (NIMS) Database of COVID-19 vaccination; they identified 250 BP cases and found no association with BNT162b2 IRR 1.06, 95% CI: 0.80–1.25) (Patone et al., 2021).

**TABLE 3-4** Epidemiological Studies in the Bell's Palsy Evidence Review

| Author | Study Design and Control Group | Location | Data Source | Vaccine(s) | Age Range | N | Number of Events | Results (95% CI) |
|---|---|---|---|---|---|---|---|---|
| Ab Rahman et al. (2022) | Self-controlled case series | Malaysia | EMR | BNT162b2 | ≥12 years | Dose 1: 8.7 million vaccinees | Dose 1: 17 | Dose 1: IRR 1.32 (0.77–2.24) |
| | | | | | | Dose 2: 6.7 million vaccinees | Dose 2: 10 | Dose 2: IRR 0.88 (0.45–1.73) |
| Klein et al. (2021) | Cohort with vaccinated concurrent comparators | US | EMR | BNT162b2 | ≥16 years | 6.8 million doses | BNT162b2 and mRNA-1273 combined: 535 | BNT162b2 and mRNA-1273 combined: RR 1.00 (0.86–1.17) |
| | | | | mRNA-1273 | | 5.1 million doses | | |
| Li et al. (2022) | Cohort and self-controlled/ Background rates and self-controlled | UK and Spain | EMR Clinical Practice Research Datalink Aurum database (UK)/ Information System for the Development of Research in Primary Care (SIDIAP) database (Spain) | BNT162b2 (UK and Spain) | ≥18 years | **UK** Dose 1: 1.7 million vaccinees Dose 2: 1.2 million vaccinees | **UK** Dose 1: 46 Dose 2: 24 | **UK** Dose 1: SIR 0.40 (0.30–0.53) Dose 2: SIR 0.24 (0.16–0.36) SCCS IRR 0.83 (0.66–1.02) |
| | | | | | | **Spain** Dose 1: 1.9 million vaccinees Dose 2: 1.3 million vaccinees | **Spain** Dose 1:100 Dose 2: 85 | **Spain** Dose 1: SIR 0.86 (0.70–1.04) Dose 2: SIR 0.88 (0.71–1.08) SCCS: IRR 0.83 (0.66–1.02) |
| | | | | mRNA-1273 (Spain only) | | Dose 1: 244,913 vaccinees Dose 2: 160,228 vaccinees | Dose 1: 14 Dose 2: 5 | Dose 1: SIR 0.92 (0.54–1.55) Dose 2: SIR 0.44 (0.18–1.06) SCCS: IRR 0.99 (0.54–1.64) |
| | | | | Ad26.COV2.S (Spain only) | | Dose 1: 120,731 vaccinees | Dose 1: 6 | SIR 1.15 (0.52–2.56) |
| Patone et al. (2021) | Self-controlled case series | UK | EMR | BNT162b2 | ≥16 years | Dose 1: 12.1 million vaccinees | 247 | IRR 1.06 (0.90–1.26) |

*continued*

**TABLE 3-4** Continued

| Author | Study Design and Control Group | Location | Data Source | Vaccine(s) | Age Range | N | Number of Events | Results (95% CI) |
|---|---|---|---|---|---|---|---|---|
| Shasha et al. (2022) | Matched cohort vaccinated vs. unvaccinated | Israel | EMR | BNT162b2 | ≥16 years | Dose 1: 233,159 vaccinees | 23 | RR 0.96 (0.54–1.70) |
| Shemer et al. (2021) | Case control | Israel | Hospitaliza-tion data | BNT162b2 | 50.9 ± 20.2 years | 37 cases | 21 | OR 0.84 (0.37–1.90) |
| Shibli et al. (2021) | Cohort using background rate | Israel | EMR | BNT162b2 | ≥16 years | Dose 1: 2.6 million vaccinees | 132 | SIR 1.36 (1.14–1.61) |
| | | | | | | Dose 2: 2.4 million vaccinees | 152 | SIR 1.16 (0.99–1.36) |
| Shoaibi et al. (2023) | Self-controlled case series | US | Claims-based data with medical record review | BNT162b2 (booster dose) | ≥65 years | 6.2 million vaccinees | 1,674 | IRR 1.13 (0.77–1.65) |
| | | | | mRNA-1273 (booster dose) | | | 1,594 | IRR 1.02 (0.70–1.50) |
| Sturken-boom et al. (2022) | Cohort using background rate | Italy, Netherlands, UK, and Spain | EMR | BNT162b2 | Varied | 54% of 12.1 million vaccinees total | 149 | IRR 0.87 (0.69–1.10) |
| | | | | mRNA-1273 | | 6% | 27 | IRR 0.99 (0.68–1.45) |
| | | | | Ad26.COV2.S | | 2% | 6 | IRR 1.08 (0.45–2.60) |
| Takeuchi et al. (2022) | Cohort and self-controlled case series (SCCS) | Japan | EMR | mRNA (BNT162b2, mRNA-1273) | ≥18 years | Dose 1: 136,667 vaccinees  Dose 2: 127,322 vaccinees | Cohort: Dose 1: 1 Dose 2: 1 | Dose 1: IRR 1.14 (0.27–4.89) Dose 2: IRR 0.60 (0.08–4.49) |
| | | | | | | | SCCS: Dose 1: 15 Dose 2: 15 | Dose 1: IRR 1.03 (0.20–5.31) Dose 2: IRR 0.47 (0.05–4.18) |

**TABLE 3-4** Continued

| Author | Study Design and Control Group | Location | Data Source | Vaccine(s) | Age Range | N | Number of Events | Results (95% CI) |
|--------|-------------------------------|----------|-------------|------------|-----------|---|------------------|------------------|
| Walker et al. (2022) | Self-controlled case series | England | EMR | BNT162b2 | 18–105 years | 5,729,152 | 3,609 | Dose 1: IRR 0.88 (0.76–1.02) Dose 2: IRR 0.92 (0.78–1.10) |
| | | | | mRNA-1273 | | 255,446 | 78 | Dose 1: IRR 0.80 (0.24–2.62) |

NOTES: BNT162b2 refers to the COVID-19 vaccine manufactured by Pfizer-BioNTech under the name Comirnaty®. mRNA-1273 refers to the COVID-19 vaccine manufactured by Moderna under the name Spikevax®. Ad26.COV2.S refers to the COVID-19 vaccine manufactured by Janssen. The primary series for Ad26.COV2.S is one dose. Number of events refers to events in vaccinees only. CI: confidence interval; EMR: electronic medical record; IRR: incidence rate ratio; OR: odds ratio; RR: relative risk; SCCS: self-controlled case series; SIR: standardized incidence ratio.
SOURCES: Ab Rahman et al., 2022; Klein et al., 2021; Li et al., 2022; Patone et al., 2021; Shasha et al., 2022; Shemer et al., 2021; Shibli et al., 2021; Shoaibi et al., 2023; Sturkenboom et al., 2022; Takeuchi et al., 2022; Walker et al., 2022.

Walker et al. (2022) analyzed primary care data from more than 17 million patients in England linked to emergency care, hospital admission, and mortality records in the OpenSAFELY platform (Walker et al., 2022). They excluded BP cases that occurred before the study start date. Cases were determined from any primary care, emergency department, hospital admission, or mortality records. They used an SCCS analytical approach where the risk interval was 4–28 days after vaccination. Among 5.7 million recipients of BNT162b2, 3,609 BP cases were identified, and among 255,446 recipients of mRNA-1273, 78 BP cases were identified. They found no association between the first dose of BNT162b2 and BP (IRR 0.89, 95% CI: 0.76–1.03) or the second dose (IRR 0.92, 95% CI: 0.78–1.10). Similarly, no association appeared with mRNA-1273 after the first or second dose (IRR 0.59, 95% CI: 0.13–2.62 and IRR 0.80, 95% CI: 0.24–2.62, respectively) (Walker et al., 2022).

Ab Rahman et al. (2022) conducted an SCCS study among hospitalized BP cases in Malaysia. Vaccination status was determined from the national COVID-19 register data. The incidence of BP was assessed during a 21-day risk interval after vaccination relative to a control period using conditional Poisson regression with adjustment for calendar time. After more than 15 million doses of BNT162b2, 27 cases of BP were identified in the risk interval. Compared with the control interval, no significant increased risk of BP occurred after the first (IRR 1.32, 95% CI: 0.77–2.24) or second (IRR 0.88, 95% CI: 0.45–1.73) dose. The IRR after any dose was 1.11 (95% CI: 0.77–1.75) (Ab Rahman et al., 2022).

Li et al. (2022) evaluated the association between vaccination and BP using two study designs: a population-based cohort design where they compared rates of BP identified through medical records among vaccinees with historical background rates and an SCCS analysis. They used CPRD Aurum and SIDIAP. The study included 3.6 million people who received BNT162b2, 244,913 who received mRNA-1273, 120,731 who received Ad26.COV2.S, and 14.3 million people from the general population. Of the BNT162b2 vaccinees, 46 and 24 BP cases occurred after a first and second dose, respectively, in CPRD Aurum, compared with 116.4 and 99.5 expected. The standardized incidence ratio (SIR) was 0.40 (95% CI: 0.30–0.53) for the first and 0.24 (95% CI: 0.16–0.36) for the second dose. SIDIAP had 100 and 85 BP cases after the first and second dose, respectively, of BNT162b2, compared with 116.7 and 97.1 expected. SIR was 0.86 (95% CI: 0.70–1.04) for the first and 0.88 (95% CI: 0.71–1.08) for the second dose. For mRNA-1273, 14 and 5 cases occurred after the first and second dose, respectively, compared with 15.2 and 11.3 expected. The corresponding SIRs are 0.92 (95% CI: 0.54–1.55) and 0.4 (95% CI: 0.18–1.06). For Ad26.COV2.S, six BP cases were identified compared with 5.2 expected, corresponding to an SIR of 1.15 (95% CI: 0.52–2.56) (Li et al., 2022). The SCCS analysis was only sufficiently powered to study those with a first dose of BNT162b2 and mRNA-1273. In CPRD Aurum, the adjusted IRR of BP 1–21 days after vaccination was 0.83 (95% CI: 0.61–1.10) for BNT162b2. In SIDIAP, the adjusted IRR was 0.83 (95% CI: 0.66–1.02) for BNT162b2 and 0.99 (95% CI: 0.54–1.64) for mRNA-1273 (Li et al., 2022).

Shibli et al. (2021) used data from the computerized database of Clalit Health Services, which provides inclusive health care for more than half of the Israeli population, to assess whether BNT162b2 was associated with increased risk by comparing BP rates in vaccinees with historical rates in the general population. They assessed rates 21 days after the first dose and 30 days after the second dose. Overall, 132 cases of BP were reported in 2.6 million vaccinees with the first dose compared with 97.1 expected, and 152 cases in 2.4 million vaccinees were reported compared with 130.49 expected after the second dose. The age- and sex-weighted SIRs were 1.36 (95% CI: 1.14–1.61) and 1.16 (95% CI: 0.99–1.36) after the first and second doses, respectively. Although more cases were observed than expected, the attributable risk fraction was 0.26 for the first and 0.14 for the second dose. The attributable risk per 100,000 vaccinees was 1.35 for the first and 0.86 for the second dose (Shibli et al., 2021).

Shasha et al. (2022) conducted a matched cohort study in which they compared risk of BP in 233,159 BNT162b2 vaccinees with that in 233,159 age- and sex-matched unvaccinated individuals. BP cases were identified by ICD-10 code and confirmed by chart review. Of the 123 cases identified by ICD-10 codes, 76 were excluded because they were not incident cases or not consistent with BP. Vaccinated and unvaccinated individuals had 23 versus 24 cases, respectively, of BP (RR 0.96, 95% CI: 0.54–1.70).

Sturkenboom et al. (2022) conducted a cross-national multi-database retrospective dynamic cohort study using primary and/or secondary health care data from four European countries: Italy, the Netherlands, the United Kingdom, and Spain. Individuals were required to have at least 365 days of data availability before cohort entry. The end of follow-up was the earliest dates of BP occurrence, last data collection, or death. Person-time after the start of the study was divided in two main periods, nonvaccinated and vaccinated; the latter started at the first dose of any of the COVID-19 vaccines and lasted for a maximum of 28 days after dose 1 and 28 days after dose 2 or until the date of last data available. Of the 25.7 million people included, 149 BP cases were identified after BNT162b2, 27 after mRNA-1273, and 6 after Ad26.COV2.S. They found no increased risk of BP 28 days after BNT162b2 (IRR 0.87, 95% CI: 0.69–1.10), mRNA-1273 (IRR 0.99, 95% CI: 0.68–1.45), or Ad26.COV2.S (IRR 1.08, 95% CI: 0.45–2.60) (Sturkenboom et al., 2022).

Shemer et al. (2021) conducted a case-control study using data from the emergency department of a tertiary referral center in central Israel. Patients admitted for facial nerve palsy (37 confirmed BP cases) were matched by age, sex, and date of admission with 72 controls admitted for other reasons and assessed against the odds of BNT162b2 vaccination. The odds of vaccination were not different between cases and controls. The odds ratio for vaccination was 0.84 (95% CI: 0.37–1.90) (Shemer et al., 2021).

Shoaibi et al. (2023) conducted an SCCS study of BNT162b2 and mRNA-1273 among U.S. Medicare beneficiaries aged 65+ to evaluate association with BP after only a booster dose (Shoaibi et al., 2023). The study included 6.2 million individuals. Of 79 cases identified through electronic health records, chart reviews determined that 10 were confirmed or probable, for a positive predictive value of 12.66 percent. After adjusting for outcome misclassification, they found no significant association between BNT162b2 and BP (IRR 1.13, 95% CI: 0.77–1.65) or mRNA-1273 and BP (IRR 1.02, 95% CI: 0.70–1.50) (Shoaibi et al., 2023).

In addition to these studies that evaluated individual vaccines, two studies evaluated the association of mRNA vaccines with risk of BP. Takeuchi et al. (2022) evaluated BP risk after any BNT162b2 and mRNA-1273 in administrative claims data using a cohort study design and an SCCS design. BP was defined by ICD codes from hospitalized claims data. The study included 136,644 people who received one dose, 127,268 who received two doses, and 183,990 unvaccinated. The vaccinees had two BP cases 21 days after dose 1 and one BP case after dose 2 compared with 18 cases among the unvaccinated. The adjusted IRR of BP was 1.14 (95% CI: 0.27–4.89) and 0.60 (95% CI: 0.08–4.49) after dose 1 and dose 2, respectively, compared with unvaccinated. The results of the SCCS analysis indicated no increased risk of BP after dose 1 (IRR 1.03, 95% CI: 0.20–5.31) or dose 2 (IRR 0.47, 95% CI: 0.05–4.18) (Takeuchi et al., 2022).

Klein et al. (2021) conducted a surveillance study within VSD. They compared incidence of BP 1–21 days after either dose 1 or 2 of an mRNA vaccine with that of concurrent comparators who, on the same calendar day, had received their most recent dose 22–42 days earlier. After 11.8 million doses, 535 BP cases were identified in the risk interval compared with 301 in the controlled interval. The adjusted IRR was 1.00 (95% CI: 0.86–1.17). In a supplemental analysis comparing vaccinated with unvaccinated people, they found no risk association with an mRNA vaccine (RR 1.06, 95% CI: 0.95–1.17) (Klein et al., 2021).

## From Evidence to Conclusions

Among the 11 epidemiology studies reviewed, only one reported a significantly increased risk of BP after the first dose of BNT162b2 (Shibli et al., 2021). Its results are prone to confounding because it used historical BP rate as the comparator. Factors associated with that rate may be very different from those during the pandemic. Furthermore, comparing vaccinated with unvaccinated is problematic because, without randomization, it is practically impossible to balance their confounding factors. Although informative, this study weakly contributed to the final conclusion because of its limitations including using historical background rates as comparators; studies using concurrent comparators did not find an association between BP and mRNA vaccines. The main limitation is that most of the studies relied on ICD codes from electronic data without chart confirmation. Some cases of BP identified by the ICD codes might not be true or incident cases, which could have biased the measure of association. Studies may have missed cases because they were not based on active surveillance, and the majority of the cases included are likely more severe, as those with mild symptoms may not have sought medical attention during the pandemic. Furthermore, some studies may have incompletely measured or adjusted for some confounding.

**Conclusion 3-9: The evidence favors rejection of a causal relationship between the BNT162b2 vaccine and Bell's palsy.**

**Conclusion 3-10: The evidence favors rejection of a causal relationship between the mRNA-1273 vaccine and Bell's palsy.**

Only two of the 11 studies evaluated the relationship between Ad26.COV2.S and BP; neither showed an increased risk. No studies evaluated the relationship between BP and NVX-CoV2373.

**Conclusion 3-11: The evidence is inadequate to accept or reject a causal relationship between the Ad26.COV2.S vaccine and Bell's palsy.**

**Conclusion 3-12: The evidence is inadequate to accept or reject a causal relationship between the NVX-CoV2373 vaccine and Bell's palsy.**

## TRANSVERSE MYELITIS

---

### BOX 3-4
### Conclusions for Transverse Myelitis

**Conclusion 3-13: The evidence is inadequate to accept or reject a causal relationship between the BNT162b2 vaccine and transverse myelitis.**

**Conclusion 3-14: The evidence is inadequate to accept or reject a causal relationship between the mRNA-1273 vaccine and transverse myelitis.**

**Conclusion 3-15: The evidence is inadequate to accept or reject a causal relationship between the Ad26.COV2.S vaccine and transverse myelitis.**

**Conclusion 3-16: The evidence is inadequate to accept or reject a causal relationship between the NVX-CoV2373 vaccine and transverse myelitis.**

---

## Background

Spinal cord dysfunction of any cause is referred to as "myelopathy"; "myelitis" designates inflammation of the spinal cord. Acute TM refers to a group of acquired, acute-onset, focal inflammatory myelopathies. Consensus diagnostic criteria that rely on clinical and radiographic features have been published, and the diagnosis requires bilateral (although not necessarily symmetric) weakness and sensory deficits, with a clearly defined sensory level; evidence of inflammation by CSF or MRI gadolinium enhancement; and clinical progression to nadir between 4 hours and 21 days (Transverse Myelitis Consortium Working Group, 2002). This clinicoradiologic syndrome can be a manifestation of other inflammatory central nervous system disorders (disease-associated TM), including demyelinating disorders, such as neuromyelitis optica spectrum disorder; acute disseminated encephalomyelitis (ADEM), where up to 50 percent of patients have antibodies to myelin oligodendrocyte glycoprotein; and multiple sclerosis (MS) (Lopez Chiriboga and Flanagan, 2021). Spinal cord infections, paraneoplastic autoimmune syndromes, and systemic inflammatory disorders can also present as disease-associated TM (Flanagan et al., 2016; Jain et al., 2023). When the etiology is unknown, it is called "idiopathic TM." Confusingly, noninflammatory causes of myelopathy, such as ischemic or hemorrhagic stroke, nutritional deficiencies, and neoplasms, can mimic this clinical and radiographic picture. In one study, 70 percent of patients referred to a tertiary care center with a diagnosis of idiopathic TM had a more specific disease-associated TM, such as myelin oligodendrocyte glycoprotein antibody–associated disease or MS, but a quarter of them did not have an inflammatory myelopathy at all (Zalewski et al., 2019). Idiopathic TM is therefore a diagnosis of exclusion (of known causes of disease-associated TM and noninflammatory myelopathies that can mimic TM). Another study, based on retrospective review of Veterans Health Administration electronic medical records, found that 57.6 percent of patients assigned an ICD code of TM lacked CSF testing, which is a core feature of current diagnostic criteria (Abbatemarco et al., 2021). As the aforementioned studies suggest, existing criteria lack specificity, which can affect the accuracy of epidemiological studies, especially those relying on ICD codes.

Idiopathic TM is rare, with a reported incidence of 1.34–4.6 per million per year, with bimodal peaks between ages 10–19 and 30–39 years and no sex predisposition (Bhat et al., 2010). It has been reported a few weeks after vaccination, although a large retrospective cohort study from VSD, a collaboration between the Centers for Disease Control and Prevention's Immunization Safety Office and several integrated health care systems across the United States, did not find an increased risk in association with routine vaccines (Baxter et al., 2016).

## Mechanisms

The pathophysiology of idiopathic TM is unknown, but postinfectious immune-mediated injury is the most widely accepted mechanism. This could be due to bystander activation, epitope spreading, or polyclonal activation of previously dormant self-reactive lymphocytes (see Chapter 2). Up to 40 percent of TM cases follow an infection, most commonly coxsackie viruses and mycoplasma pneumoniae, and infectious agents have sometimes been isolated from the spinal fluid (Bhat et al., 2010; Krishnan et al., 2004). TM has also been reported after a variety of vaccines, including hepatitis B, rabies, and rubella (Agmon-Levin et al., 2009). The fact that TM has been associated with many different viruses and vaccines argues against molecular mimicry as a mechanism. In England in 1922–1923, over 200 cases of encephalomyelitis were reported after smallpox and rabies vaccination, and autopsy studies revealed inflammatory cells and demyelination in the spinal cord (Krishnan et al., 2004; Rivers, 1932). More recent pathological studies demonstrate focal infiltrates of monocytes and lymphocytes in the spinal cord and perivascular space, astroglial and microglial activation, and involvement of both white and gray matter (Krishnan et al., 2004). In the acute phase, heavy infiltration by CD4+ and CD8+ T cells and monocytes is found, whereas the subacute phase is characterized by macrophage infiltration and demyelination (Krishnan et al., 2004). Most patients with TM have CSF pleocytosis, suggesting breakdown of the blood–brain barrier (Bhat et al., 2010; Krishnan et al., 2004).

Patients with TM have been shown to have elevated levels of IL-6 in their CSF, and in acute TM, CSF IL-6 levels correlate with the ultimate level of clinical disability (Kaplin et al., 2005). In an animal model, IL-6 can be shown to mediate cord injury by inducing nitric oxide production, which is associated with oligodendrocyte injury, demyelination, and axonal injury (Kaplin et al., 2005).

## Epidemiological Evidence

Clinical trial results submitted to FDA for Emergency Use Authorization and/or full approval do not indicate a signal regarding TM and any of the vaccines under study (FDA, 2021, 2023a,b,c). Table 3-5 presents five studies that contributed to the causality assessment.

**TABLE 3-5** Epidemiological Studies in the Transverse Myelitis Evidence Review

| Author | Study Design and Control Group | Location | Data Source | Vaccine(s) | Age Range | N | Number of Events | Results (95% CI) |
|---|---|---|---|---|---|---|---|---|
| Klein et al. (2021) | Cohort/ vaccinated concurrent comparators | US | VSD/EMR | BNT162b2 | ≥16 years | 6.8 million doses | BNT162b2 and mRNA-1273 combined: 2 | BNT162b2 and mRNA-1273 combined: RR 1.45 (0.10–47.73) |
| | | | | mRNA-1273 | | 5.1 million doses | | |
| Li et al. (2022) | Cohort/self-controlled and historical background | UK and Spain | Primary care databases linked to hospital data/ EMR | BNT162b2 (UK and Spain) | ≥18 years | 3.6 million vaccinees | UK: Dose 1: <5 Dose 2: No cases  Spain: Dose 1: <5 Dose 2: No cases | SIR not calculated |
| | | | | mRNA-1273 (Spain only) | | 244,913 vaccinees | Dose 1: No cases Dose 2: <5 | |
| | | | | Ad26.COV2.S (Spain only) | | 120,731 vaccinees | Dose 1: No cases | |
| Patone et al. (2021) | Cohort/self-controlled | UK | English immunization records/EMR | BNT162b2 | ≥16 years | 12.1 million vaccinees | 68 | BNT162b2 IRR 1.02 (0.75–1.40) |
| Sturkenboom et al. (2022) | Cohort/ background rate | European countries | Primary and secondary care databases/ EMR | BNT162b2 | Varied | 6.5 million doses | 9 | BNT162b2 IRR 1.88 (0.37–9.60) |
| | | | | mRNA-1273 | | 727,047 doses | No cases | N/A |
| | | | | Ad26.COV2.S | | 242,349 doses | No cases | N/A |
| Walker et al. (2022) | Cohort/Self-controlled | UK | EMR | BNT162b2 | ≥18 | 5.7 million doses | 109 | IRR 1.49 (0.71–3.10) |
| | | | | mRNA-1273 | | 255,446 doses | No cases | N/A |

NOTES: BNT162b2 refers to the COVID-19 vaccine manufactured by Pfizer-BioNTech under the name Comirnaty®. mRNA-1273 refers to the COVID-19 vaccine manufactured by Moderna under the name Spikevax®. Ad26.COV2.S refers to the COVID-19 vaccine manufactured by Janssen. The primary series for Ad26.COV2.S is one dose. Number of events refers to events in vaccinees only. CI: confidence interval; EMR: electronic medical record; IRR: incidence rate ratio; N/A: not applicable; RR: risk ratio; SIR: standardized incidence ratio; VSD: Vaccine Safety Datalink.
SOURCES: Klein et al., 2021; Li et al., 2022; Patone et al., 2021; Sturkenboom et al., 2022; Walker et al., 2022.

Klein et al. (2021) conducted a surveillance study within VSD comparing TM incidence 1–21 days after either dose 1 or 2 of a mRNA vaccine with that of vaccinated concurrent comparators who, on the same calendar day, had received their most recent dose 22–42 days earlier. After 11.8 million doses (57 percent BNT162b2), two cases were identified in the risk interval compared with one in the controlled interval, with an adjusted rate ratio of 1.45 (95% CI: 0.10–47.73) and excess cases of 0.1 (95% CI: −1.6–0.2) risk interval per million doses (Klein et al., 2021).

Li et al. (2022) compared TM rates identified through medical records among vaccinees with historical background rates and conducted an SCCS analysis. They used data from CPRD Aurum and SIDIAP. The study included 3.6 million people who received BNT162b2, 244,913 who received mRNA-1273, 120,731 who received Ad26.COV2.S, and 14.3 million people from the general population. Of the BNT162b2 vaccinees, fewer than five cases occurred within 1–21 days after a first dose in CPRD Aurum, compared with 4.7 expected. SIDIAP had <5 cases after the first dose of BNT162b2, compared with 0.9 expected. For mRNA-1273, <5 cases were diagnosed after the second dose compared with 0.1 expected. No cases were observed with the second dose of BNT162b2, first dose of mRNA-1273, or Ad26.COV2.S.

Walker et al. (2022) analyzed primary care data from more than 17 million patients in England linked to emergency care, hospital admission, and mortality records in OpenSAFELY. They used an SCCS analytical approach where the risk interval was 4–28 days after vaccination. Among 5.7 million recipients of BNT162b2, 109 TM cases were identified during the risk and controlled periods, and none were identified among 255,446 recipients of mRNA-1273. They found no significant association between the first dose of BNT162b2 and TM (IRR 1.62, 95% CI: 0.86–3.03). Few events were observed, so they were unable to precisely estimate the risk association. Adjusting for calendar time or history of COVID-19 infection did not significantly change the measure of association (IRR 1.49, 95% CI: 0.71–3.10) (Walker et al., 2022).

Sturkenboom et al. (2022) conducted a cross-national multi-database retrospective dynamic cohort study using primary and/or secondary health care data from four European countries: Italy, the Netherlands, the United Kingdom, and Spain. They compared TM incidence in vaccine recipients with nonvaccinated persons in 2020 within 28 days after each dose. Of 25.7 million people, nine cases were identified after BNT162b2 (IRR 1.88, 95% CI: 0.37–9.6) and none after mRNA-1273 and Ad26.COV2.S (Sturkenboom et al., 2022). The results are consistent with an increased risk, but few events were observed, and the authors were unable to precisely estimate risk and results; this could also be consistent with no or decreased risk.

Patone et al. (2021) investigated the association between BNT162b2 with potential neurological harms among 32.6 million vaccinees, 12.1 million of whom received BNT162b2 (Patone et al., 2021). An ICD-10 code for TM was included in the category "acute demyelinating events," which contained ICD-10 codes for other demyelinating syndromes, such as ADEM. This retrospective self-controlled cohort study compared the incidence rate at several intervals (1–7, 8–14, 15–21, 22–28, and 1–28 days) after vaccination with that during periods outside of this interval. Sixty-eight events were observed after BNT162b2 during the risk period. They found no association for BNT162b2 at any interval, including in the 1–28 days period (IRR 1.02, 95% CI: 0.75–1.40). Few events were observed, so the authors were unable to precisely estimate the risk; the results would be consistent with no increased risk but also with slightly increased risk.

## From Evidence to Conclusions

The main limitation of the reviewed studies is their reliance on ICD codes from electronic data without chart confirmation. In addition, the studies used varying nomenclature when designating cases of vaccine-associated myelitis. Most had TM as a stand-alone adverse event, but one (Patone et al., 2021) included ICD codes for TM within the larger category "acute demyelinating events," which also included ICD codes for other central nervous system inflammatory disorders. Three studies (Klein et al., 2021; Li et al., 2022; Patone et al., 2021) included a separate category "encephalitis/myelitis/encephalomyelitis," and cases clinically and radiographically consistent with TM may have been classed within this category based on their ICD code, resulting in a lower number of total reported events.

None of the five epidemiology studies suggested a causal association between TM and BNT162b2, and no evidence suggests a large association. However, the limited number of studies, along with the overall low number of events reported, raises the concern that a small association may have been missed, given that TM is a very rare disorder. Four studies included a few mRNA-1273 recipients, with no TM cases reported in two of the studies. Only one study included patients who received Ad26.COV2.S, with a comparatively low number of vaccinees and no cases reported (Li et al., 2022).

**Conclusion 3-13: The evidence is inadequate to accept or reject a causal relationship between the BNT162b2 vaccine and transverse myelitis.**

**Conclusion 3-14: The evidence is inadequate to accept or reject a causal relationship between the mRNA-1273 vaccine and transverse myelitis.**

**Conclusion 3-15: The evidence is inadequate to accept or reject a causal relationship between the Ad26.COV2.S vaccine and transverse myelitis.**

**Conclusion 3-16: The evidence is inadequate to accept or reject a causal relationship between the NVX-CoV2373 vaccine and transverse myelitis.**

## CHRONIC HEADACHE

---

**BOX 3-5**
**Conclusions for Chronic Headache**

**Conclusion 3-17: The evidence is inadequate to accept or reject a causal relationship between the BNT162b2 vaccine and chronic headache.**

**Conclusion 3-18: The evidence is inadequate to accept or reject a causal relationship between the mRNA-1273 vaccine and chronic headache.**

**Conclusion 3-19: The evidence is inadequate to accept or reject a causal relationship between the Ad26.COV2.S vaccine and chronic headache.**

**Conclusion 3-20: The evidence is inadequate to accept or reject a causal relationship between the NVX-CoV2373 vaccine and chronic headache.**

---

### Background

Headache is a frequently reported symptom of systemic illness, cerebrovascular disorders, intracranial disease, or craniocervical trauma. It is also reported commonly and can be a symptom of substance withdrawal. When a headache results from a separate medical condition, it is called a "secondary headache." Most headaches, however, occur as the principal manifestation of a primary headache disorder; these are characterized by recurrent headaches of varying characteristics, frequency, and accompanying symptoms and signs. Although the frequency and severity of individual headache episodes vary over the lifetime, primary headache disorders are usually considered lifelong conditions. They have no biological markers, and their diagnosis is made with reasonable precision based on consensus diagnostic criteria set forth in the International Classification of Headache Disorders (ICHD-3), which was last revised in 2018 (International Headache Society, 2018). Ancillary studies, mostly brain and vascular imaging and occasionally lumbar puncture, are used to rule out various forms of secondary headaches.

Tension-type headache (TTH) and migraine are by far the more common primary headache disorders, with an estimated lifetime prevalence in the general population of 46 and 14 percent, respectively (Stovner et al., 2007). Geographic variations exist, but it is unclear whether these are driven by genetic differences or methodological differences between studies. Other primary headache disorders, such as cluster headache, are much rarer, with a lifetime prevalence of 0.06–0.3 percent (Jensen and Stovner, 2008). The frequency, duration, and severity of headache varies significantly even within the same primary headache disorder: from infrequent, short, and mild to continuous and/or disabling. Migraine is more common in women compared to men, with a ratio of 2:1 to 3:1 (Jensen and Stovner, 2008). The female:male ratio for TTH is 5:4 (Jensen and Stovner, 2008). The prevalence of migraine peaks between the second and third decades of life but can affect people of all ages, including children. Data regarding age dependence in TTH are more limited, but prevalence peaks around the fourth decade of life. Cluster headache has a male:female ratio of 4.3:1 (Fischera et al., 2008), with prevalence peaking between the second and fourth decades of life.

No single consensus diagnostic criteria exist for chronic headache. Rather, ICHD-3 provides diagnostic criteria for chronic forms of individual headache subtypes based on frequency and duration. These include chronic migraine headache, chronic TTH, chronic cluster headache, hemicrania continua, new daily persistent headache, and medication overuse headache, which is a form of secondary headache (International Headache Society, 2018). In most, but not all, chronicity is based on a frequency of more than 15 headache days per month for longer than 3 months. Although ICHD-3 criteria for secondary headache do not specify measures of chronicity, they do specify that when a pre-existing primary headache becomes chronic shortly after a known causative disorder, both chronic primary headache and secondary headache diagnoses should be given (International Headache Society, 2018). Data on chronic headaches are relatively scarce, but prevalence as a group is estimated as 3–4 percent in the general population (Jensen and Stovner, 2008).

Systemic infection, including with COVID-19, can be associated with headache (Togha et al., 2022), and "headache attributed to systemic infection" is included as a subtype of secondary headache in ICHD-3. Headache was also a frequently reported symptom in the clinical trials for the various COVID-19 vaccines (Baden et al., 2021; Heath et al., 2021; Polack et al., 2020; Sadoff et al., 2021). Most of these headaches occurred within 24 hours of vaccination and were frequently accompanied by systemic symptoms, such as fatigue, fever, chills, and myalgia (Göbel et al., 2021a,b). In most, headaches lasted less than 72 hours, with only a small minority reporting more than 3 days. Pre-existing migraine was associated with more severe and long-lasting headaches in some but not all studies (Silvestro et al., 2021) and may predispose someone to postvaccine headache (Sekiguchi et al., 2022). Although ICHD-3 does include "headache attributed to use or exposure to a substance" as a subtype of secondary headache, vaccines are not listed within the known causes (International Headache Society, 2018). Evidence suggests that headache may be common with other vaccines as well, and some have proposed that post-vaccination headache should be included in the next iteration of the ICHD (Garces et al., 2022). Headache is also one of the main symptoms of cerebral venous sinus thrombosis (CVST), a manifestation of vaccine-induced immune thrombotic thrombocytopenia (VITT). VITT has been reported in association with the AV COVID-19 vaccines and is discussed elsewhere in this report (See et al., 2021). Unlike the more common post-vaccination headache, which occurs shortly after vaccination, the headache secondary to VITT-associated CVST is approximately a week after vaccination (García-Azorín et al., 2021).

## Mechanisms

The pathophysiology of primary headache disorders remains ill-defined and is different for individual disorders. Post-vaccination headache is not included as a type of secondary headache in ICHD-3; however, it may bear some resemblance to "headache attributed to systemic infection," which is included. The more widely accepted hypothesis is that post-vaccination headache is secondary to downstream effects stemming from the immune response to the vaccine (Garces et al., 2022). Vaccines, including COVID-19 vaccines, are associated with the release of inflammatory mediators, such as prostaglandin E, and proinflammatory cytokines. It is conjectured that these are responsible for the headache and frequently associated systemic symptoms. Some have proposed that inflammatory mediators may modulate the release of calcitonin gene–related peptide (CGRP), which plays an important role in migraine via activation of the trigeminovascular system. Similarly, substance P, a nociceptive neuropeptide released by trigeminal sensory fibers and implicated in migraine, is also produced by mast cells, suggesting a link between immune activation and migraines (Suvas, 2017). Data supporting this hypothesis are limited. One study found increased levels of inflammatory and nociceptive molecules in COVID-19 hospitalized patients with headache compared to those without; CGRP levels, however, did not differ significantly between the two groups (Bolay et al., 2021). Finally, some have hypothesized direct modulation of the trigeminal nerve when the spike protein, which is either synthetized intracellularly or introduced directly after vaccination, binds the angiotensin-converting enzyme 2 (ACE2) receptor. However, it remains unclear whether ACE2 is expressed in the relevant neural structures (Caronna et al., 2023), and some studies suggest that headache is more common after the second dose (Ceccardi et al., 2022), which appears counterintuitive given the probable presence of neutralizing antibodies against the spike protein.

## Epidemiological Evidence

Chronic headache is not a single diagnostic entity with widely accepted diagnostic criteria. The committee relied on ICHD-3, which provides diagnostic criteria for the subtypes. Although a self-limited headache was a commonly reported symptom after BNT162b2, mRNA-1273, Ad26.COV2.S, and NVX-CoV2373, none of the studies reviewed included a stand-alone category for chronic headache, nor did they include chronic headache subtypes as defined in ICHD-3. Clinical trial results submitted to FDA for Emergency Use Authorization and/or full approval do not indicate a signal regarding chronic headache and any of the vaccines under study (FDA, 2021, 2023a,b,c). None were included in the final report for analysis.

## From Evidence to Conclusions

The epidemiological and mechanistic literature are absent regarding the relationship between COVID-19 vaccines and chronic headache.

**Conclusion 3-17: The evidence is inadequate to accept or reject a causal relationship between the BNT162b2 vaccine and chronic headache.**

**Conclusion 3-18: The evidence is inadequate to accept or reject a causal relationship between the mRNA-1273 vaccine and chronic headache.**

**Conclusion 3-19: The evidence is inadequate to accept or reject a causal relationship between the Ad26.COV2.S vaccine and chronic headache.**

**Conclusion 3-20: The evidence is inadequate to accept or reject a causal relationship between the NVX-CoV2373 vaccine and chronic headache.**

## POSTURAL ORTHOSTATIC TACHYCARDIA SYNDROME

---

**BOX 3-6**
**Conclusions for Postural Orthostatic Tachycardia Syndrome**

**Conclusion 3-21: The evidence is inadequate to accept or reject a causal relationship between the BNT162b2 vaccine and postural orthostatic tachycardia syndrome.**

**Conclusion 3-22: The evidence is inadequate to accept or reject a causal relationship between the mRNA-1273 vaccine and postural orthostatic tachycardia syndrome.**

**Conclusion 3-23: The evidence is inadequate to accept or reject a causal relationship between the Ad26.COV2.S vaccine and postural orthostatic tachycardia syndrome.**

**Conclusion 3-24: The evidence is inadequate to accept or reject a causal relationship between the NVX-CoV2373 vaccine and postural orthostatic tachycardia syndrome.**

---

## Background

POTS is marked by symptoms of orthostatic intolerance despite relative preservation of autonomic reflexes. The hallmark is an exaggerated increase in heart rate in response to standing or tilt without a drop in blood pressure as seen in classic autonomic failure (Cutsforth-Gregory, 2020). POTS is defined as a sustained heart rate increase of 30 beats per minute (bpm) or increase to 120 bpm within the first 10 minutes of orthostasis, along with symptoms of orthostatic intolerance, including dizziness, palpitations, weakness, and tremulousness. For children and adolescents (12–19 years), the required increment is 40 bpm (Vernino et al., 2021).

POTS predominantly affects a younger and primarily female (at a ratio of 4:1) demographic, with the typical age range of onset being 12–50 (Vernino et al., 2021). Epidemiologically, it is a relatively common condition in developed countries, with prevalence estimates of 0.2–1.0 percent of the U.S. population, which represents 1–3 million people (Cutsforth-Gregory, 2020; Vernino et al., 2021).

Orthostatic symptoms are probably driven by both cerebral hypoperfusion (dizziness, lightheadedness, and vision and hearing changes) and sympathoexcitation (palpitations, chest pain, difficulty breathing, tremulousness, sweating, and coldness of the extremities) (Cutsforth-Gregory, 2020). Particularly, tachycardia can be triggered either directly by influencing the sinus rate control system via adrenergic and muscarinic receptors or indirectly as a compensatory response to peripheral vasodilation. This indirect response may involve adrenergic, angiotensin, and other potential vasoactive receptors (see Figure 3-2). POTS patients, however, frequently experience other symptoms as well, including sleep disturbances, headache, fatigue, cognitive impairment, gastrointestinal complaints, urinary frequency, and exercise intolerance (Vernino et al., 2021). The sheer variety and nonspecificity of these symptoms make it difficult to attribute all of them to a single clinical entity sharing the same underlying mechanism. Various comorbid conditions are associated with POTS, including migraine, somatic hypervigilance,

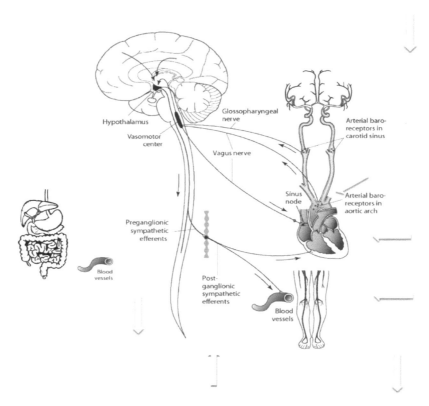

**FIGURE 3-2** Postulated mechanisms of orthostatic intolerance and tachycardia in postural orthostatic tachycardia syndrome.
SOURCE: Fedorowski et al., 2017. CC BY NC-ND.

irritable bowel syndrome, hypermobile Ehlers-Danlos syndrome, mast cell activation syndrome, systemic auto-immune disease, small-fiber neuropathy, and fibromyalgia and chronic fatigue syndrome (Gradin et al., 1987; Low et al., 2009; Shibao et al., 2005). It is unclear whether the presence of these diagnoses defines unique patho-physiological subsets (Vernino et al., 2021). In either case, the diagnostic criteria emphasize symptoms *and* heart rate increment *in response to* an orthostatic challenge as the core feature, which is appropriate, as an excessive heart rate is the most consistent and reproducible of various indexes of orthostatic intolerance (Vernino et al., 2021). Symptoms alone in the absence of orthostatic tachycardia cannot be used to make the diagnosis, and the syndrome must be present for at least 3 months (Vernino et al., 2021). The diagnostic approach begins with a comprehensive clinical assessment focused on orthostatic intolerance symptoms. Excessive increase in heart rate without orthostatic hypotension within 3–10 minutes from standing should be confirmed at bedside or with a tilt-table test (Freeman et al., 2011; Vernino et al., 2021). Laboratory tests play an important role in excluding other conditions that might mimic POTS symptoms. Further autonomic testing and/or skin biopsy may be warranted to explore the full spectrum of autonomic dysfunction and assess for underlying small-fiber neuropathy (Vernino et al., 2021). A 12-lead electrocardiography should be performed in all patients, but expanded cardiac evaluation may be indicated in some (Cutsforth-Gregory, 2020).

Between 20 and 50 percent of patients report a viral illness before the onset of symptoms. In these cases, POTS symptoms appear to arise abruptly weeks after the acute illness, but in others, the symptoms appear slowly (Thieben et al., 2007). Other triggers include surgery and head trauma, although these are less well established (Olshansky et al., 2020). Patients have developed POTS symptoms at the time of or within 6 weeks of acute SARS-CoV-2 infection (Goodman et al., 2021), but latency can be longer, and POTS is considered a phenotype of postacute or "long" COVID-19 (Fedorowski and Sutton, 2023). POTS has also been reported in association with the COVID-19 vaccine (Kwan et al., 2022).

## Mechanisms

The pathophysiology of POTS remains ill defined, and it is unlikely that it is a single disorder. Rather, it is probably a heterogeneous syndrome that can arise in various clinical scenarios resulting from distinct but over-lapping pathophysiologic mechanisms (Benarroch, 2012). Several mechanisms have been proposed and account for some of its phenotypic variability. These include catecholamine excess (hyperadrenergic POTS), sympathetic denervation leading to impaired vasoconstriction of the lower limbs (neuropathic POTS), volume dysregulation, and deconditioning (Vernino et al., 2021).

The clinical picture with hyperadrenergic POTS is dominated by palpitations, sweating, tremulousness, and orthostatic hypertension. Some of these patients have high plasma norepinephrine concentrations during orthostasis (Fedorowski and Sutton, 2023), although in others, the hyperadrenergic state may be secondary to medications, such a tricyclic antidepressants or methylphenidate (Cheshire, 2016). Neuropathic POTS may be secondary to a length-dependent autonomic neuropathy leading to impaired vasomotor tone in the lower limbs. Autonomic test-ing in some patients demonstrates loss of sweating in the feet and reduced increment of norepinephrine in the lower limbs when standing, which is consistent with a length-dependent autonomic neuropathy. The etiology of this autonomic neuropathy is not usually evident, although several lines of evidence suggest a potential immune-mediated mechanism in some cases. Reports of an earlier viral illness in up to one-half of patients suggests a postinfectious autoimmune process (Sandroni et al., 1999; Vernino et al., 2021). In addition, several small studies have demonstrated higher levels of functionally active antibodies to G-protein-coupled adrenergic receptors α1 and α2 in individuals with POTS than in healthy controls (Fedorowski and Sutton, 2023; Kharraziha et al., 2020; Li et al., 2014; Vernino et al., 2021). These findings, plus reports of the successful treatment of POTS with IVIG (Rodriguez et al., 2021; Weinstock et al., 2018), suggest an autoimmune etiology, at least in a subset of patients. However, a recent randomized controlled trial of IVIG in POTS found no difference in symptom response com-pared to albumin infusion (Vernino et al., 2023).

Most patients have some degree of hypovolemia. Studies have demonstrated that many of them have low levels of plasma-renin activity and aldosterone compared with controls (Raj et al., 2005), and some have reduced ACE2 activity (Stewart et al., 2009). The excessive venous pooling that occurs with vasomotor impairment in neurogenic POTS can lead to reduced cardiac preload and capillary leakage upon standing with associated net loss of plasma volume (Cutsforth-Gregory, 2020). In those with poor oral intake or excess fluid loss, such as in irritable bowel syndrome, managing the primary disorder will improve orthostatic intolerance. Finally, physical deconditioning can lead to orthostatic intolerance. Many patients show evidence of deconditioning: reduced stroke volume and left ventricular mass and persistent tachycardia and reduced peak oxygen when standing or exercising (Fu et al., 2010; Masuki et al., 2007).

POTS has been reported in association with SARS-CoV-2 infection (Kwan et al., 2022; Miglis et al., 2020), including in patients with post-acute COVID-19 (Fedorowski and Sutton, 2023). However, caution is needed when assessing the literature because although orthostatic intolerance is commonly reported in patients with post-acute COVID-19, many may not meet diagnostic criteria for POTS. In one study of patients with de novo orthostatic intolerance after COVID-19, only 22 percent fulfilled criteria for POTS (Shouman et al., 2021); the symptoms may be driven by deconditioning in some of these patients. In addition to POTS, small-fiber neuropathy, which can cause autonomic dysfunction and a POTS phenotype, has been described after COVID-19, including in post-acute COVID-19 (Abrams et al., 2022; Oaklander et al., 2022). POTS has also been reported after COVID-19 vaccination (Kwan et al., 2022). Many of these reports postulate an immune-mediated mechanism, but definitive evidence is lacking. One study demonstrated elevated inflammatory cytokines and markers of autoimmunity in patients presenting with POTS after COVID-19, although this study did not include relevant controls. One in silico study identified a variety of SARS-CoV-2 amino acid sequences, including in the spike protein, that are also present in vagal nuclei and ganglia (Marino Gammazza et al., 2020). This raises the theoretical possibility that molecular mimicry could induce cross-reactive immune responses resulting in low vagal tone after infection or vaccination.

**Epidemiological Evidence**

Clinical trial results submitted to FDA for Emergency Use Authorization and/or full approval do not indicate a signal regarding POTS and any of the vaccines under study (FDA, 2021, 2023a,b,c). Table 3-6 summarizes one study that contributed to the causality assessment.

Kwan et al. (2022) derived cohorts from the diverse patient population of the Cedars-Sinai Health System in Los Angeles County, California. The authors identified patients who had at least one COVID-19 vaccination between 2020 and 2022 and excluded those with a documented COVID-19 infection 90 days before or after vaccination ($n = 5{,}070$). The final sample was 284,592 patients (age $52 \pm 20$ years; 57 percent female; 63 percent White, 10 percent Asian, 8.9 percent African American, and 12 percent Hispanic). Among the sample, 62 percent received BNT162b2, 31 percent mRNA-1273, 6.9 percent Ad26.COV2.S, and less than 0.1 percent other vaccines. POTS was identified using diagnosis codes (ICD-9 I49.8; ICD-10 G90.9) and modeled as both a single diagnosis and a combination of POTS-associated diagnoses (POTS diagnosis codes, Fatigue, Dysautonomia, Ehlers-Danlos syndrome, and mast cell disorders). Only outpatient encounters were used. From the 90-day prevaccination to 90-day post-vaccination periods, the incidence of new diagnoses of POTS increased from 176 per 100,000 to 268 per 100,000 vaccinees (the authors did not report incidence per 100,000 for the combined diagnoses). Relative to the prevaccination period, the odds of a new diagnosis of POTS and POTS-associated diagnoses increased 52 percent, odds ratio (OR) 1.52 (95% CI: 1.36–1.71) and 33 percent, OR 1.33 (95% CI: 1.25–1.41) in the post-vaccination period, respectively. Limitations exist from unmeasured confounding, lack of inclusion of COVID-19 infection, and open nature of the dataset, as patients could have had encounters in other health systems as well. In addition, the measure of effect was calculated for all vaccines combined, and conclusions cannot be drawn regarding a potential association between POTS and individual vaccines or platforms.

The committee also reviewed a case series (Eldokla and Numan, 2022) of five patients who developed de novo POTS within 21 days of an mRNA vaccine (four BNT162b2, one mRNA-1273). All five underwent detailed autonomic testing and met diagnostic criteria for POTS. Two had elevated proinflammatory cytokines, and two had mildly elevated autoantibodies (thyroid peroxidase antibodies and antinuclear antibodies), without other signs or symptoms of systemic autoimmune disease. One had a low titer of acetylcholine receptor ganglionic antibodies; at higher titers, this has been associated with autoimmune autonomic failure.

**TABLE 3-6** Epidemiological Study in the Postural Orthostatic Tachycardia Syndrome Evidence Review

| Author | Study Design and Control Group | Location | Data Source | Vaccine(s) | Age Range | Sample Size | Number of Events | Results (95% CI) |
|---|---|---|---|---|---|---|---|---|
| Kwan et al. (2022) | Cohort/self-controlled | US | EMR | BNT162b2 | ≥12 years | 284,592 patients (62.2%) | 763 events per 100,000 POTS cases during exposure period compared to 501 per 100,000 pre-exposure | OR 1.52 (1.36–1.71) |
| | | | | mRNA-1273 | | 31% | | |
| | | | | Ad26.COV 2.S | | 6.9% | | |
| | | | | NVX-CoV2373 | | <0.1% other* | | |

NOTES: BNT162b2 refers to the COVID-19 vaccine manufactured by Pfizer-BioNTech under the name Comirnaty®. mRNA-1273 refers to the COVID-19 vaccine manufactured by Moderna under the name Spikevax®. Ad26.COV2.S refers to the COVID-19 vaccine manufactured by Janssen. NVX-CoV2373 refers to the COVID-19 vaccine manufactured by Novavax. *<0.1% of other vaccines includes ChAdOx1-S, NVX-CoV2373, and CoronaVac. Number of events refers to events in vaccinees only. CI: confidence interval; EMR: electronic medical record; OR: odds ratio.
SOURCE: Kwan et al., 2022.

### From Evidence to Conclusions

The totality of the evidence included one epidemiological study with methodological limitations and one case series with adequate case identification but no comparator group. No definitive mechanism was identified in the literature.

**Conclusion 3-21: The evidence is inadequate to accept or reject a causal relationship between the BNT162b2 vaccine and postural orthostatic tachycardia syndrome.**

**Conclusion 3-22: The evidence is inadequate to accept or reject a causal relationship between the mRNA-1273 vaccine and postural orthostatic tachycardia syndrome.**

**Conclusion 3-23: The evidence is inadequate to accept or reject a causal relationship between the Ad26.COV2.S vaccine and postural orthostatic tachycardia syndrome.**

**Conclusion 3-24: The evidence is inadequate to accept or reject a causal relationship between the NVX-CoV2373 vaccine and postural orthostatic tachycardia syndrome.**

### REFERENCES

Ab Rahman, N., M. T. Lim, F. Y. Lee, S. C. Lee, A. Ramli, S. N. Saharudin, T. L. King, E. B. Anak Jam, N. A. Ayub, R. K. Sevalingam, R. Bahari, N. N. Ibrahim, F. Mahmud, S. Sivasampu, and K. M. Peariasamy. 2022. Risk of serious adverse events after the BNT162b2, CoronaVac, and ChAdOx1 vaccines in Malaysia: A self-controlled case series study. *Vaccine* 40(32):4394–4402. https://doi.org/10.1016/j.vaccine.2022.05.075.
Abara, W. E., J. Gee, P. Marquez, J. Woo, T. R. Myers, A. DeSantis, J. A. G. Baumblatt, E. J. Woo, D. Thompson, N. Nair, J. R. Su, T. T. Shimabukuro, and D. K. Shay. 2023. Reports of Guillain-Barré syndrome after COVID-19 vaccination in the United States. *JAMA Network Open* 6(2):e2253845. https://doi.org/10.1001/jamanetworkopen.2022.53845.

Abbatemarco, J. R., J. R. Galli, M. L. Sweeney, N. G. Carlson, V. C. Samara, H. Davis, S. Rodenbeck, K. H. Wong, M. M. Paz Soldan, J. E. Greenlee, J. W. Rose, A. Delic, and S. L. Clardy. 2021. Modern look at transverse myelitis and inflammatory myelopathy: Epidemiology of the National Veterans Health Administration population. *Neurology Neuroimmunology & Neuroinflammation* 8(6). https://doi.org/10.1212/nxi.0000000000001071.

Abrams, R. M. C., D. M. Simpson, A. Navis, N. Jette, L. Zhou, and S. C. Shin. 2022. Small fiber neuropathy associated with SARS-CoV-2 infection. *Muscle and Nerve* 65(4):440–443. https://doi.org/10.1002/mus.27458.

Agmon-Levin, N., S. Kivity, M. Szyper-Kravitz, and Y. Shoenfeld. 2009. Transverse myelitis and vaccines: A multi-analysis. *Lupus* 18(13):1198–1204. https://doi.org/10.1177/0961203309345730.

Arunachalam, P. S., M. K. D. Scott, T. Hagan, C. Li, Y. Feng, F. Wimmers, L. Grigoryan, M. Trisal, V. V. Edara, L. Lai, S. E. Chang, A. Feng, S. Dhingra, M. Shah, A. S. Lee, S. Chinthrajah, S. B. Sindher, V. Mallajosyula, F. Gao, N. Sigal, S. Kowli, S. Gupta, K. Pellegrini, G. Tharp, S. Maysel-Auslender, S. Hamilton, H. Aoued, K. Hrusovsky, M. Roskey, S. E. Bosinger, H. T. Maecker, S. D. Boyd, M. M. Davis, P. J. Utz, M. S. Suthar, P. Khatri, K. C. Nadeau, and B. Pulendran. 2021. Systems vaccinology of the BNT162b2 mRNA vaccine in humans. *Nature* 596(7872):410–416. https://doi.org/10.1038/s41586-021-03791-x.

Asbury, A. K., B. G. Arnason, and R. D. Adams. 1969. The inflammatory lesion in idiopathic polyneuritis. Its role in pathogenesis. *Medicine* 48(3):173–215. https://doi.org/10.1097/00005792-196905000-00001.

Baden, L. R., H. M. El Sahly, B. Essink, K. Kotloff, S. Frey, R. Novak, D. Diemert, S. A. Spector, N. Rouphael, C. B. Creech, J. McGettigan, S. Khetan, N. Segall, J. Solis, A. Brosz, C. Fierro, H. Schwartz, K. Neuzil, L. Corey, P. Gilbert, H. Janes, D. Follmann, M. Marovich, J. Mascola, L. Polakowski, J. Ledgerwood, B. S. Graham, H. Bennett, R. Pajon, C. Knightly, B. Leav, W. Deng, H. Zhou, S. Han, M. Ivarsson, J. Miller, and T. Zaks. 2021. Efficacy and safety of the mRNA-1273 SARS-CoV-2 vaccine. *New England Journal of Medicine* 384(5):403–416. https://doi.org/10.1056/NEJMoa2035389.

Baker, A. T., R. J. Boyd, D. Sarkar, A. Teijeira-Crespo, C. K. Chan, E. Bates, K. Waraich, J. Vant, E. Wilson, C. D. Truong, M. Lipka-Lloyd, P. Fromme, J. Vermaas, D. Williams, L. Machiesky, M. Heurich, B. M. Nagalo, L. Coughlan, S. Umlauf, P. L. Chiu, P. J. Rizkallah, T. S. Cohen, A. L. Parker, A. Singharoy, and M. J. Borad. 2021. ChAdOx1 interacts with CAR and PF4 with implications for thrombosis with thrombocytopenia syndrome. *Science Advances* 7(49):eabl8213. https://doi.org/10.1126/sciadv.abl8213.

Baugh, R. F., G. J. Basura, L. E. Ishii, S. R. Schwartz, C. M. Drumheller, R. Burkholder, N. A. Deckard, C. Dawson, C. Driscoll, M. B. Gillespie, R. K. Gurgel, J. Halperin, A. N. Khalid, K. A. Kumar, A. Micco, D. Munsell, S. Rosenbaum, and W. Vaughan. 2013. Clinical practice guideline: Bell's palsy executive summary. *Otolaryngology—Head and Neck Surgery* 149(5):656–663. https://doi.org/10.1177/0194599813506835.

Baxter, R., E. Lewis, K. Goddard, B. Fireman, N. Bakshi, F. DeStefano, J. Gee, H. F. Tseng, A. L. Naleway, and N. P. Klein. 2016. Acute demyelinating events following vaccines: A case-centered analysis. *Clinical Infectious Diseases* 63(11):1456–1462. https://doi.org/10.1093/cid/ciw607.

Benarroch, E. E. 2012. Postural tachycardia syndrome: A heterogeneous and multifactorial disorder. *Mayo Clinic Proceedings* 87(12):1214–1225. https://doi.org/10.1016/j.mayocp.2012.08.013.

Bhat, A., S. Naguwa, G. Cheema, and M. E. Gershwin. 2010. The epidemiology of transverse myelitis. *Autoimmunity Reviews* 9(5):A395–A399. https://doi.org/10.1016/j.autrev.2009.12.007.

Bolay, H., Ö. Karadas, B. Oztürk, R. Sonkaya, B. Tasdelen, T. D. S. Bulut, Ö. Gülbahar, A. Özge, and B. Baykan. 2021. HMGB1, NLRP3, IL-6 and ACE2 levels are elevated in COVID-19 with headache: A window to the infection-related headache mechanism. *Journal of Headache and Pain* 22(1):94. https://doi.org/10.1186/s10194-021-01306-7.

Bragazzi, N. L., A. A. Kolahi, S. A. Nejadghaderi, P. Lochner, F. Brigo, A. Naldi, P. Lanteri, S. Garbarino, M. J. M. Sullman, H. Dai, J. Wu, J. D. Kong, H. Jahrami, M. R. Sohrabi, and S. Safiri. 2021. Global, regional, and national burden of Guillain-Barré syndrome and its underlying causes from 1990 to 2019. *Journal of Neuroinflammation* 18(1):264. https://doi.org/10.1186/s12974-021-02319-4.

Caronna, E., T. C. van den Hoek, H. Bolay, D. Garcia-Azorin, A. B. Gago-Veiga, M. Valeriani, T. Takizawa, K. Messlinger, R. E. Shapiro, P. J. Goadsby, M. Ashina, C. Tassorelli, H. C. Diener, G. M. Terwindt, and P. Pozo-Rosich. 2023. Headache attributed to SARS-CoV-2 infection, vaccination and the impact on primary headache disorders of the COVID-19 pandemic: A comprehensive review. *Cephalalgia* 43(1). https://doi.org/10.1177/03331024221131337.

Ceccardi, G., F. Schiano di Cola, M. Di Cesare, P. Liberini, M. Magoni, C. Perani, R. Gasparotti, R. Rao, and A. Padovani. 2022. Post COVID-19 vaccination headache: A clinical and epidemiological evaluation. *Frontiers in Pain Research* 3:994140. https://doi.org/10.3389/fpain.2022.994140.

Chen, Y., Z. Xu, P. Wang, X. M. Li, Z. W. Shuai, D. Q. Ye, and H. F. Pan. 2022a. New-onset autoimmune phenomena post-COVID-19 vaccination. *Immunology* 165(4):386–401. https://doi.org/10.1111/imm.13443.

Chen, Y. J., P. L. Cheng, W. N. Huang, H. H. Chen, H. W. Chen, J. P. Chen, C. T. Lin, K. T. Tang, W. T. Hung, T. Y. Hsieh, Y. H. Chen, Y. M. Chen, and T. H. Hsiao. 2022b. Single-cell RNA sequencing to decipher the immunogenicity of ChAdOx1 NCOV-19/AZD1222 and mRNA-1273 vaccines in patients with autoimmune rheumatic diseases. *Frontiers in Immunology* 13:920865. https://doi.org/10.3389/fimmu.2022.920865.

Cheshire, W. P. 2016. Stimulant medication and postural orthostatic tachycardia syndrome: A tale of two cases. *Clinical Autonomic Research* 26(3):229–233. https://doi.org/10.1007/s10286-016-0347-9.

Cutsforth-Gregory, J. K. 2020. Postural tachycardia syndrome and neurally mediated syncope. *Continuum* 26(1):93–115. https://doi.org/10.1212/con.0000000000000818.

Dalakas, M. C. 2011. Advances in the diagnosis, pathogenesis and treatment of CIDP. *Nature Reviews: Neurology* 7(9):507–517. https://doi.org/10.1038/nrneurol.2011.121.

Dalakas, M. C., and W. K. Engel. 1980. Immunoglobulin and complement deposits in nerves of patients with chronic relapsing polyneuropathy. *Archives of Neurology* 37(10):637–640. https://doi.org/10.1001/archneur.1980.00500590061010.

Dowling, P., J. Menonna, and S. Cook. 1977. Cytomegalovirus complement fixation antibody in Guillain-Barré syndrome. *Neurology* 27(12):1153–1156. https://doi.org/10.1212/wnl.27.12.1153.

Eldokla, A. M., and M. T. Numan. 2022. Postural orthostatic tachycardia syndrome after mRNA COVID-19 vaccine. *Clinical Autonomic Research* 32(4):307–311. https://doi.org/10.1007/s10286-022-00880-3.

FDA (Food and Drug Administration). 2021. *Emergency use authorization (EUA) amendment for an unapproved product review memorandum.* Food and Drug Administration. https://www.fda.gov/media/153439/download (accessed May 3, 2023).

FDA. 2023a. *BLA clinical review memorandum—COMIRNATY.* Food and Drug Administration. https://www.fda.gov/media/172333/download?attachment (accessed December 5, 2023).

FDA. 2023b. *BLA clinical review memorandum—SPIKEVAX.* Food and Drug Administration. https://www.fda.gov/media/172357/download?attachment (accessed December 5, 2023).

FDA. 2023c. *Emergency use authorization (EUA) for an unapproved product review memorandum.* Food and Drug Administration. https://www.fda.gov/media/168233/download?attachment (accessed December 5, 2023).

Fedorowski, A., H. Li, X. Yu, K. A. Koelsch, V. M. Harris, C. Liles, T. A. Murphy, S. M. S. Quadri, R. H. Scofield, R. Sutton, O. Melander, and D. C. Kem. 2017. Antiadrenergic autoimmunity in postural tachycardia syndrome. *Europace: European Pacing, Arrhythmias, and Cardiac Electrophysiology* 19(7):1211–1219. https://doi.org/10.1093/europace/euw154.

Fedorowski, A., and R. Sutton. 2023. Autonomic dysfunction and postural orthostatic tachycardia syndrome in post-acute COVID-19 syndrome. *Nature Reviews: Cardiology* 20(5):281–282. https://doi.org/10.1038/s41569-023-00842-w.

Felipe Cuspoca, A., P. Isaac Estrada, and A. Velez-van-Meerbeke. 2022. Molecular mimicry of SARS-CoV-2 spike protein in the nervous system: A bioinformatics approach. *Computational and Structural Biotechnology Journal* 20:6041–6054. https://doi.org/10.1016/j.csbj.2022.10.022.

Fischera, M., M. Marziniak, I. Gralow, and S. Evers. 2008. The incidence and prevalence of cluster headache: A meta-analysis of population-based studies. *Cephalalgia* 28(6):614–618. https://doi.org/10.1111/j.1468-2982.2008.01592.x.

Flanagan, E. P., T. J. Kaufmann, K. N. Krecke, A. J. Aksamit, S. J. Pittock, B. M. Keegan, C. Giannini, and B. G. Weinshenker. 2016. Discriminating long myelitis of neuromyelitis optica from sarcoidosis. *Annals of Neurology* 79(3):437–447. https://doi.org/10.1002/ana.24582.

Fokke, C., B. van den Berg, J. Drenthen, C. Walgaard, P. A. van Doorn, and B. C. Jacobs. 2014. Diagnosis of Guillain-Barré syndrome and validation of Brighton criteria. *Brain* 137(Pt 1):33–43. https://doi.org/10.1093/brain/awt285.

Freeman, R., W. Wieling, F. B. Axelrod, D. G. Benditt, E. Benarroch, I. Biaggioni, W. P. Cheshire, T. Chelimsky, P. Cortelli, C. H. Gibbons, D. S. Goldstein, R. Hainsworth, M. J. Hilz, G. Jacob, H. Kaufmann, J. Jordan, L. A. Lipsitz, B. D. Levine, P. A. Low, C. Mathias, S. R. Raj, D. Robertson, P. Sandroni, I. Schatz, R. Schondorff, J. M. Stewart, and J. G. van Dijk. 2011. Consensus statement on the definition of orthostatic hypotension, neurally mediated syncope and the postural tachycardia syndrome. *Clinical Autonomic Research* 21(2):69–72. https://doi.org/10.1007/s10286-011-0119-5.

Fu, Q., T. B. Vangundy, M. M. Galbreath, S. Shibata, M. Jain, J. L. Hastings, P. S. Bhella, and B. D. Levine. 2010. Cardiac origins of the postural orthostatic tachycardia syndrome. *Journal of the American College of Cardiology* 55(25):2858–2868. https://doi.org/10.1016/j.jacc.2010.02.043.

Garces, K. N., A. N. Cocores, P. J. Goadsby, and T. S. Monteith. 2022. Headache after vaccination: An update on recent clinical trials and real-world reporting. *Current Pain and Headache Reports* 26(12):895–918. https://doi.org/10.1007/s11916-022-01094-y.

García-Azorín, D., T. P. Do, A. R. Gantenbein, J. M. Hansen, M. N. P. Souza, M. Obermann, H. Pohl, C. J. Schankin, H. W. Schytz, A. Sinclair, G. G. Schoonman, and E. S. Kristoffersen. 2021. Delayed headache after COVID-19 vaccination: A red flag for vaccine induced cerebral venous thrombosis. *Journal of Headache and Pain* 22(1):108. https://doi.org/10.1186/s10194-021-01324-5.

García-Grimshaw, M., J. A. Galnares-Olalde, O. Y. Bello-Chavolla, A. Michel-Chávez, A. Cadena-Fernández, M. E. Briseño-Godínez, N. E. Antonio-Villa, I. Núñez, A. Gutiérrez-Romero, L. Hernández-Vanegas, M. Del Mar Saniger-Alba, R. Carrillo-Mezo, S. E. Ceballos-Liceaga, G. Carbajal-Sandoval, F. D. Flores-Silva, J. L. Díaz-Ortega, R. Cortes-Alcalá, J. R. Pérez-Padilla, H. López-Gatell, E. Chiquete, G. Reyes-Terán, A. Arauz, and S. I. Valdés-Ferrer. 2022. Incidence of Guillain-Barré syndrome following SARS-CoV-2 immunization: Analysis of a nationwide registry of recipients of 81 million doses of seven vaccines. *European Journal of Neurology* 29(11):3368–3379. https://doi.org/10.1111/ene.15504.

Göbel, C. H., A. Heinze, S. Karstedt, M. Morscheck, L. Tashiro, A. Cirkel, Q. Hamid, R. Halwani, M. H. Temsah, M. Ziemann, S. Görg, T. Münte, and H. Göbel. 2021a. Clinical characteristics of headache after vaccination against COVID-19 (coronavirus SARS-CoV-2) with the BNT162b2 mRNA vaccine: A multicentre observational cohort study. *Brain Communications* 3(3):fcab169. https://doi.org/10.1093/braincomms/fcab169.

Göbel, C. H., A. Heinze, S. Karstedt, M. Morscheck, L. Tashiro, A. Cirkel, Q. Hamid, R. Halwani, M. H. Temsah, M. Ziemann, S. Görg, T. Münte, and H. Göbel. 2021b. Headache attributed to vaccination against COVID-19 (coronavirus SARS-CoV-2) with the ChAdOx1 NCOV-19 (AZD1222) vaccine: A multicenter observational cohort study. *Pain Therapy* 10(2):1309–1330. https://doi.org/10.1007/s40122-021-00296-3.

Goodman, B. P., J. A. Khoury, J. E. Blair, and M. F. Grill. 2021. COVID-19 dysautonomia. *Frontiers in Neurology* 12:624968. https://doi.org/10.3389/fneur.2021.624968.

Gradin, K., J. Hedner, T. Hedner, A. C. Towle, A. Pettersson, and B. Persson. 1987. Effects of chronic salt loading on plasma atrial natriuretic peptide (ANP) in the spontaneously hypertensive rat. *Acta Physiologica Scandinavica* 129(1):67–72. https://doi.org/10.1111/j.1748-1716.1987.tb08041.x.

Ha, J., S. Park, H. Kang, T. Kyung, N. Kim, D. K. Kim, H. Kim, K. Bae, M. C. Song, K. J. Lee, E. Lee, B. S. Hwang, J. Youn, J. M. Seok, and K. Park. 2023. Real-world data on the incidence and risk of Guillain-Barré syndrome following SARS-CoV-2 vaccination: A prospective surveillance study. *Scientific Reports* 13(1):3773. https://doi.org/10.1038/s41598-023-30940-1.

Hafsteinsdottir, B., and E. Olafsson. 2016. Incidence and natural history of idiopathic chronic inflammatory demyelinating polyneuropathy: A population-based study in Iceland. *European Neurology* 75(5–6):263–268. https://doiorg/10.1159/000445884.

Hanson, K. E., K. Goddard, N. Lewis, B. Fireman, T. R. Myers, N. Bakshi, E. Weintraub, J. G. Donahue, J. C. Nelson, S. Xu, J. M. Glanz, J. T. B. Williams, J. D. Alpern, and N. P. Klein. 2022. Incidence of Guillain-Barré syndrome after COVID-19 vaccination in the Vaccine Safety Datalink. *JAMA Network Open* 5(4):e228879. https://doi.org/10.1001/jamanetworkopen.2022.8879.

Heath, P. T., E. P. Galiza, D. N. Baxter, M. Boffito, D. Browne, F. Burns, D. R. Chadwick, R. Clark, C. Cosgrove, J. Galloway, A. L. Goodman, A. Heer, A. Higham, S. Iyengar, A. Jamal, C. Jeanes, P. A. Kalra, C. Kyriakidou, D. F. McAuley, A. Meyrick, A. M. Minassian, J. Minton, P. Moore, I. Munsoor, H. Nicholls, O. Osanlou, J. Packham, C. H. Pretswell, A. San Francisco Ramos, D. Saralaya, R. P. Sheridan, R. Smith, R. L. Soiza, P. A. Swift, E. C. Thomson, J. Turner, M. E. Viljoen, G. Albert, I. Cho, F. Dubovsky, G. Glenn, J. Rivers, A. Robertson, K. Smith, and S. Toback. 2021. Safety and efficacy of NVX-CoV2373 COVID-19 vaccine. *New England Journal of Medicine* 385(13):1172–1183. https://doi.org/10.1056/NEJMoa2107659.

Hemsath, J. R., A. M. Liaci, J. D. Rubin, B. J. Parrett, S. C. Lu, T. V. Nguyen, M. A. Turner, C. Y. Chen, K. Cupelli, V. S. Reddy, T. Stehle, M. K. Liszewski, J. P. Atkinson, and M. A. Barry. 2022. Ex vivo and in vivo CD46 receptor utilization by Species D human adenovirus serotype 26 (HADV26). *Journal of Virology* 96(3):e0082621. https://doi.org/10.1128/JVI.00826-21.

Hwang, I., T. B. Calvit, B. D. Cash, and K. C. Holtzmuller. 2004. Bell's palsy: A rare complication of interferon therapy for hepatitis C. *Digestive Diseases and Sciences* 49(4):619–620. https://doi.org/10.1023/b:ddas.0000026389.56819.0c.

International Headache Society. 2018. Headache classification committee of the International Headache Society (IHS): The International Classification of Headache Disorders, 3rd edition. *Cephalalgia* 38(1):1–211. https://doi.org/10.1177/0333102417738202.

Jacobs, B. C., M. P. Hazenberg, P. A. van Doorn, H. P. Endtz, and F. G. van der Meché. 1997. Cross-reactive antibodies against gangliosides and *Campylobacter jejuni* lipopolysaccharides in patients with Guillain-Barré or Miller Fisher syndrome. *Journal of Infectious Diseases* 175(3):729–733. https://doi.org/10.1093/infdis/175.3.729.

Jain, S., A. Khormi, S. R. Sangle, and D. P. D'Cruz. 2023. Transverse myelitis associated with systemic lupus erythematosus (SLE-TM): A review article. *Lupus* 32(9):1033–1042. https://doi.org/10.1177/09612033231185612.

Jensen, R., and L. J. Stovner. 2008. Epidemiology and comorbidity of headache. *Lancet Neurology* 7(4):354–361. https://doi.org/10.1016/s1474-4422(08)70062-0.

Kadkhoda, K. 2022. Post-adenoviral-based vaccines Guillain-Barré syndrome: A proposed mechanism. *Medical Hypotheses* 160:110792. https://doi.org/10.1016/j.mehy.2022.110792.

Kaplin, A. I., D. M. Deshpande, E. Scott, C. Krishnan, J. S. Carmen, I. Shats, T. Martinez, J. Drummond, S. Dike, M. Pletnikov, S. C. Keswani, T. H. Moran, C. A. Pardo, P. A. Calabresi, and D. A. Kerr. 2005. IL-6 induces regionally selective spinal cord injury in patients with the neuroinflammatory disorder transverse myelitis. *Journal of Clinical Investigation* 115(10):2731–2741. https://doi.org/10.1172/JCI25141.

Keddie, S., J. Pakpoor, C. Mousele, M. Pipis, P. M. Machado, M. Foster, C. J. Record, R. Y. S. Keh, J. Fehmi, R. W. Paterson, V. Bharambe, L. M. Clayton, C. Allen, O. Price, J. Wall, A. Kiss-Csenki, D. P. Rathnasabapathi, R. Geraldes, T. Yermakova, J. King-Robson, M. Zosmer, S. Rajakulendran, S. Sumaria, S. F. Farmer, R. Nortley, C. R. Marshall, E. J. Newman, N. Nirmalananthan, G. Kumar, A. A. Pinto, J. Holt, T. M. Lavin, K. M. Brennan, M. S. Zandi, D. L. Jayaseelan, J. Pritchard, R. D. M. Hadden, H. Manji, H. J. Willison, S. Rinaldi, A. S. Carr, and M. P. Lunn. 2021. Epidemiological and cohort study finds no association between COVID-19 and Guillain-Barré syndrome. *Brain* 144(2):682–693. https://doi.org/10.1093/brain/awaa433.

Keh, R. Y. S., S. Scanlon, P. Datta-Nemdharry, K. Donegan, S. Cavanagh, M. Foster, D. Skelland, J. Palmer, P. M. Machado, S. Keddie, A. S. Carr, M. P. Lunn, and BPNS/ABN COVID-19 Study Group. 2023. COVID-19 vaccination and Guillain-Barré syndrome: Analyses using the National Immunoglobulin Database. *Brain* 146(2):739–748. https://doi.org/10.1093/brain/awac067.

Kharraziha, I., J. Axelsson, F. Ricci, G. Di Martino, M. Persson, R. Sutton, A. Fedorowski, and V. Hamrefors. 2020. Serum activity against G protein–coupled receptors and severity of orthostatic symptoms in postural orthostatic tachycardia syndrome. *Journal of the American Heart Association* 9(15):e015989. https://doi.org/10.1161/jaha.120.015989.

Kim, M. H., and S. Y. Park. 2021. Population-based study and a scoping review for the epidemiology and seasonality in and effect of weather on Bell's palsy. *Scientific Reports* 11(1):16941. https://doi.org/10.1038/s41598-021-96422-4.

Klein, N. P., N. Lewis, K. Goddard, B. Fireman, O. Zerbo, K. E. Hanson, J. G. Donahue, E. O. Kharbanda, A. Naleway, J. C. Nelson, S. Xu, W. K. Yih, J. M. Glanz, J. T. B. Williams, S. J. Hambidge, B. J. Lewin, T. T. Shimabukuro, F. DeStefano, and E. S. Weintraub. 2021. Surveillance for adverse events after COVID-19 mRNA vaccination. *JAMA* 326(14):1390–1399. https://doi.org/10.1001/jama.2021.15072.

Krishnan, C., A. I. Kaplin, D. M. Deshpande, C. A. Pardo, and D. A. Kerr. 2004. Transverse myelitis: Pathogenesis, diagnosis and treatment. *Frontiers in Bioscience* 9:1483–1499. https://doi.org/10.2741/1351.

Kwan, A. C., J. E. Ebinger, J. Wei, C. N. Le, J. R. Oft, R. Zabner, D. Teodorescu, P. G. Botting, J. Navarrette, D. Ouyang, M. Driver, B. Claggett, B. N. Weber, P. S. Chen, and S. Cheng. 2022. Apparent risks of postural orthostatic tachycardia syndrome diagnoses after COVID-19 vaccination and SARS-CoV-2 infection. *Nature Cardiovascular Research* 1(12):1187–1194. https://doi.org/10.1038/s44161-022-00177-8.

Laughlin, R., P. Dyck, L. R. Melton, C. Leibson, J. Ransom, and P. Dyck. 2009. Incidence and prevalence of CIDP and the association of diabetes mellitus. *Neurology* 73(1):39–45.

Leibowitz, U. 1969. Epidemic incidence of Bell's palsy. *Brain* 92(1):109–114. https://doi.org/10.1093/brain/92.1.109.

Leonhard, S. E., A. A. van der Eijk, H. Andersen, G. Antonini, S. Arends, S. Attarian, F. A. Barroso, K. J. Bateman, M. R. Batstra, L. Benedetti, B. van den Berg, P. Van den Bergh, J. Bürmann, M. Busby, C. Casasnovas, D. R. Cornblath, A. Davidson, A. Y. Doets, P. A. van Doorn, C. Dornonville de la Cour, T. E. Feasby, J. Fehmi, T. Garcia-Sobrino, J. M. Goldstein, K. C. Gorson, V. Granit, R. D. M. Hadden, T. Harbo, H. P. Hartung, I. Hasan, J. V. Holbech, J. K. L. Holt, I. Jahan, Z. Islam, S. Karafiath, H. D. Katzberg, R. P. Kleyweg, N. Kolb, K. Kuitwaard, M. Kuwahara, S. Kusunoki, L. W. G. Luijten, S. Kuwabara, E. Lee Pan, H. C. Lehmann, M. Maas, L. Martín-Aguilar, J. A. L. Miller, Q. D. Mohammad, S. Monges, V. Nedkova-Hristova, E. Nobile-Orazio, J. Pardo, Y. Pereon, L. Querol, R. Reisin, W. Van Rijs, S. Rinaldi, R. C. Roberts, J. Roodbol, N. Shahrizaila, S. H. Sindrup, B. Stein, T. Cheng-Yin, H. Tankisi, A. P. Tio-Gillen, M. J. Sedano Tous, C. Verboon, F. H. Vermeij, L. H. Visser, R. Huizinga, H. J. Willison, and B. C. Jacobs. 2022. An international perspective on preceding infections in Guillain-Barré syndrome: The IGOS-1000 cohort. *Neurology* 99(12):e1299–e1313. https://doi.org/10.1212/wnl.0000000000200885.

Li, H., X. Yu, C. Liles, M. Khan, M. Vanderlinde-Wood, A. Galloway, C. Zillner, A. Benbrook, S. Reim, D. Collier, M. A. Hill, S. R. Raj, L. E. Okamoto, M. W. Cunningham, C. E. Aston, and D. C. Kem. 2014. Autoimmune basis for postural tachycardia syndrome. *Journal of the American Heart Association* 3(1):e000755. https://doi.org/10.1161/jaha.113.000755.

Li, X., B. Raventos, E. Roel, A. Pistillo, E. Martinez-Hernandez, A. Delmestri, C. Reyes, V. Strauss, D. Prieto-Alhambra, E. Burn, and T. Duarte-Salles. 2022. Association between COVID-19 vaccination, SARS-CoV-2 infection, and risk of immune mediated neurological events: Population-based cohort and self-controlled case series analysis. *British Medical Journal* 376:e068373. https://doi.org/10.1136/bmj-2021-068373.

Liston, S. L., and M. S. Kleid. 1989. Histopathology of Bell's palsy. *Laryngoscope* 99(1):23–26. https://doi.org/10.1288/00005537-198901000-00006.

Loo, L. K., O. Salim, D. Liang, A. Goel, S. Sumangala, A. S. Gowda, B. Davies, and Y. A. Rajabally. 2022. Acute-onset polyradiculoneuropathy after SARS-COV2 vaccine in the west and north Midlands, United Kingdom. *Muscle and Nerve* 65(2):233–237. https://doi.org/10.1002/mus.27461.

Lopez Chiriboga, S., and E. P. Flanagan. 2021. Myelitis and other autoimmune myelopathies. *Continuum (Minneap Minn)* 27(1):62–92. https://doi.org/10.1212/CON.0000000000000900.

Low, P. A., P. Sandroni, M. Joyner, and W. K. Shen. 2009. Postural tachycardia syndrome (POTS). *Journal of Cardiovascular Electrophysiology* 20(3):352–358. https://doi.org/10.1111/j.1540-8167.2008.01407.x.

Marino Gammazza, A., S. Légaré, G. Lo Bosco, A. Fucarino, F. Angileri, E. Conway de Macario, A. J. Macario, and F. Cappello. 2020. Human molecular chaperones share with SARS-CoV-2 antigenic epitopes potentially capable of eliciting autoimmunity against endothelial cells: Possible role of molecular mimicry in COVID-19. *Cell Stress and Chaperones* 25(5):737–741. https://doi.org/10.1007/s12192-020-01148-3.

Masuki, S., J. H. Eisenach, W. G. Schrage, C. P. Johnson, N. M. Dietz, B. W. Wilkins, P. Sandroni, P. A. Low, and M. J. Joyner. 2007. Reduced stroke volume during exercise in postural tachycardia syndrome. *Journal of Applied Physiology* 103(4):1128–1135. https://doi.org/10.1152/japplphysiol.00175.2007.

McCombe, P. A., J. G. McLeod, J. D. Pollard, Y. P. Guo, and T. J. Ingall. 1987. Peripheral sensorimotor and autonomic neuropathy associated with systemic lupus erythematosus. Clinical, pathological and immunological features. *Brain* 110(Pt 2):533–549. https://doi.org/10.1093/brain/110.2.533.

Miglis, M. G., T. Prieto, R. Shaik, S. Muppidi, D. I. Sinn, and S. Jaradeh. 2020. A case report of postural tachycardia syndrome after COVID-19. *Clinical Autonomic Research* 30(5):449–451. https://doi.org/10.1007/s10286-020-00727-9.

Morciano, C., S. Spila Alegiani, F. Menniti Ippoliti, V. Belleudi, G. Trifirò, G. Zanoni, A. Puccini, E. Sapigni, N. Mores, O. Leoni, G. Monaco, E. Clagnan, C. Zappetti, E. Bovo, R. Da Cas, and M. Massari. 2023. Post-marketing active surveillance of Guillan Barré syndrome following vaccination with anti-COVID-19 vaccines in persons aged ≥12 years in Italy: A multi-database self-controlled case series study. *medRxiv*:2023.2001.2017.23284585. https://doi.org/10.1101/2023.01.17.23284585.

Morsy, S. 2020. NCAM protein and SARS-CoV-2 surface proteins: In-silico hypothetical evidence for the immunopathogenesis of Guillain-Barre syndrome. *Medical Hypotheses* 145:110342. https://doi.org/10.1016/j.mehy.2020.110342.

NORD (National Organization for Rare Disorders). 2022. Bell's palsy. https://rarediseases.org/rare-diseases/bells-palsy (accessed February 20, 2024).

Oaklander, A. L., A. J. Mills, M. Kelley, L. S. Toran, B. Smith, M. C. Dalakas, and A. Nath. 2022. Peripheral neuropathy evaluations of patients with prolonged long COVID. *Neuroimmunology & Neuroinflammation* 9(3). https://doi.org/10.1212/nxi.0000000000001146.

Olshansky, B., D. Cannom, A. Fedorowski, J. Stewart, C. Gibbons, R. Sutton, W. K. Shen, J. Muldowney, T. H. Chung, S. Feigofsky, H. Nayak, H. Calkins, and D. G. Benditt. 2020. Postural orthostatic tachycardia syndrome (POTS): A critical assessment. *Progress in Cardiovascular Diseases* 63(3):263–270. https://doi.org/10.1016/j.pcad.2020.03.010.

Patone, M., L. Handunnetthi, D. Saatci, J. Pan, S. V. Katikireddi, S. Razvi, D. Hunt, X. W. Mei, S. Dixon, F. Zaccardi, K. Khunti, P. Watkinson, C. A. C. Coupland, J. Doidge, D. A. Harrison, R. Ravanan, A. Sheikh, C. Robertson, and J. Hippisley-Cox. 2021. Neurological complications after first dose of COVID-19 vaccines and SARS-CoV-2 infection. *Nature Medicine* 27(12):2144–2153. https://doi.org/10.1038/s41591-021-01556-7.

Pegat, A., A. Vogrig, C. Khouri, K. Masmoudi, T. Vial, and E. Bernard. 2022. Adenovirus COVID-19 vaccines and Guillain-Barré syndrome with facial paralysis. *Annals of Neurology* 91(1):162–163. https://doi.org/10.1002/ana.26258.

Polack, F. P., S. J. Thomas, N. Kitchin, J. Absalon, A. Gurtman, S. Lockhart, J. L. Perez, G. Pérez Marc, E. D. Moreira, C. Zerbini, R. Bailey, K. A. Swanson, S. Roychoudhury, K. Koury, P. Li, W. V. Kalina, D. Cooper, R. W. Frenck, Jr., L. L. Hammitt, Ö. Türeci, H. Nell, A. Schaefer, S. Ünal, D. B. Tresnan, S. Mather, P. R. Dormitzer, U. Şahin, K. U. Jansen, and W. C. Gruber. 2020. Safety and efficacy of the BNT162b2 mRNA COVID-19 vaccine. *New England Journal of Medicine* 383(27):2603–2615. https://doi.org/10.1056/NEJMoa2034577.

Rafati, A., Y. Pasebani, M. Jameie, Y. Yang, M. Jameie, S. Ilkhani, M. Amanollahi, D. Sakhaei, M. Rahimlou, and A. Kheradmand. 2023. Association of SARS-CoV-2 vaccination or infection with Bell palsy: A systematic review and meta-analysis. *JAMA Otolaryngology—Head & Neck Surgery* 149(6):493–504. https://doi.org/10.1001/jamaoto.2023.0160.

Raj, S. R., I. Biaggioni, P. C. Yamhure, B. K. Black, S. Y. Paranjape, D. W. Byrne, and D. Robertson. 2005. Renin-aldosterone paradox and perturbed blood volume regulation underlying postural tachycardia syndrome. *Circulation* 111(13):1574–1582. https://doi.org/10.1161/01.Cir.0000160356.97313.5d.

Rivers, T. M. 1932. Viruses. *Science* 75(1956):654–656. https://doi.org/10.1126/science.75.1956.654.

Rodriguez, B., R. Hoepner, A. Salmen, N. Kamber, and W. J. Z'Graggen. 2021. Immunomodulatory treatment in postural tachycardia syndrome: A case series. *European Journal of Neurology* 28(5):1692–1697. https://doi.org/10.1111/ene.14711.

Rzymski, P. 2023. Guillain-Barré syndrome and COVID-19 vaccines: Focus on adenoviral vectors. *Frontiers in Immunology* 14:1183258. https://doi.org/10.3389/fimmu.2023.1183258.

Sadoff, J., G. Gray, A. Vandebosch, V. Cárdenas, G. Shukarev, B. Grinsztejn, P. A. Goepfert, C. Truyers, H. Fennema, B. Spiessens, K. Offergeld, G. Scheper, K. L. Taylor, M. L. Robb, J. Treanor, D. H. Barouch, J. Stoddard, M. F. Ryser, M. A. Marovich, K. M. Neuzil, L. Corey, N. Cauwenberghs, T. Tanner, K. Hardt, J. Ruiz-Guiñazú, M. Le Gars, H. Schuitemaker, J. Van Hoof, F. Struyf, and M. Douoguih. 2021. Safety and efficacy of single-dose Ad26.COV2.S vaccine against COVID-19. *New England Journal of Medicine* 384(23):2187–2201. https://doi.org/10.1056/NEJMoa2101544.

Sandroni, P., T. L. Opfer-Gehrking, B. R. McPhee, and P. A. Low. 1999. Postural tachycardia syndrome: Clinical features and follow-up study. *Mayo Clinic Proceedings* 74(11):1106–1110. https://doi.org/10.4065/74.11.1106.

See, I., J. R. Su, A. Lale, E. J. Woo, A. Y. Guh, T. T. Shimabukuro, M. B. Streiff, A. K. Rao, A. P. Wheeler, S. F. Beavers, A. P. Durbin, K. Edwards, E. Miller, T. A. Harrington, A. Mba-Jonas, N. Nair, D. T. Nguyen, K. R. Talaat, V. C. Urrutia, S. C. Walker, C. B. Creech, T. A. Clark, F. DeStefano, and K. R. Broder. 2021. U.S. case reports of cerebral venous sinus thrombosis with thrombocytopenia after Ad26.COV2.S vaccination, March 2 to April 21, 2021. *JAMA* 325(24):2448–2456. https://doi.org/10.1001/jama.2021.7517.

Sejvar, J. J., K. S. Kohl, J. Gidudu, A. Amato, N. Bakshi, R. Baxter, D. R. Burwen, D. R. Cornblath, J. Cleerbout, K. M. Edwards, U. Heininger, R. Hughes, N. Khuri-Bulos, R. Korinthenberg, B. J. Law, U. Munro, H. C. Maltezou, P. Nell, J. Oleske, R. Sparks, P. Velentgas, P. Vermeer, and M. Wiznitzer. 2011. Guillain-Barré syndrome and Fisher syndrome: Case definitions and guidelines for collection, analysis, and presentation of immunization safety data. *Vaccine* 29(3):599–612. https://doi.org/10.1016/j.vaccine.2010.06.003.

Sekiguchi, K., N. Watanabe, N. Miyazaki, K. Ishizuchi, C. Iba, Y. Tagashira, S. Uno, M. Shibata, N. Hasegawa, R. Takemura, J. Nakahara, and T. Takizawa. 2022. Incidence of headache after COVID-19 vaccination in patients with history of headache: A cross-sectional study. *Cephalalgia* 42(3):266–272. https://doi.org/10.1177/03331024211038654.

Shahrizaila, N., H. C. Lehmann, and S. Kuwabara. 2021. Guillain-Barré syndrome. *Lancet* 397(10280):1214–1228. https://doi.org/10.1016/S0140-6736(21)00517-1.

Shasha, D., R. Bareket, F. H. Sikron, O. Gertel, J. Tsamir, D. Dvir, D. Mossinson, A. D. Heymann, and G. Zacay. 2022. Real-world safety data for the Pfizer BNT162b2 SARS-CoV-2 vaccine: Historical cohort study. *Clinical Microbiology and Infection* 28(1):130–134. https://doi.org/10.1016/j.cmi.2021.09.018.

Sheerin, D., C. Dold, D. O'Connor, A. J. Pollard, and C. S. Rollier. 2021. Distinct patterns of whole blood transcriptional responses are induced in mice following immunisation with adenoviral and poxviral vector vaccines encoding the same antigen. *BMC Genomics* 22(1):777. https://doi.org/10.1186/s12864-021-08061-8.

Sheikh, K. A., I. Nachamkin, T. W. Ho, H. J. Willison, J. Veitch, H. Ung, M. Nicholson, C. Y. Li, H. S. Wu, B. Q. Shen, D. R. Cornblath, A. K. Asbury, G. M. McKhann, and J. W. Griffin. 1998. *Campylobacter jejuni* lipopolysaccharides in Guillain-Barré syndrome: Molecular mimicry and host susceptibility. *Neurology* 51(2):371–378. https://doi.org/10.1212/wnl.51.2.371.

Shemer, A., E. Pras, A. Einan-Lifshitz, B. Dubinsky-Pertzov, and I. Hecht. 2021. Association of COVID-19 vaccination and facial nerve palsy: A case-control study. *JAMA Otolaryngology—Head & Neck Surgery* 147(8):739–743. https://doi.org/10.1001/jamaoto.2021.1259.

Shibao, C., C. Arzubiaga, L. J. Roberts, II, S. Raj, B. Black, P. Harris, and I. Biaggioni. 2005. Hyperadrenergic postural tachycardia syndrome in mast cell activation disorders. *Hypertension* 45(3):385–390. https://doi.org/10.1161/01.Hyp.0000158259.68614.40.

Shibli, R., O. Barnett, Z. Abu-Full, N. Gronich, R. Najjar-Debbiny, I. Doweck, G. Rennert, and W. Saliba. 2021. Association between vaccination with the BNT162b2 mRNA COVID-19 vaccine and Bell's palsy: A population-based study. *Lancet Regional Health—Europe* 11:100236. https://doi.org/10.1016/j.lanepe.2021.100236.

Shoaibi, A., P. C. Lloyd, H. L. Wong, T. C. Clarke, Y. Chillarige, R. Do, M. Hu, Y. Jiao, A. Kwist, A. Lindaas, K. Matuska, R. McEvoy, M. Ondari, S. Parulekar, X. Shi, J. Wang, Y. Lu, J. Obidi, C. K. Zhou, J. A. Kelman, R. A. Forshee, and S. A. Anderson. 2023. Evaluation of potential adverse events following COVID-19 mRNA vaccination among adults aged 65 years and older: Two self-controlled studies in the U.S. *Vaccine* 41(32):4666–4678. https://doi.org/10.1016/j.vaccine.2023.06.014.

Shouman, K., G. Vanichkachorn, W. P. Cheshire, M. D. Suarez, S. Shelly, G. J. Lamotte, P. Sandroni, E. E. Benarroch, S. E. Berini, J. K. Cutsforth-Gregory, E. A. Coon, M. L. Mauermann, P. A. Low, and W. Singer. 2021. Autonomic dysfunction following COVID-19 infection: An early experience. *Clinical Autonomic Research* 31(3):385–394. https://doi.org/10.1007/s10286-021-00803-8.

Silvestro, M., A. Tessitore, I. Orologio, P. Sozio, G. Napolitano, M. Siciliano, G. Tedeschi, and A. Russo. 2021. Headache worsening after COVID-19 vaccination: An online questionnaire-based study on 841 patients with migraine. *Journal of Clinical Medicine* 10(24). https://doi.org/10.3390/jcm10245914.

Steiner, I., and Y. Mattan. 1999. Bell's palsy and herpes viruses: To (acyclo)vir or not to (acyclo)vir? *Journal of the Neurological Sciences* 170(1):19–23. https://doi.org/10.1016/s0022-510x(99)00187-2.

Stewart, J. M., A. J. Ocon, D. Clarke, I. Taneja, and M. S. Medow. 2009. Defects in cutaneous angiotensin-converting enzyme 2 and angiotensin-(1-7) production in postural tachycardia syndrome. *Hypertension* 53(5):767–774. https://doi.org/10.1161/hypertensionaha.108.127357.

Stovner, L., K. Hagen, R. Jensen, Z. Katsarava, R. Lipton, A. Scher, T. Steiner, and J. A. Zwart. 2007. The global burden of headache: A documentation of headache prevalence and disability worldwide. *Cephalalgia* 27(3):193–210. https://doi.org/10.1111/j.1468-2982.2007.01288.x.

Sturkenboom, M., D. Messina, O. Paoletti, A. de Burgos-Gonzalez, R. Zabner, P. García-Poza, C. Huerta, A. Llorente García, M. Martin-Perez, M. Martinez, I. Martin, J. Overbeek, M. Padros-Goossens, P. Souverein, K. Swart, O. Klungel, and R. Gini. 2022. Cohort monitoring of 29 adverse events of special interest prior to and after COVID-19 vaccination in four large European electronic health care data sources. *medRxiv*:2022.2008.2017.22278894. https://doi.org/10.1101/2022.08.17.22278894.

Sullivan, F. M., I. R. Swan, P. T. Donnan, J. M. Morrison, B. H. Smith, B. McKinstry, R. J. Davenport, L. D. Vale, J. E. Clarkson, V. Hammersley, S. Hayavi, A. McAteer, K. Stewart, and F. Daly. 2007. Early treatment with prednisolone or acyclovir in Bell's palsy. *New England Journal of Medicine* 357(16):1598–1607. https://doi.org/10.1056/NEJMoa072006.

Suvas, S. 2017. Role of substance P neuropeptide in inflammation, wound healing, and tissue homeostasis. *Journal of Immunology* 199(5):1543–1552. https://doi.org/10.4049/jimmunol.1601751.

Takeuchi, Y., M. Iwagami, S. Ono, N. Michihata, K. Uemura, and H. Yasunaga. 2022. A post-marketing safety assessment of COVID-19 mRNA vaccination for serious adverse outcomes using administrative claims data linked with vaccination registry in a city of Japan. *Vaccine* 40(52):7622–7630. https://doi.org/10.1016/j.vaccine.2022.10.088.

Takuva, S., A. Takalani, I. Seocharan, N. Yende-Zuma, T. Reddy, I. Engelbrecht, M. Faesen, K. Khuto, C. Whyte, V. Bailey, V. Trivella, J. Peter, J. Opie, V. Louw, P. Rowji, B. Jacobson, P. Groenewald, R. E. Dorrington, R. Laubscher, D. Bradshaw, H. Moultrie, L. Fairall, I. Sanne, L. Gail-Bekker, G. Gray, A. Goga, and N. Garrett. 2022. Safety evaluation of the single-dose Ad26.COV2.S vaccine among healthcare workers in the Sisonke study in South Africa: A phase 3b implementation trial. *PLoS Medicine* 19(6):e1004024. https://doi.org/10.1371/journal.pmed.1004024.

Thieben, M. J., P. Sandroni, D. M. Sletten, L. M. Benrud-Larson, R. D. Fealey, S. Vernino, V. A. Lennon, W. K. Shen, and P. A. Low. 2007. Postural orthostatic tachycardia syndrome: The Mayo Clinic experience. *Mayo Clinic Proceedings* 82(3):308–313. https://doi.org/10.4065/82.3.308.

Thomas, P. K., R. W. Walker, P. Rudge, J. A. Morgan-Hughes, R. H. King, J. M. Jacobs, K. R. Mills, I. E. Ormerod, N. M. Murray, and W. I. McDonald. 1987. Chronic demyelinating peripheral neuropathy associated with multifocal central nervous system demyelination. *Brain* 110(Pt 1):53–76. https://doi.org/10.1093/brain/110.1.53.

Togha, M., S. M. Hashemi, N. Yamani, F. Martami, and Z. Salami. 2022. A review on headaches due to COVID-19 infection. *Frontiers in Neurology* 13:942956. https://doi.org/10.3389/fneur.2022.942956.

Transverse Myelitis Consortium Working Group. 2002. Proposed diagnostic criteria and nosology of acute transverse myelitis. *Neurology* 59(4):499–505. https://doi.org/10.1212/wnl.59.4.499.

Van den Bergh, P. Y., R. D. Hadden, P. Bouche, D. R. Cornblath, A. Hahn, I. Illa, C. L. Koski, J. M. Léger, E. Nobile-Orazio, and J. Pollard. 2010. European Federation of Neurological Societies/Peripheral Nerve Society guideline on management of chronic inflammatory demyelinating polyradiculoneuropathy: Report of a joint task force of the European Federation of Neurological Societies and the Peripheral Nerve Society—first revision. *European Journal of Neurology* 17(3):356–363.

Van den Bergh, P. Y. K., P. A. van Doorn, R. D. M. Hadden, B. Avau, P. Vankrunkelsven, J. A. Allen, S. Attarian, P. H. Blomkwist-Markens, D. R. Cornblath, F. Eftimov, H. S. Goedee, T. Harbo, S. Kuwabara, R. A. Lewis, M. P. Lunn, E. Nobile-Orazio, L. Querol, Y. A. Rajabally, C. Sommer, and H. A. Topaloglu. 2021. European Academy of Neurology/Peripheral Nerve Society guideline on diagnosis and treatment of chronic inflammatory demyelinating polyradiculoneuropathy: Report of a joint task force—second revision. *Journal of the Peripheral Nervous System* 26(3):242–268. https://doi.org/10.1111/jns.12455.

Vellozzi, C., S. Iqbal, and K. Broder. 2014. Guillain-Barré syndrome, influenza, and influenza vaccination: The epidemiologic evidence. *Clinical Infectious Diseases* 58(8):1149–1155. https://doi.org/10.1093/cid/ciu005.

Vernino, S., K. M. Bourne, L. E. Stiles, B. P. Grubb, A. Fedorowski, J. M. Stewart, A. C. Arnold, L. A. Pace, J. Axelsson, J. R. Boris, J. P. Moak, B. P. Goodman, K. R. Chémali, T. H. Chung, D. S. Goldstein, A. Diedrich, M. G. Miglis, M. M. Cortez, A. J. Miller, R. Freeman, I. Biaggioni, P. C. Rowe, R. S. Sheldon, C. A. Shibao, D. M. Systrom, G. A. Cook, T. A. Doherty, H. I. Abdallah, A. Darbari, and S. R. Raj. 2021. Postural orthostatic tachycardia syndrome (POTS): State of the science and clinical care from a 2019 National Institutes of Health expert consensus meeting—part 1. *Autonomic Neuroscience* 235:102828. https://doi.org/10.1016/j.autneu.2021.102828.

Vernino, S., S. Hopkins, M. Bryarly, R. Hernandez, and A. Salter. 2023. Randomized controlled trial of intravenous immunoglobulin for autoimmune postural tachycardia syndrome (ISTAND). *Clinical Autonomic Research* 34(1):153–163.

Walker, J. L., A. Schultze, J. Tazare, A. Tamborska, B. Singh, K. Donegan, J. Stowe, C. E. Morton, W. J. Hulme, H. J. Curtis, E. J. Williamson, A. Mehrkar, R. M. Eggo, C. T. Rentsch, R. Mathur, S. Bacon, A. J. Walker, S. Davy, D. Evans, P. Inglesby, G. Hickman, B. MacKenna, L. Tomlinson, A. Ca Green, L. Fisher, J. Cockburn, J. Parry, F. Hester, S. Harper, C. Bates, S. J. Evans, T. Solomon, N. J. Andrews, I. J. Douglas, B. Goldacre, L. Smeeth, and H. I. McDonald. 2022. Safety of COVID-19 vaccination and acute neurological events: A self-controlled case series in England using the OpenSafely platform. *Vaccine* 40(32):4479–4487. https://doi.org/10.1016/j.vaccine.2022.06.010.

Wanschitz, J., H. Maier, H. Lassmann, H. Budka, and T. Berger. 2003. Distinct time pattern of complement activation and cytotoxic T cell response in Guillain-Barré syndrome. *Brain* 126(Pt 9):2034–2042. https://doi.org/10.1093/brain/awg207.

Weinstock, L. B., J. B. Brook, T. L. Myers, and B. Goodman. 2018. Successful treatment of postural orthostatic tachycardia and mast cell activation syndromes using naltrexone, immunoglobulin and antibiotic treatment. *BMJ Case Reports*. https://doi.org/10.1136/bcr-2017-221405.

Wratten, S. J., D. J. Faulkner, K. Hirotsu, and J. Clardy. 1977. Trimethylenemethane. A reversible, temperature dependent transformation from higher to lower symmetry as observed by electron spin resonance spectroscopy. *Journal of the American Chemical Society* 99(8):2824–2825. https://doi.org/10.1021/ja00450a083.

Yılmaz, M., M. Tarakcioglu, N. Bayazit, Y. A. Bayazit, M. Namiduru, and M. Kanlikama. 2002. Serum cytokine levels in Bell's palsy. *Journal of the Neurological Sciences* 197(1–2):69–72. https://doi.org/10.1016/s0022-510x(02)00049-7.

Yuki, N., T. Taki, F. Inagaki, T. Kasama, M. Takahashi, K. Saito, S. Handa, and T. Miyatake. 1993. A bacterium lipopolysaccharide that elicits Guillain-Barré syndrome has a GM1 ganglioside-like structure. *Journal of Experimental Medicine* 178(5):1771–1775. https://doi.org/10.1084/jem.178.5.1771.

Yuki, N., K. Susuki, M. Koga, Y. Nishimoto, M. Odaka, K. Hirata, K. Taguchi, T. Miyatake, K. Furukawa, T. Kobata, and M. Yamada. 2004. Carbohydrate mimicry between human ganglioside GM1 and *Campylobacter jejuni* lipooligosaccharide causes Guillain-Barré syndrome. *Proceedings of the National Academy of Sciences of the United States of America* 101(31):11404–11409. https://doi.org/10.1073/pnas.0402391101.

Zalewski, N. L., A. A. Rabinstein, K. N. Krecke, R. D. Brown, Jr., E. F. M. Wijdicks, B. G. Weinshenker, T. J. Kaufmann, J. M. Morris, A. J. Aksamit, J. D. Bartleson, G. Lanzino, M. M. Blessing, and E. P. Flanagan. 2019. Characteristics of spontaneous spinal cord infarction and proposed diagnostic criteria. *JAMA Neurology* 76(1):56–63. https://doi.org/10.1001/jamaneurol.2018.2734.

Zhang, W., L. Xu, T. Luo, F. Wu, B. Zhao, and X. Li. 2020. The etiology of Bell's palsy: A review. *Journal of Neurology* 267(7):1896–1905. https://doi.org/10.1007/s00415-019-09282-4.

Zussy, C., F. Loustalot, F. Junyent, F. Gardoni, C. Bories, J. Valero, M. G. Desarmenien, F. Bernex, D. Henaff, N. Bayo-Puxan, J. W. Chen, N. Lonjon, Y. de Koninck, J. O. Malva, J. M. Bergelson, M. di Luca, G. Schiavo, S. Salinas, and E. J. Kremer. 2016. Coxsackievirus adenovirus receptor loss impairs adult neurogenesis, synapse content, and hippocampus plasticity. *Journal of Neuroscience* 36(37):9558–9571. https://doi.org/10.1523/JNEUROSCI.0132-16.2016.

# 4

# Sensorineural Hearing Loss, Tinnitus, and COVID-19 Vaccines

This chapter describes the potential relationship between COVID-19 vaccines and sudden sensorineural hearing loss (SSNHL) and tinnitus (see Boxes 4-1 and 4-2 for all conclusions in this chapter).

## SENSORINEURAL HEARING LOSS

---

**BOX 4-1**
**Conclusions for Sensorineural Hearing Loss**

**Conclusion 4-1: The evidence is inadequate to accept or reject a causal relationship between the BNT162b2 vaccine and sensorineural hearing loss.**

**Conclusion 4-2: The evidence is inadequate to accept or reject a causal relationship between the mRNA-1273 vaccine and sensorineural hearing loss.**

**Conclusion 4-3: The evidence is inadequate to accept or reject a causal relationship between the Ad26.COV2.S vaccine and sensorineural hearing loss.**

**Conclusion 4-4: The evidence is inadequate to accept or reject a causal relationship between the NVX-CoV2373 vaccine and sensorineural hearing loss.**

---

### Background

The whole auditory system is how humans access and make sense of environmental sounds. It is a multistage system characterized by encoding of environmental auditory stimuli by peripheral structures and decoding of the stimuli by central structures in the brainstem and cerebral cortex (Pickles, 2013). Peripherally, auditory energy is funneled into the pinna toward the tympanic membrane (eardrum), where it is converted to mechanical energy and moves along the ossicles in the middle ear to the cochlea, which contains the organ of Corti, which acts to encode auditory signals as neuroelectric signals (e.g., action potentials) that are transmitted to the temporal lobe via the eighth nerve and brainstem for decoding and processing (Pickles, 2013).

Damage can occur at any step in this process, resulting in different types of hearing loss. Conductive hearing loss is characterized by an inability for the outer and middle ear to transmit signals to the inner ear (e.g., rupture in the tympanic membrane, fluid in the middle ear) and is often transient (e.g., fluid drains from the ear) or can be addressed via medical or surgical interventions (Lee, 2013; Pickles, 2013). Sensorineural hearing loss is distinguished by disruption in encoding auditory information in the cochlea or along the eighth nerve and is usually permanent. Central hearing loss or auditory processing disorders (Martin and Jerger, 2005; Task Force on Central Auditory Processing Consensus Development, 1996), although more poorly understood and considered rare, especially among adults, occur when sound is encoded normally in the peripheral ear (e.g., no sign of sensorineural or conductive loss but deficits in the neural processing of auditory information mean that individuals struggle with understanding it despite functioning peripheral hearing [Katz et al., 2015]).

Audiologists and otolaryngologists diagnose hearing loss using a comprehensive assessment battery, including various measures assessing different processes of the auditory system (Katz et al., 2015). The criterion standard for peripheral hearing is pure-tone audiometry, which identifies the softest volume at which tones at different frequencies can be detected. A combination of methods of presenting the tone via air conduction (e.g., traditional headphones that stimulate the entire outer, middle, and inner ears) and bone conduction (e.g., oscillator that directly stimulates the cochlea) distinguish different types of hearing loss (Katz et al., 2015).

Self-reported hearing has relatively poor agreement with the criterion standard, with sensitivity and specificity reported as 41–65 percent and 81–88 percent among U.S. adults over 20 years old, respectively (Agrawal et al., 2008). Moreover, accuracy and the direction of misclassification (e.g., directional difference between self-report and criterion-measured degree of hearing loss) differ by key demographic variables, including age, race, and sex; older White men are more likely to underestimate their level of hearing loss relative to younger Black women (Kamil et al., 2015). The relatively poor accuracy of self-reported hearing can be attributed to the insidious onset of age-related hearing loss masking the change, perceived normalcy for a given age group, stigma, or projection (believing that others are mumbling or speaking poorly). Moreover, understanding speech requires both an auditory (e.g., accessing sound) and cognitive (e.g., making sense of the information) component, and listening with hearing loss can contribute to fatigue from cognitive load placed on the brain when decoding poor peripheral signals (Hornsby et al., 2016; Wingfield et al., 2005). Some may misattribute hearing loss to cognitive processes and vice versa when considering their own hearing levels.

Although the procedures are standardized, the actual clinical cut points vary by professional organizations and are at the discretion of the provider. Population estimates vary by the definition and whether hearing loss estimates are limited to bilateral or unilateral (estimates increase when including unilateral loss) (Lin et al., 2011). Using the commonly cited World Health Organization (WHO) cutoffs from before 2021, estimates suggest that 23 percent of U.S. individuals over age 12 have bilateral hearing loss and that prevalence increases with age, from less than 1 percent at 20–29 years to more than 80 percent over 80 years (Goman and Lin, 2016). WHO suggests approximately 20 percent of the global population has hearing loss (WHO, 2024). Among the types of hearing loss, specific reliable national estimates are not reported. Permanent conductive hearing loss is relatively rare (Cruickshanks et al., 1998), and sensorineural hearing loss is the overwhelmingly most common permanent form, with the majority of cases being attributed to age (Reed et al., 2023; Yamasoba et al., 2013). However, estimates vary by definition of hearing loss and global region and are limited due to the often-transient nature of conductive hearing loss, relatively low uptake of hearing assessment within health systems, and lack of feasibility for comprehensive hearing assessment in epidemiological studies (Chadha et al., 2021; Katz et al., 2015; Powell et al., 2021).

Known individual risk factors for sensorineural hearing loss include congenital and progressive genetic conditions, excessive noise, certain medications and chemicals, health behaviors (e.g., smoking), chronic cardiovascular conditions, viral infections, and age-related cellular degeneration (Agrawal et al., 2008; Eggermont, 2017; Van Eyken et al., 2007). The majority of adult hearing loss is often labeled as "age-related" and attributed to a combination of exposures that insidiously degrades hearing acuity such that changes are so subtle they often go unnoticed until they are more pronounced (Lin et al., 2011; Yamasoba et al., 2013).

SSNHL is characterized as an acute change (e.g., within a 72-hour period). The specific mechanisms are poorly characterized as several risk factors and potential causes have been reported including infection, trauma, autoimmune disease, certain medications (e.g., aminoglycosides), and certain disorders of the inner ear (e.g., Meniere's) (Kuhn et al., 2011; Schreiber et al., 2010; Stachler et al., 2012). It is relatively rare (approximately 5–20 of 100,000 people yearly), but estimates are mostly reliant on high-income countries (Stachler et al., 2012). Estimates suggest that approximately 40–60 percent of cases will recover to normal levels in a few weeks of follow-up (Kuhn et al., 2011; Mattox and Simmons, 1977; Wilson et al., 1980). However, the incidence and recovery rate are not well documented in low- and middle-income countries. Moreover, there is variation in the literature of the different definitions for risk-windows and specific change in audiometric thresholds.

## Mechanisms

The mechanistic evidence for a biologically plausible association between hearing loss and COVID-19 vaccination is limited; a paucity of work offers direct evidence. Similarly, there is little mechanistic evidence whether COVID-19 infection causes hearing loss. Much of the relevant literature is theoretical or postulated based on adjacent research. Moreover, no literature offers substantive discussion of the potential for increased risk of an association by comorbid conditions, genetic predisposition, concurrent pharmacologic agent, or environmental exposures.

The initial consideration is the possible direct viral involvement of the inner ear or the vestibulocochlear nerve (Kaliyappan et al., 2022). The inflammatory response, possibly cochleitis or neuritis, could be an effect of the immune activation by the vaccine. The hyperproduction of proinflammatory cytokines in response to the vaccine could inadvertently affect the audio vestibular system, leading to symptoms such as vertigo, tinnitus, and hearing loss. Such a hyperinflammatory state is known to cause tissue damage and could be particularly detrimental to the sensitive structures of the ear (Kamogashira et al., 2022). Specifically, the response to BNT162b2[1] provides a hypothetical framework. Studies demonstrate that this vaccine elicits a strong immune response, characterized by high levels of neutralizing antibodies and robust T cell responses, including antigen-specific CD8+ and Th1-type CD4+ T cells (Sadarangani et al., 2021). Although this is crucial for protective immunity, it also raises the potential for unintended auditory effects. The inflammatory environment can indirectly inflict damage on the intricate anatomy of the ear, affecting or occluding small areas within it. The vigorous immune response, especially the aspects involving cell-mediated immunity and cytokine production, could inadvertently affect the ear through either direct inflammatory damage or secondary effects, such as vascular complications.

Others have postulated about molecular mimicry and immunological considerations, such as an autoimmune-like response, where antibodies or T cells, activated by the vaccine, might erroneously recognize inner ear antigens as viral epitopes and trigger an immune attack (Ahmed et al., 2022). Given the specificity and sensitivity of the immune response, particularly the adaptive immunity involving antigen-specific T cell and B cell responses, this cross-reactivity could be a plausible mechanism for vaccine-induced auditory damage.

Last, the unique anatomical and physiological characteristics of the cochlea and semicircular canals, notably their isolated blood supply, make them particularly vulnerable to ischemic events (Tabuchi et al., 2010). Vaccine-induced alterations in the cardiovascular system, either directly or through an immune-mediated pathway, could lead to thrombosis or hypoxia in these areas, resulting in auditory dysfunction.

## Epidemiological Evidence

Clinical trial results submitted to the Food and Drug Administration (FDA) for Emergency Use Authorization and/or full approval do not indicate a signal regarding sensorineural hearing loss and any of the vaccines under study (FDA, 2021, 2023a,b,c). Table 4-1 presents five studies that contributed to the causality assessment.

Nieminen et al. (2023) compared the incidence rate (IR) of SSNHL in the 30-day window preceding vaccination and 0–54 days and more than 54 days after vaccination to that between January 1, 2019, and March 1, 2020, using a national Finnish electronic health database (*n* = 5.5 million people), excluding those with pre-existing

---

[1] The COVID-19 vaccine manufactured by Pfizer-BioNTech under the name Comirnaty®.

**TABLE 4-1** Epidemiological Studies in the Sensorineural Hearing Loss Evidence Review

| Author | Study Design and Control Group | Location | Data Source | Vaccine(S) | Age Range | N | Number of Events | Results (95% CI) |
|---|---|---|---|---|---|---|---|---|
| Formeister et al. (2022) | Surveillance; single arm | USA | VAERS | BNT162b2 | 15–93 years | 185.4 million doses | 305 | All vaccines: IR 0.6 (probable; minimum estimate) and 28.0 (maximum estimate) cases of SSNHL per 100,000 people per year |
| | | | | mRNA-1273 | | | 222 | |
| | | | | Ad26.COV2.S | | | 28 | |
| Frontera et al. (2022) | Surveillance; single arm | USA | VAERS | BNT162b2 | ≥12 years | 167.0 million doses | Not reported | 3.20 per 1 million doses |
| | | | | mRNA-1273 | | 128.1 million doses | | 3.08 per 1 million doses |
| | | | | Ad26.COV2.S | | 11.6 million doses | | 6.29 per 1 million doses |
| Leong et al. (2023) | Clinical convenience sample; single arm | New York, NY, USA | Otology clinic at an academic center | BNT162b2 | 16–101 years | 244 vaccinees | 10 | 1.7% of all vaccinated individuals had adjudicated new hearing loss |
| | | | | mRNA-1273 | | 123 vaccinees | 9 | |
| | | | | Ad26.COV2.S | | 16 vaccinees | 1 | |
| Nieminen et al. (2023) | Population-based cohort; pre and post | Finland | Finnish Population Information System | BNT162b2 | 0 to ≥80 years | 5.5 million individuals (total cohort) | Dose 1: 111 Dose 2: 104 | IRR 0.8 (0.6–1.0) IRR 0.8 (0.6–1.2) |
| | | | | mRNA-1273 | | | Dose 1: 15 Dose 2: 20 | IRR 0.8 (0.5–1.4) IRR 1.2 (0.7–1.9) |
| Yanir et al. (2022) | Population-based cohort; pre and post | Israel | Clalit Health Services | BNT162b2 | 16 to ≥65 years | Dose 1: 2.6 million vaccinees | 91 | SIR 1.35 (1.09–1.65) |
| | | | | | | Dose 2: 2.4 million vaccinees | 79 | SIR 1.23 (0.98–1.53) |

NOTES: BNT162b2 refers to the COVID-19 vaccine manufactured by Pfizer-BioNTech under the name Comirnaty®. mRNA-1273 refers to the COVID-19 vaccine manufactured by Moderna under the name Spikevax®. Ad26.COV2.S refers to the COVID-19 vaccine manufactured by Janssen. The three approved COVID-19 vaccines in the United Kingdom are BNT162b2, mRNA-1273, and ChAdOx1-S. Number of events refers to events in vaccinees only. CI: confidence interval; IR: incidence rate; IRR: incidence rate ratio; SIR: standardized incidence ratio; VAERS: Vaccine Adverse Event Reporting System.
SOURCES: Formeister et al., 2022; Frontera et al., 2022; Leong et al., 2023; Nieminen et al., 2023; Yanir et al., 2022.

recent diagnosis of SSNHL from the period immediately before the study (2015–2018). Finland's national vaccination register provided the vaccination dates and product names. SSNHL was identified using an International Classification of Diseases (ICD-10) diagnostic code for specialized care visits and from hospital wards. Comorbid conditions were identified from multiple sources. Models were adjusted for calendar time, coronavirus-2 (SARS-CoV-2) infection, demographic, cardiovascular, chronic comorbidities, and health care use covariates. Relative to the incidence before March 2020, adjusted models suggest no increased risk in the initial 0–54-day risk period after the first dose or second dose with BNT162b2 (Dose 1: IR 0.8, 95% confidence interval [CI]: 0.6–1.0; Dose 2: incidence rate ratio [IRR] 0.8, 95% CI: 0.6–1.2), or mRNA-1273[2] (Dose 1: IR 0.8, 95% CI: 0.5–1.4; Dose 2: IRR 1.2, 95% CI: 0.7–1.9). Secondary models examining risk after 54 days post-vaccination and after a third dose likewise yielded no associations.

Yanir et al. (2022) used the Clalit Health Services database in Israel to estimate the incidence of SSNHL after first and second doses of BNT162b2 from December 20, 2020, to April 30, 2021. Subsequent analysis compared estimates to the incidence of SSNHL from the same database in 2018 and 2019 and developed age- and sex-standardized incidence ratios. SSNHL was identified using a broad array of ICD-9 codes for hearing loss (388.2, 389.1, 389.10–389.13, 389.15–389.18, 389.8, and 389.9) and concurrent prednisone use within 30 days of diagnosis. The authors reported that 2.6 million people (mean standard deviation age, 46.8 [19.6] years; 51.5 percent female) received the first dose, with 91 cases of SSNHL reported. Of these, 2.4 million (93.8 percent) received the second dose, with 79 cases of SSNHL reported. The age- and sex-weighted standardized incidence ratios were 1.35 (95% CI: 1.09–1.65) after the first dose and 1.23 (95% CI: 0.98–1.53) after the second dose when using 2018 data as a reference (the sensitivity analysis was similar when using 2019 data).

Leong et al. (2023) leveraged a clinical convenience sample from an otology clinic (New York City, New York) (rather than prospective outreach) from May to July 2021 to characterize the incidence of hearing loss after COVID-19 vaccination. Among 500 individuals who completed screening (median age 56.6 years; 59.4 percent female), 420 reported being vaccinated (58.4 percent BNT162b2, 29.1 percent mRNA-1273, 3.3 percent Ad26.COV2.S); 21 (5 percent) reported hearing loss within 4 weeks of vaccination. However, after comprehensive audiologic and otologic evaluation, only seven cases (1.7 percent of vaccinated individuals) were deemed to be SSNHL; the rest represented new or exacerbated symptoms of known pathologies of hearing loss that did not represent SSNHL definition or were unrelated to vaccination. The study did not compare vaccinated to unvaccinated individuals. Despite concerns with selection bias, recall bias, and confounding, a key finding from this paper was that self-reported declines in hearing after vaccination may be unreliable, as a majority of cases were attributable to other etiologies. Inaccurate reporting of tinnitus may lead to overestimation of observed associations.

Two included studies used data from the U.S. Vaccine Adverse Event Reporting System (VAERS). For denominators, each of these studies utilized publicly available data from the Centers for Disease Control and Prevention on the total number of individuals vaccinated with COVID-19 vaccines and the total number of doses administered in the United States during the time frames of interest. As part of a larger analysis of neurologic events after COVID-19 vaccination, Frontera et al. (2022) reported an IR of 3.26 cases of hearing loss identified by free text or automated coding per 1,000,000 vaccines (IR per 1,000,000 by vaccine type: 3.20 BNT162b2, 3.08 mRNA-1273, 6.29 Ad26.COV2.S) between January 1, 2021, and June 14, 2021 (306.9 million COVID-19 vaccine doses; 314,610 total adverse events). The number of hearing loss events is not specifically reported (Frontera et al., 2022). Formeister et al. (2022) described the incidence rate of SSNHL in the initial 7-month period of the U.S. vaccination campaign (December 14, 2020, to July 16, 2021). The authors identified 2,170 reports of hearing loss after vaccination in VAERS (search terms: *sudden hearing loss*, *deafness*, *deafness neurosensory*, *deafness unilateral*, *deafness bilateral*, and *hypoacusis*). Of those, the authors deemed 555 events as credible because they occurred within 21 days of vaccination and had one of the following: reference to an audiologic assessment; evaluation by an otolaryngologist, audiologist, or other physician resulting in diagnosis of SSNHL; or evaluation by an otolaryngologist resulting in magnetic resonance imaging and/or treatment with systemic or intratympanic steroid medication. The resultant estimates of annual incidence of SSNHL after COVID-19 vaccination in VAERS data were between 0.6 (probable; minimum estimate) and 28.0 (maximum estimate) cases per 100,000 people

---

[2] Refers to the COVID-19 vaccine manufactured by Moderna under the name Spikevax®.

per year. The authors note that this is lower than or similar to the estimated annual U.S. incidence (11–77 per 100,000 people per year) (Formeister et al., 2022). In a secondary analysis, the authors note that the reports per 100,000 doses in VAERS decreased from 1.10 in December 2020 to 0.01 in June 2021, despite large increases in the absolute number of vaccines administered.

## From Evidence to Conclusions

The broader academic literature includes a handful of published articles reporting SSNHL in individuals receiving COVID-19 vaccination; however, this level of evidence does not support an association between vaccination and SSNHL (Formeister et al., 2022; Jeong and Choi, 2021; Tsetsos et al., 2021). However, the committee found that the majority of the literature was limited to single case reports, unadjusted descriptive reports lacking a comparison or without thoughtful adjudication of hearing loss, or publications with potential bias; these did not meet its inclusion criteria during screening. Only one of the studies included in this review suggested an association between COVID-19 vaccination and SSNHL. However, the magnitude of the effect was small, with potential for confounding from unmeasured variables. In contrast, the most methodologically rigorous analysis that included potential confounders (e.g., infection status, comorbidities, and health care use patterns) in models found no association. Using pharmacovigilance data without comparators offers low-level evidence to support a conclusion. Nonetheless, one article used VAERS data and offered compelling evidence that incidence of SSNHL was similar to expected rates and much lower after an adjudication procedure to assess the credibility of the reported hearing loss. Moreover, the same report showed that the weekly number of reports of SSNHL did not change over time despite large increases in the number of vaccines administered.

An emergent theme is heterogeneity in identification of SSNHL and potential for misclassification. First, self-reported data may be unreliable. Insights from the reviewed literature may reflect this. Formeister et al. (2022) offered insights that many reports of SSNHL in the VAERS data may not be true cases, and Leong et al. (2023) found that the majority of self-reported new cases from vaccination were attributable to exacerbating known etiologies of hearing loss. Another consideration may be that hearing includes peripheral encoding and central processing of information in the brain, and cognitive processes play a key role in how individuals understand speech. The role of cognition in the potential association between self-reported hearing and COVID-19 infection or vaccination may be highly overlooked, as it is plausible that existing age-related hearing loss, which is highly prevalent, could be perceived as "new" due to fatigue or "brain fog." Second, studies varied in definitions of SSNHL, including using different risk-windows. Moreover, different and unverified approaches to diagnosis codes were used. Two studies used diagnosis codes. Yanir et al. (2022) took a wide approach by looking for many different ICD codes for hearing loss with concurrent prednisone usage; Nieminen et al. (2023) used a single SSNHL code. Given the acute nature of SSNHL, diagnosis codes may be accurate and reliable with some suggestion that an audiological test battery occurred. However, it is unknown if concurrent ICD codes for more general hearing loss paired with prednisone use is reliable. No studies examined the relationship between NVX-CoV2373[3] and SSNHL.

Overall, we found that the literature on vaccination and sensorineural hearing loss focused almost exclusively on SSNHL. Our review of said literature resulted in weak evidence and concerns about the measurement of SSNHL. Although the combination of the more methodologically rigorous evidence suggesting no association and lack of identified potential mechanisms beyond hypotheses may hint at no relationship between vaccination and SSNHL, the literature is inadequate to offer a decision on the acceptance or rejection of a causal relationship. Future epidemiological evidence is required.

**Conclusion 4-1: The evidence is inadequate to accept or reject a causal relationship between the BNT162b2 vaccine and sensorineural hearing loss.**

**Conclusion 4-2: The evidence is inadequate to accept or reject a causal relationship between the mRNA-1273 vaccine and sensorineural hearing loss.**

---

[3] Refers to the COVID-19 vaccine manufactured by Novavax.

**Conclusion 4-3: The evidence is inadequate to accept or reject a causal relationship between the Ad26.COV2.S vaccine and sensorineural hearing loss.**

**Conclusion 4-4: The evidence is inadequate to accept or reject a causal relationship between the NVX-CoV2373 vaccine and sensorineural hearing loss.**

## TINNITUS

---

### BOX 4-2
### Conclusions for Tinnitus

**Conclusion 4-5: The evidence is inadequate to accept or reject a causal relationship between the BNT162b2 vaccine and tinnitus.**

**Conclusion 4-6: The evidence is inadequate to accept or reject a causal relationship between the mRNA-1273 vaccine and tinnitus.**

**Conclusion 4-7: The evidence is inadequate to accept or reject a causal relationship between the Ad26.COV2.S vaccine and tinnitus.**

**Conclusion 4-8: The evidence is inadequate to accept or reject a causal relationship between the NVX-CoV2373 vaccine and tinnitus.**

---

### Background

Tinnitus is the phenomenon of perceiving sound without an external stimulus. The sound can be continuous or intermittent. Reported descriptions vary (e.g., ringing, buzzing, hissing, pulsation, clicks), and reported acoustic characteristics range in amplitude (volume) and frequency (pitch) (Baguley et al., 2013; Lockwood et al., 2002). Prevalence estimates vary (4.6–30 percent) due to heterogeneity in measures, and studies are mostly limited to North America and Europe (Baguley et al., 2013; Lockwood et al., 2002; McCormack et al., 2016). A meta-analysis of 113 articles estimated the pooled prevalence of tinnitus and suggests that 14.4 percent of adults report it (Jarach et al., 2022). However, this estimate varied by definition of tinnitus and dropped to 3.4 percent for diagnosed tinnitus (as opposed to self-reported). Prevalence increases with age; 23.6 percent of older adults report tinnitus. The pooled incidence rate of any tinnitus was 1,164 per 100,000 person-years (Jarach et al., 2022).

Tinnitus is considered a symptom of an underlying condition rather than a disease. Risk factors are broad and include occupational (e.g., noise exposure), muscular tension, neurological, trauma, cardiovascular, rheumatological, psychological, endocrinological, metabolic, and pharmacological conditions and factors (Baguley et al., 2013; Koning, 2021; Lockwood et al., 2002; Pezzoli et al., 2015). Overarching hypotheses (Roberts et al., 2013) on the cause are that a lack of sensory stimulation due to hearing loss (bottom-up) leads to reorganization and changes in neural firing/synchrony in neural networks that are responsible for limbic, attention, and audition (top-down), resulting in perceived sound. Clinical consensus is that peripheral hearing loss, particularly when the origin is noise-induced, is the most common source of tinnitus (Baguley et al., 2013; Lockwood et al., 2002; Piccirillo et al., 2020).

Without an objective measure, tinnitus diagnosis relies on a combination of patient-reported perceived sound characteristics, subjective impact on quality of life and well-being, medical history review, and accompanying assessments to uncover the etiology (Baguley et al., 2013; Bhatt et al., 2016; Langguth et al., 2013). Validated tinnitus questionnaires play a key role in offering a standardized characterization, and comprehensive audiometric testing should be performed to assess the function of the auditory system for potential sources of the symptom (e.g., hearing loss). Imaging is employed to investigate the source of tinnitus in complex cases, especially for asymmetric tinnitus, concurrent associated neurological symptoms, and pulsatile tinnitus (Baguley et al., 2013; Bhatt et al., 2016; Langguth et al., 2013).

## Mechanisms

Tinnitus etiology is multifactorial, encompassing neural, vascular, muscular, and metabolic processes, and often influenced by environmental factors. Moreover, tinnitus may differ by predisposing risk factors, and the individual reactions to it differ by anxiety levels, which may influence reporting of the symptom and perceived impact.

An important consideration is that tinnitus is a symptom of other conditions. It primarily involves the peripheral and central auditory systems, with the prevailing theory that it results from altered neuronal activity within the auditory pathway secondary to peripheral hearing loss, leading to a reduction in afferent input to the central auditory system. The brain compensates for this loss by increasing the gain in the central auditory pathways, a phenomenon known as "central gain." This heightened sensitivity and neuronal hyperactivity can manifest as the perception of sound (Makar, 2021). Therefore, a proposed mechanistic relationship between tinnitus and vaccination includes potential for it as a secondary symptom of vaccine-induced hearing loss. However, as noted, mechanistic evidence linking hearing loss and COVID-19 vaccination is limited.

Vaccines can occasionally lead to adverse effects, including reported cases of tinnitus. Little direct evidence exists for a direct link, but hypotheses appear in the literature; these mechanisms are not fully understood but thought to involve immune-mediated responses. One hypothesis is molecular mimicry, where the immune response against vaccine components cross-reacts with inner ear antigens, leading to inflammation and damage. Similarly, an autoimmune response triggered by the vaccine (e.g., type 3 hypersensitivity) may manifest as autoimmune inner ear disease in susceptible individuals (Kamogashira et al., 2022). Less-well-described mechanisms involve toxic responses from vaccine components or restricted cochlear blood flow (Ahmed et al., 2022).

Although the previous mechanisms focus on a bottom-up insult leading to tinnitus, top-down changes resulting from vaccination are hypothetical. In common theories of tinnitus, neuroplastic changes occur in the neuronal activity of the auditory cortex, thalamus, and other related brain areas after peripheral injury that reduces sensory input. These changes can include increased spontaneous firing rates, enhanced neural synchrony, and reorganization of the auditory cortex. These neural alterations are thought to contribute to the persistence and severity of tinnitus (Ahmed et al., 2022; Baguley et al., 2013; Ciorba et al., 2018; Piccirillo et al., 2020). Proinflammatory cytokines, immune responses, and other inflammatory mediators could exacerbate neural damage (Becker et al., 2022) and contribute to the development of vaccine-mediated tinnitus.

## Epidemiological Evidence

Clinical trial results submitted to FDA for Emergency Use Authorization and/or full approval do not indicate a signal regarding tinnitus and any of the vaccines under study (FDA, 2021, 2023a,b,c). Table 4-2 presents four studies that contributed to the causality assessment.

Leong et al. (2023) leveraged a convenience sample from an otology clinic in a large, urban medical center (New York City, New York) from May to July 2021 to characterize the incidence of hearing loss after COVID-19 vaccination. Among 500 individuals who completed screening (median age 56.6 years; 40.2 percent female), 420 reported being vaccinated (58.4 percent BNT162b2, 29.1 percent mRNA-1273, 3.8 percent Ad26.COV2.S), and 26 of these (all vaccines) (6.2 percent) reported tinnitus. However, after audiologic and medical evaluation, 10 cases were attributed to hearing loss and eight to other conditions (e.g., temporomandibular joint syndrome, otitis media, and earwax), resulting in eight (1.9 percent) individuals with subjective tinnitus as the primary diagnosis.

Whittaker et al. (2021) conducted a population-based study using electronic health records data from 1,392 general practices in England contributing to the Clinical Practice Research Datalink Aurum database (August 2020–May 2021) to describe rates of consulting a general practitioner for new symptoms, diseases, prescriptions, and health care use among adults after diagnosis of COVID-19. Adults with evidence of outcomes of interest before COVID-19 diagnosis were excluded. In the study, 267,993 individuals who had a COVID-19 diagnosis and were managed in the community were vaccinated during the follow-up period. Among this group, the estimated

**TABLE 4-2** Epidemiological Studies in the Tinnitus Evidence Review

| Author | Study Design and Control Group | Location | Data Source | Vaccine(S) | Age Range | N | Number of Events | Results (95% CI) |
|---|---|---|---|---|---|---|---|---|
| Frontera et al. (2022) | Surveillance; single arm | US | VAERS | BNT162b2 | Median age = 50 years IQR 35–64 for all neurologic adverse events | 167.0 million doses | Not reported | 13.53 per 1 million doses |
| | | | | mRNA-1273 | | 128.1 million doses | | 13.90 per 1 million doses |
| | | | | Ad26.COV2.S | | 11.6 million doses | | 51.52 per 1 million doses |
| Kant et al. (2022) | Surveillance; single arm | Netherlands | The Netherlands Pharmaco-vigilance Centre Lareb | BNT162b2 | 12 to >80 years | 12,888 | 1 serious, 18 non-serious | Relatively low incidence of tinnitus cases reported but no comparison group included for inference |
| | | | | mRNA-1273 | | 3,426 | 7 non-serious | |
| | | | | Ad26.COV2.S | | 2,458 | 8 non-serious | |
| Leong et al. (2023) | Clinical convenience sample; single arm | New York, NY, USA | Otology clinic at academic center | BNT162b2 | 16–101 years | 244 | 16 | 1.9% of vaccinated individuals had adjudicated new or not otherwise explained tinnitus |
| | | | | mRNA-1273 | | 123 | 8 | |
| | | | | Ad26.COV2.S | | 16 | 1 | |
| Whittaker et al. (2021) | Population-based retrospective cohort; pre and post | England, UK | Electronic health records from Clinical Practice Research Datalink Aurum database | Unspecified percentages but included any of three approved COVID-19 vaccines in the UK | 18 to >80 years | 267,993 | Pre-vaccination: 294 events Post-vaccination: 69 events | Prevaccination: 100.8 (89.6–113.0) per 100,000 person-weeks Post-vaccination: 41.8 (32.5–52.8) per 100,000 person-weeks |

NOTES: BNT162b2 refers to the COVID-19 vaccine manufactured by Pfizer-BioNTech under the name Comirnaty®. mRNA-1273 refers to the COVID-19 vaccine manufactured by Moderna under the name Spikevax®. Ad26.COV2.S refers to the COVID-19 vaccine manufactured by Janssen. Number of events refers to events in vaccinees only. IQR: interquartile range; VAERS: Vaccine Adverse Event Reporting System.
SOURCES: Frontera et al., 2022; Kant et al., 2022; Leong et al., 2023; Whittaker et al., 2021.

incidence of tinnitus events dropped from 100.8 (range 89.6–113.0) prevaccination to 41.8 (range 32.5–52.8) post-vaccination per 100,000 person-weeks; an analysis adjusted for age, sex, smoking, body mass index, and the Charlson Comorbidity Index found a decrease in incidence of tinnitus events after vaccination (IRR 0.39, 95% CI: 0.25–0.59, $p < 0.001$).

Two surveillance studies were included in the review. Frontera et al. (2022) used VAERS to examine adverse events after vaccination between January 1, 2021, and June 14, 2021 (306.9 million COVID-19 vaccine doses; 314,610 adverse events [71 percent female]). They reported an incidence of 15.14 cases of tinnitus identified by free text or automated coding per 1,000,000 vaccines (13.53 BNT162b2, 13.90 mRNA-1273, 51.52 Ad26.COV2.S).

Kant et al. (2022) recruited participants within 2 days of vaccination at sites across the Netherlands for a Web-based surveillance study of self-reported adverse events using closed and open questionnaires. They analyzed adverse events within 7 days of first and second doses (if applicable). Among the 27,554 events, one serious and 33 nonserious occurrences of tinnitus were reported. Events were coded as serious or not according to the Council for International Organizations of Medical Sciences criteria (Macrae, 2007; CIOMS, 2010).

Dorney et al. (2023) used data from a large, deidentified electronic health record database (TriNetX Analytics Network) from December 15, 2020, to March 1, 2022, to compare the prevalence of new-onset tinnitus (within 21 days) after COVID-19 vaccination relative to other common vaccines that are not suspected of causing tinnitus. Even though this paper did not use an unvaccinated control (and is therefore not included in Table 4-2), it is informative. Tinnitus was identified based on electronic health records data. The authors reported an estimated 0.038 percent (95% CI: 0.036–0.041) prevalence and 0.031 percent (95% CI: 0.029–0.034) prevalence of new tinnitus after the first ($n$ = 2.6 million) and second ($n$ = 1.5 million) doses. The authors used propensity matching (age at vaccination, sex, race, and ethnicity) to compare the relative risk (RR) of new-onset tinnitus after other vaccines to a first COVID-19 vaccine. The authors reported a higher RR of new-onset tinnitus after the influenza vaccine (998,991 vs. 1,009,935 first dose COVID-19 vaccine patients; mean age: 43.0 vs. 45.6 years; RR 1.95, 95% CI: 1.72–2.21), Tdap (444,708 vs. 444,721 first dose COVID-19 vaccine patients; mean age: 39.4 vs. 40.3 years; RR 2.36, 95% CI: 1.93–2.89), and polysaccharide pneumococcus (154,344 vs. 154,825 first dose COVID-19 vaccine patients; mean age: 59.3 vs. 59.5 years; RR 1.97, 95% CI: 1.48–2.64) vaccines, respectively. While these data do not offer direct evidence of any of the aforementioned vaccines being associated with new onset tinnitus, they do suggest that COVID-19 vaccination does not have any higher risk of new onset tinnitus compared to common vaccines that are not suspected of causing tinnitus.

## From Evidence to Conclusions

Several case reports appear in the academic literature and media of tinnitus after COVID-19 vaccination. However, the epidemiological evidence review offered limited insight. Three surveillance and clinical sample studies suggest relatively low incidence after vaccination but lack comparator groups for inferential conclusions and suffer from biases, particularly selection, and confounding. Other studies offered valuable insights but were limited in scope and indirectly addressed the question. Dorney et al. (2023) found onset of tinnitus was lower after COVID-19 vaccination relative to other common vaccinations, and Whittaker et al. (2021) found that vaccination reduced the incidence of tinnitus as a reason for general practitioner visits among individuals who had been diagnosed with COVID-19. However, while these studies met inclusion criteria, inherent flaws in the study designs or limitations to the reference group limit any conclusive evidence.

Of further concern, the heterogeneity in tinnitus etiology, pathophysiology, and characteristics combined with no objective diagnostic measure or standardized subjective measure make it difficult to assess a relationship with vaccination. Despite several hypotheses, no definitive mechanistic evidence was identified in the literature. The nature of tinnitus as a symptom of other conditions further complicates a review of the data, as it is plausible for it to be a symptom of conditions potentially caused by vaccination, but it is unclear how this is reflected in the measurement of tinnitus across studies. Leong et al. (2023) do offer some insight into this: 18 of 26 cases were attributable to other conditions after medical evaluation.

> **Conclusion 4-5: The evidence is inadequate to accept or reject a causal relationship between the BNT162b2 vaccine and tinnitus.**

> **Conclusion 4-6: The evidence is inadequate to accept or reject a causal relationship between the mRNA-1273 vaccine and tinnitus.**

> **Conclusion 4-7: The evidence is inadequate to accept or reject a causal relationship between the Ad26.COV2.S vaccine and tinnitus.**

> **Conclusion 4-8: The evidence is inadequate to accept or reject a causal relationship between the NVX-CoV2373 vaccine and tinnitus.**

# REFERENCES

Agrawal, Y., E. A. Platz, and J. K. Niparko. 2008. Prevalence of hearing loss and differences by demographic characteristics among U.S. adults: Data from the National Health and Nutrition Examination Survey, 1999–2004. *Archives of Internal Medicine* 168(14):1522–1530. https://doi.org/10.1001/archinte.168.14.1522.

Ahmed, S. H., S. Waseem, T. G. Shaikh, N. A. Qadir, S. A. Siddiqui, I. Ullah, A. Waris, and Z. Yousaf. 2022. SARS-CoV-2 vaccine-associated-tinnitus: A review. *Annals of Medicine and Surgery* 75:103293. https://doi.org/10.1016/j.amsu.2022.103293.

Baguley, D., D. McFerran, and D. Hall. 2013. Tinnitus. *Lancet* 382(9904):1600–1607. https://doi.org/10.1016/s0140-6736(13)60142-7.

Becker, L., A. Keck, N. Rohleder, and N. Muller-Voggel. 2022. Higher peripheral inflammation is associated with lower orbitofrontal gamma power in chronic tinnitus. *Frontiers in Behavioral Neuroscience* 16:883926. https://doi.org/10.3389/fnbeh.2022.883926.

Bhatt, J. M., H. W. Lin, and N. Bhattacharyya. 2016. Prevalence, severity, exposures, and treatment patterns of tinnitus in the United States. *JAMA Otolaryngology—Head & Neck Surgery* 142(10):959–965. https://doi.org/10.1001/jamaoto.2016.1700.

Chadha, S., K. Kamenov, and A. Cieza. 2021. The world report on hearing, 2021. *Bulletin of the World Health Organization* 99(4):242–242a. https://doi.org/10.2471/blt.21.285643.

CIOMS (Council for International Organizations of Medical Sciences) Working Group VIII. 2010. Practical aspects of signal detection in pharmacovigilance: Report of CIOMS working group VIII. Geneva.

Ciorba, A., V. Corazzi, C. Bianchini, C. Aimoni, S. Pelucchi, P. H. Skarżyński, and S. Hatzopoulos. 2018. Autoimmune inner ear disease (AIED): A diagnostic challenge. *International Journal of Immunopathology and Pharmacology* 32:2058738418808680. https://doi.org/10.1177/2058738418808680.

Cruickshanks, K. J., T. L. Wiley, T. S. Tweed, B. E. Klein, R. Klein, J. A. Mares-Perlman, and D. M. Nondahl. 1998. Prevalence of hearing loss in older adults in Beaver Dam, Wisconsin. The epidemiology of hearing loss study. *American Journal of Epidemiology* 148(9):879–886. https://doi.org/10.1093/oxfordjournals.aje.a009713.

Dorney, I., L. Bobak, T. Otteson, and D. C. Kaelber. 2023. Prevalence of new-onset tinnitus after COVID-19 vaccination with comparison to other vaccinations. *Laryngoscope* 133(7):1722–1725. https://doi.org/10.1002/lary.30395.

Eggermont, J. J. 2017. Chapter 6—causes of acquired hearing loss. In *Hearing loss*, edited by J. J. Eggermont. Academic Press. Pp. 177–208.

FDA (Food and Drug Administration). 2021. *Emergency use authorization (EUA) amendment for an unapproved product review memorandum*. Food and Drug Administration. https://www.fda.gov/media/153439/download (accessed May 3, 2023).

FDA. 2023a. *BLA clinical review memorandum—COMIRNATY*. Food and Drug Administration. https://www.fda.gov/media/172333/download?attachment (accessed December 5, 2023).

FDA. 2023b. *BLA clinical review memorandum—SPIKEVAX*. Food and Drug Administration. https://www.fda.gov/media/172357/download?attachment (accessed December 5, 2023).

FDA. 2023c. *Emergency use authorization (EUA) for an unapproved product review memorandum*. Food and Drug Administration. https://www.fda.gov/media/168233/download?attachment (accessed December 5, 2023).

Formeister, E. J., M. J. Wu, D. A. Chari, R. Meek, III, S. D. Rauch, A. K. Remenschneider, A. M. Quesnel, R. de Venecia, D. J. Lee, W. Chien, C. M. Stewart, D. Galaiya, E. D. Kozin, and D. Q. Sun. 2022. Assessment of sudden sensorineural hearing loss after COVID-19 vaccination. *JAMA Otolaryngology—Head & Neck Surgery* 148(4):307–315. https://doi.org/10.1001/jamaoto.2021.4414.

Frontera, J. A., A. A. Tamborska, M. F. Doheim, D. García-Azorin, H. Gezegen, A. Guekht, A. H. K. Yusof Khan, M. Santacatterina, J. Sejvar, K. T. Thakur, E. Westenberg, A. S. Winkler, and E. Beghi. 2022. Neurological events reported after COVID-19 vaccines: An analysis of VAERS. *Annals of Neurology* 91(6):756–771. https://doi.org/10.1002/ana.26339.

Goman, A. M., and F. R. Lin. 2016. Prevalence of hearing loss by severity in the United States. *American Journal of Public Health* 106(10):1820–1822. https://doi.org/10.2105/ajph.2016.303299.

Hornsby, B. W., G. Naylor, and F. H. Bess. 2016. A taxonomy of fatigue concepts and their relation to hearing loss. *Ear and Hearing* 37(Suppl 1):136s–144s. https://doi.org/10.1097/aud.0000000000000289.

Jarach, C. M., A. Lugo, M. Scala, P. A. van den Brandt, C. R. Cederroth, A. Odone, W. Garavello, W. Schlee, B. Langguth, and S. Gallus. 2022. Global prevalence and incidence of tinnitus: A systematic review and meta-analysis. *JAMA Neurology* 79(9):888–900. https://doi.org/10.1001/jamaneurol.2022.2189.

Jeong, J., and H. S. Choi. 2021. Sudden sensorineural hearing loss after COVID-19 vaccination. *International Journal of Infectious Diseases* 113:341–343. https://doi.org/10.1016/j.ijid.2021.10.025.

Kaliyappan, K., Y. C. Chen, and V. P. Krishnan Muthaiah. 2022. Vestibular cochlear manifestations in COVID-19 cases. *Frontiers in Neurology* 13:850337. https://doi.org/10.3389/fneur.2022.850337.

Kamil, R. J., D. J. Genther, and F. R. Lin. 2015. Factors associated with the accuracy of subjective assessments of hearing impairment. *Ear and Hearing* 36(1):164–167. https://doi.org/10.1097/aud.0000000000000075.

Kamogashira, T., H. Funayama, S. Asakura, and S. Ishimoto. 2022. Vestibular neuritis following COVID-19 vaccination: A retrospective study. *Cureus* 14(4):e24277. https://doi.org/10.7759/cureus.24277.

Kant, A., J. Jansen, L. van Balveren, and F. van Hunsel. 2022. Description of frequencies of reported adverse events following immunization among four different COVID-19 vaccine brands. *Drug Safety* 45(4):319–331. https://doi.org/10.1007/s40264-022-01151-w.

Katz, J., M. Chasin, K. M. English, L. J. Hood, and K. L. Tillery. 2015. *Handbook of clinical audiology* Vol. 7. Philadelphia, PA: Wolters Kluwer Health.

Koning, H. M. 2021. Cervical nerve projections to the auditory pathway in tinnitus. *International Tinnitus Journal* 24(2):70–74. https://doi.org/10.5935/0946-5448.20200011.

Kuhn, M., S. E. Heman-Ackah, J. A. Shaikh, and P. C. Roehm. 2011. Sudden sensorineural hearing loss: A review of diagnosis, treatment, and prognosis. *Trends Amplify* 15(3):91–105. https://doi.org/10.1177/1084713811408349.

Langguth, B., P. M. Kreuzer, T. Kleinjung, and D. De Ridder. 2013. Tinnitus: Causes and clinical management. *Lancet Neurology* 12(9):920–930. https://doi.org/10.1016/s1474-4422(13)70160-1.

Lee, K. Y. 2013. Pathophysiology of age-related hearing loss (peripheral and central). *Korean Journal of Audiology* 17(2):45–49. https://doi.org/10.7874/kja.2013.17.2.45.

Leong, S., B. Teh, and A. H. Kim. 2023. Characterization of otologic symptoms appearing after COVID-19 vaccination. *American Journal of Otolaryngology* 44(2):103725. https://doi.org/10.1016/j.amjoto.2022.103725.

Lin, F. R., J. K. Niparko, and L. Ferrucci. 2011. Hearing loss prevalence in the United States. *Archives of Internal Medicine* 171(20):1851–1852. https://doi.org/10.1001/archinternmed.2011.506.

Lockwood, A. H., R. J. Salvi, and R. F. Burkard. 2002. Tinnitus. *New England Journal of Medicine* 347(12):904–910. https://doi.org/10.1056/NEJMra013395.

Macrae, D. J. 2007. The Council for International Organizations and Medical Sciences (CIOMS) guidelines on ethics of clinical trials. *Proceedings of the American Thoracic Society* 4(2):176–178, discussion 178–179. https://doi.org/10.1513/pats.200701-011GC.

Makar, S. K. 2021. Etiology and pathophysiology of tinnitus—a systematic review. *International Tinnitus Journal* 25(1):76–86. https://doi.org/10.5935/0946-5448.20210015.

Martin, J. S., and J. F. Jerger. 2005. Some effects of aging on central auditory processing. *Journal of Rehabilitation Research and Development* 42(4 Suppl 2):25–44. https://doi.org/10.1682/jrrd.2004.12.0164.

Mattox, D. E., and F. B. Simmons. 1977. Natural history of sudden sensorineural hearing loss. *Annals of Otology, Rhinology and Laryngology* 86(4 Pt 1):463–480. https://doi.org/10.1177/000348947708600406.

McCormack, A., M. Edmondson-Jones, S. Somerset, and D. Hall. 2016. A systematic review of the reporting of tinnitus prevalence and severity. *Hearing Research* 337:70–79. https://doi.org/10.1016/j.heares.2016.05.009.

Nieminen, T. A., I. Kivekäs, M. Artama, H. Nohynek, J. Kujansivu, and P. Hovi. 2023. Sudden hearing loss following vaccination against COVID-19. *JAMA Otolaryngology—Head & Neck Surgery* 149(2):133–140. https://doi.org/10.1001/jamaoto.2022.4154.

Pezzoli, M., A. Ugolini, E. Rota, L. Ferrero, C. Milani, L. Pezzoli, G. Pecorari, and F. Mongini. 2015. Tinnitus and its relationship with muscle tenderness in patients with headache and facial pain. *Journal of Laryngology and Otology* 129(7):638–643. https://doi.org/10.1017/S0022215115001425.

Piccirillo, J. F., T. L. Rodebaugh, and E. J. Lenze. 2020. Tinnitus. *JAMA* 323(15):1497–1498. https://doi.org/10.1001/jama.2020.0697.

Pickles, J. 2013. *An introduction to the physiology of hearing: Fourth edition*. Brill.

Powell, D. S., E. S. Oh, N. S. Reed, F. R. Lin, and J. A. Deal. 2021. Hearing loss and cognition: What we know and where we need to go. *Frontiers in Aging Neuroscience* 13:769405. https://doi.org/10.3389/fnagi.2021.769405.

Reed, N. S., E. E. Garcia-Morales, C. Myers, A. R. Huang, J. R. Ehrlich, O. J. Killeen, J. E. Hoover-Fong, F. R. Lin, M. L. Arnold, E. S. Oh, J. A. Schrack, and J. A. Deal. 2023. Prevalence of hearing loss and hearing aid use among U.S. Medicare beneficiaries aged 71 years and older. *JAMA Network Open* 6(7):e2326320. https://doi.org/10.1001/jamanetworkopen.2023.26320.

Roberts, L. E., F. T. Husain, and J. J. Eggermont. 2013. Role of attention in the generation and modulation of tinnitus. *Neuroscience and Biobehavioral Reviews* 37(8):1754–1773. https://doi.org/10.1016/j.neubiorev.2013.07.007.

Sadarangani, M., A. Marchant, and T. R. Kollmann. 2021. Immunological mechanisms of vaccine-induced protection against COVID-19 in humans. *Nature Reviews: Immunology* 21(8):475–484. https://doi.org/10.1038/s41577-021-00578-z.

Schreiber, B. E., C. Agrup, D. O. Haskard, and L. M. Luxon. 2010. Sudden sensorineural hearing loss. *Lancet* 375(9721):1203–1211. https://doi.org/10.1016/s0140-6736(09)62071-7.

Stachler, R. J., S. S. Chandrasekhar, S. M. Archer, R. M. Rosenfeld, S. R. Schwartz, D. M. Barrs, S. R. Brown, T. D. Fife, P. Ford, T. G. Ganiats, D. B. Hollingsworth, C. A. Lewandowski, J. J. Montano, J. E. Saunders, D. L. Tucci, M. Valente, B. E. Warren, K. L. Yaremchuk, and P. J. Robertson. 2012. Clinical practice guideline: Sudden hearing loss. *Otolaryngology and Head and Neck Surgery* 146(3 Suppl):S1–S35. https://doi.org/10.1177/0194599812436449.

Tabuchi, K., B. Nishimura, S. Tanaka, K. Hayashi, Y. Hirose, and A. Hara. 2010. Ischemia-reperfusion injury of the cochlea: Pharmacological strategies for cochlear protection and implications of glutamate and reactive oxygen species. *Current Neuropharmacology* 8(2):128–134. https://doi.org/10.2174/157015910791233123.

Task Force on Central Auditory Processing Consensus Development. 1996. Current status of research and implications for clinical practice. *American Journal of Audiology* 5(2):11. https://doi.org/doi.org/10.1044/1059-0889.0502.41.

Tsetsos, N., A. Poutoglidis, K. Vlachtsis, A. Kilmpasanis, and S. Gougousis. 2021. Sudden sensorineural hearing loss following the second dose of COVID-19 vaccine. *Cureus* 13(8):e17435. https://doi.org/10.7759/cureus.17435.

Van Eyken, E., G. Van Camp, and L. Van Laer. 2007. The complexity of age-related hearing impairment: Contributing environmental and genetic factors. *Audiology and Neuro-Otology* 12(6):345–358. https://doi.org/10.1159/000106478.

Whittaker, H. R., C. Gulea, A. Koteci, C. Kallis, A. D. Morgan, C. Iwundu, M. Weeks, R. Gupta, and J. K. Quint. 2021. GP consultation rates for sequelae after acute COVID-19 in patients managed in the community or hospital in the U.K.: Population-based study. *British Journal of Medicine* 375:e065834. https://doi.org/10.1136/bmj-2021-065834.

WHO (World Health Organization). 2024. *Deafness and hearing loss*. https://www.who.int/health-topics/hearing-loss#tab=tab_2 (accessed February 14, 2024).

Wilson, W. R., F. M. Byl, and N. Laird. 1980. The efficacy of steroids in the treatment of idiopathic sudden hearing loss. A double-blind clinical study. *Archives of Otolaryngology* 106(12):772–776. https://doi.org/10.1001/archotol.1980.00790360050013.

Wingfield, A., P. A. Tun, and S. L. McCoy. 2005. Hearing loss in older adulthood: What it is and how it interacts with cognitive performance. *Current Directions in Psychological Science* 14(3):144–148. https://doi.org/10.1111/j.0963-7214.2005.00356.x.

Yamasoba, T., F. R. Lin, S. Someya, A. Kashio, T. Sakamoto, and K. Kondo. 2013. Current concepts in age-related hearing loss: Epidemiology and mechanistic pathways. *Hearing Research* 303:30–38. https://doi.org/10.1016/j.heares.2013.01.021.

Yanir, Y., I. Doweck, R. Shibli, R. Najjar-Debbiny, and W. Saliba. 2022. Association between the BNT162b2 messenger RNA COVID-19 vaccine and the risk of sudden sensorineural hearing loss. *JAMA Otolaryngology—Head & Neck Surgery* 148(4):299–306. https://doi.org/10.1001/jamaoto.2021.4278.

# 5

# Thrombosis with Thrombocytopenia Syndrome, Immune Thrombocytopenic Purpura, Capillary Leak Syndrome, and COVID-19 Vaccines

This chapter describes the potential relationship of COVID-19 vaccines and thrombosis with thrombocytopenia syndrome (TTS), immune thrombocytopenic purpura (ITP), and capillary leak syndrome (CLS) (see Boxes 5-1 through 5-3 for all conclusions in this chapter).

## THROMBOSIS WITH THROMBOCYTOPENIA SYNDROME

---

**BOX 5-1**
**Conclusions for Thrombosis with Thrombocytopenia Syndrome**

**Conclusion 5-1: The evidence favors rejection of a causal relationship between the BNT162b2 vaccine and thrombosis with thrombocytopenia syndrome.**

**Conclusion 5-2: The evidence favors rejection of a causal relationship between the mRNA-1273 vaccine and thrombosis with thrombocytopenia syndrome.**

**Conclusion 5-3: The evidence favors acceptance of a causal relationship between the Ad26.COV2.S vaccine and thrombosis with thrombocytopenia syndrome.**

**Conclusion 5-4: The evidence is inadequate to accept or reject a causal relationship between the NVX-CoV2373 vaccine and thrombosis with thrombocytopenia syndrome.**

---

## Background

Within months of the introduction of ChAdOx1-S[1] in Europe and the United Kingdom, three reports appeared of an unusual safety signal characterized by the acute onset of unusual thrombotic events and thrombocytopenia 6–24 days after the first dose (Greinacher et al., 2021; Schultz et al., 2021; Scully et al., 2021). The events

---
[1] Refers to the COVID-19 vaccine manufactured by Oxford-AstraZeneca.

89

predominantly affected the cerebral venous sinus circulation and/or the splanchnic venous circulation; less commonly, pulmonary embolism (PE) and other venous beds were involved. Thrombocytopenia was usually significant, frequently in the range of $10–20 \times 10^9$ per liter (L), and D-dimer levels were markedly elevated. It was rapidly recognized that these patients had developed antibodies to platelet factor 4 (PF4), which provided the first insights into a potential mechanism for this rare event. Mortality was high if the patients were not treated with a non-heparin anticoagulant and intravenous immunoglobulin (Greinacher et al., 2021; Schultz et al., 2021; Scully et al., 2021). Because of the association between thrombotic events and thrombocytopenia, the syndrome became known as "thrombosis with thrombocytopenia syndrome" or "vaccine-induced immune thrombotic thombocytopenia" (VITT). Diagnostic criteria for VITT have been proposed, with a definite diagnosis consisting of all five of the following criteria: (1) onset of symptoms 5–30 days after vaccination against severe acute respiratory syndrome coronavirus-2 (SARS-CoV-2) (or $\le 42$ days in patients with isolated deep vein thrombosis [DVT] or PE); (2) presence of thrombosis; (3) platelet count $<150 \times 10^9$ per L; (4) D-dimer level $>4,000$ fibrinogen equivalent units; and (5) positive anti-PF4 antibodies on ELISA (Pavord et al., 2021).

## Mechanisms

Similarities in the clinical presentation of TTS to spontaneous, or autoimmune, heparin-induced thrombocytopenia (HIT) quickly led to the recognition that an immune response to PF4 was an important component of TTS. HIT develops in patients within the first 1–2 weeks of therapy with heparin, characterized by thrombocytopenia with or without thrombotic complications. The diagnosis is confirmed by identifying anti-PF4 IgG antibodies that activate platelets in the presence of heparin through binding to the Fcg receptor IIa on platelet surfaces. Epitope mapping studies identified key amino acids on PF4 that form the antibody binding site, which are spatially distinct from its heparin-binding site (Huynh et al., 2019).

Spontaneous HIT was first described in 2008, characterized by an acute presentation with thrombotic complications, thrombocytopenia, and antibodies to PF4 but no prior exposure to heparin (Jay and Warkentin, 2008; Warkentin et al., 2008). As of 2022, fewer than 40 patients with spontaneous HIT had been reported (Warkentin, 2022). Most occurred after an orthopedic surgical procedure with no exposure to heparin, but some developed after an infection. Cerebral venous sinus thrombosis was observed in 6 of 15 patients with spontaneous HIT in nonsurgical settings, a presentation infrequently seen in patients with HIT receiving heparin (Warkentin, 2022). In addition, serum samples from a subset of patients with spontaneous HIT were capable of activating platelets without heparin (Warkentin, 2022).

All three initial reports describing the development of TTS in patients vaccinated with ChAdOx1-S/nCoV-19 noted that with a single exception, anti-PF4 antibodies were present in serum samples (Greinacher et al., 2021; Schultz et al., 2021; Scully et al., 2021). The antibodies could activate platelets, and this effect could be enhanced by the addition of PF4 and blocked by the addition of heparin (Greinacher et al., 2021). In addition, TTS antibodies from some patients were able to activate platelets without heparin (Schultz et al., 2021). Epitope mapping studies found that binding of anti-PF4 antibodies from five patients with TTS after ChAdOx1-S/nCoV-19 was restricted to eight amino acids that were also located within the heparin-binding site (Huynh et al., 2023). Heparin could inhibit binding of the antibodies to PF4, explaining how it could interfere with platelet activation (Singh et al., 2022). Anti-PF4 antibodies from patients with TTS were also associated with excessive thrombus formation containing platelets, neutrophils, and fibrin in a FcgRIIa$^+$/hPF4$^+$ transgenic mouse model (Leung et al., 2022). Antibodies against PF4 did not cross-react with the SARS-CoV-2 spike protein, indicating that the desired immune response against the virus was not associated with TTS (Greinacher et al., 2021).

Fewer studies have been performed with antibodies from patients diagnosed with TTS after receiving Ad26.COV2.S.[2] Initial reports confirmed the presence of anti-PF4 antibodies detected by ELISA in most of these patients, but functional testing for anti-PF4 antibodies, using a heparin-dependent serotonin release assay, was frequently negative (See et al., 2021, 2022). In contrast, platelet activation in the presence of PF4 has been shown (Huynh et al., 2023; Kanack and Padmanabhan, 2022), and epitope mapping demonstrated that anti-PF4 antibodies from

---

[2] The COVID-19 vaccine manufactured by Janssen.

patients with TTS after Ad26.COV2.S bind to the same epitopes as anti-PF4 antibodies from patients with TTS after ChAdOx1-S/nCoV-19 (Huynh et al., 2023).

Although considerable data exist characterizing the anti-PF4 antibodies identified in these patients, very little is known about what precipitates the pathological anti-PF4 antibody response in those patients who develop TTS. That almost all cases have been reported in association with one of the two adenovirus vaccines would suggest a class effect. In contrast, the extremely small number of cases reported in patients receiving a messenger ribonucleic acid (mRNA) vaccine is less than the estimated background incidence of cerebral venous sinus thrombosis with thrombocytopenia during the years before COVID-19 (See et al., 2022).

## Epidemiological Evidence

### Clinical Trial Data

In the Phase 2/3 trial of BNT162b2,[3] one recipient presented with DVT, characterized as a nonserious adverse event, 14 days after dose 2, and two did so during the placebo-controlled follow-up period; however, none were associated with thrombocytopenia, according to the manufacturer. No study participants in either treatment group had a clinical manifestation of thrombosis similar to TTS (FDA, 2021a).

In the blinded phase of the trial evaluating mRNA-1273,[4] eight recipients and six placebo recipients developed DVT, but no events were associated with thrombocytopenia (FDA, 2022a). The Food and Drug Administration (FDA) review of the safety database and of case narratives concluded that no embolic events were suggestive of TTS.

In the Phase 3 study COV3001, one Ad26.COV2.S recipient developed venous transverse sinus thrombosis and cerebral hemorrhage, which was confirmed as TTS (FDA, 2021b), meeting Brighton Collaboration criteria Level 1 (Chen and Buttery, 2021) and Centers for Disease Control and Prevention (CDC) Criteria Tier 1. In the Phase 3 study COV3009 (FDA, 2021b), which evaluated the efficacy and safety of a booster dose of Ad26.COV2.S, one recipient presented with DVT in combination with thrombocytopenia, Brighton Collaboration criteria Level 3. No Ad26.COV2.S recipients met the Brighton Collaboration criteria Level 1 or CDC Criteria Tier 1 for TTS (Chen and Buttery, 2021) in COV3001.

In the briefing document provided on NVX-CoV2373[5] for FDA's Vaccines and Related Biological Products Advisory Committee meeting, Novavax stated that no cases of TTS had been reported in the clinical trial evaluating its vaccine (FDA, 2022a).

### Observational Studies

Table 5-1 presents three studies that contributed to the causality assessment.

Using electronic health record data from four hospitals in England and a self-controlled case series (SCCS) design, Higgins et al. (2022) evaluated the risk of TTS associated with the primary series of ChAdOx1-S and BNT162b2. TTS was defined as any acute thrombotic event associated with new onset of thrombocytopenia, defined as platelet count less than $150 \times 10^9$ per L. The study population included 170 adults admitted to a hospital between January and March 2021. They found no increased risk of TTS in days 4–13, 14–27, 28–41, or 4–27 after the first dose of BNT162b2 for the overall population or subgroups defined by age (relative incidence [RI] 0.82, 95% confidence interval [CI]: 0.38–1.75) (Higgins et al., 2022). There was an increased risk of TTS on days 4–27 after the first dose of ChAdOx1-S for the subgroup of individuals aged 18–39, but this finding was not significant for the overall study population. Strengths of the study included the definition of the outcome, based on platelet counts, and the presentation of data stratified by age group. The findings were limited by the relatively small sample size available, which may have resulted in insufficient power to detect significant differences in TTS risk associated with ChAdOx1-S in the overall population.

---

[3] Refers to the COVID-19 vaccine manufactured by Pfizer-BioNTech under the name Comirnaty®.
[4] Refers to the COVID-19 vaccine manufactured by Moderna under the name Spikevax®.
[5] Refers to the COVID-19 vaccine manufactured by Novavax.

**TABLE 5-1** Epidemiological Studies in the Thrombosis with Thrombocytopenia Evidence Review

| Author | Study Design and Control Group | Location | Data Source | Vaccine(s) | Age Range | N | Number of Events | Results (95% CI) |
|---|---|---|---|---|---|---|---|---|
| Andrews et al. (2022) | Cohort/ unvaccinated individuals | England | Hospital admissions data linked to immunization registry | BNT162b2 | 15+ years | 1.7 million person-years | Total: 45<br><br>Aged 40–64, 14–27 days: 5 | 40–64 years old, 14–27 days, RI 2.7 (1.1–7.1) |
| Higgins et al. (2022) | Self-controlled case series | England | Electronic health records | BNT162b2 | 18+ years | 170 cases | 9 | RI 0.82 (0.38–1.75) |
| Klein et al. (2021) | Cohort/ vaccinated individuals | US | Vaccine Safety Datalink (health plan data) | BNT162b2 | 12+ years | 6.8 million doses | BNT162b2 and mRNA-1273 combined: 73 | BNT162b2 and mRNA-1273 combined: RR 0.86 (0.58–1.27) |
| | | | | mRNA-1273 | | 5.1 million doses | | |

NOTES: BNT162b2 refers to the COVID-19 vaccine manufactured by Pfizer-BioNTech under the name Comirnaty®. mRNA-1273 refers to the COVID-19 vaccine manufactured by Moderna under the name Spikevax®. Number of events refers to events in vaccinees only. CI: confidence interval; RI: relative incidence; RR: risk ratio.
SOURCES: Andrews et al., 2022; Higgins et al., 2022; Klein et al., 2021.

Andrews et al. (2022) leveraged a national database of inpatient admissions in England to study the risk of TTS associated with the primary series of ChAdOx1-S and BNT162b2. TTS was defined as having a diagnosis code for thrombocytopenia and for a thrombotic event, including cerebral venous thrombosis, thrombophlebitis, deep venous thrombosis, splanchnic vein thrombosis, or PE (Andrews et al., 2022). Individuals with either diagnosis code in the year before the observation period were excluded to ensure that the study captured incident cases. Poisson regression models were used to compare the incidence of events after vaccination with that of unvaccinated individuals. The study included over 27 million individuals aged 15+ who were vaccinated between December 1, 2020, and April 18, 2021. Among those aged 15–39 and 65+, the first dose of BNT162b2 was not associated with an increased risk of TTS (Andrews et al., 2022). However, those aged 40–64 had an increased risk in days 14–27 after vaccination (RI 2.7, 95% CI: 1.1–7.1). This effect was not detected on days 0–13 or 4–13, due to insufficient number of events, or after the 28th day. There was a pronounced increase in the risk of TTS on days 4–13 and 14–37 after the first dose of ChAdOx1-S on individuals aged 15–39 and 40–64 but not for those aged 65+. The findings of the study are limited by the unavailability of platelet counts and the inclusion in the outcome definition of certain thrombotic events that are not typical manifestations of TTS, such as thrombophlebitis. Combined, these two limitations in the definition of the outcome may have resulted in an overestimation of the incidence of TTS.

Klein et al. (2021) leveraged data from the Vaccine Safety Datalink, which compiles data from eight U.S. health plans, to study the risk of 23 outcomes with BNT162b2 and mRNA-1273. TTS was defined as having an emergency room or inpatient diagnosis code for cerebral venous sinus thrombosis, splanchnic vein thrombosis, and arterial thrombosis and a platelet count less than $150 \times 10^9$ per L (Klein et al., 2021). Poisson regression compared the risk of the outcome in the 21 days after the first or the second dose with that of comparators who were in days 22–42 after their most recent vaccination. Analyses were performed for the combination of the first and second doses of both BNT162b2 and mRNA-1273 combined. The study sample included 11,845,128 doses given to individuals aged 12+; everyone under 18 received BNT162b2. Individuals who had COVID-19 in the 30 days before vaccination were excluded from analyses. No significant differences were observed in the risk in days 1–21 post-vaccination compared to days 22–42 (Klein et al., 2021). The findings are limited by the combination of the risk period after the first and second doses and the lack of reporting of separate results for BNT162b2 and mRNA-1273. The definition of the outcome was a strength of the study, as it leverages platelet counts and limits the list of thrombotic events to the common clinical manifestations of TTS.

*Pharmacovigilance Data*

Shortly after the reports on TTS with ChAdOx1-S became available, a report describing 12 U.S. patients with cerebral venous sinus thrombosis and thrombocytopenia 6–15 days after Ad26.COV2.S appeared (See et al., 2021). These patients had similar clinical manifestations as those with TTS after ChAdOx1-S and comparable platelet counts, elevated D-dimer levels, and positive testing for anti-PF4 antibodies. A follow-up study describing TTS cases reported to the U.S. Vaccine Adverse Event Reporting System (VAERS) between December 2020 and August 2021 was published in 2022. From 1,122 reports originally identified as potential TTS, 57 were determined to meet the case definition; 54 of them were after Ad26.COV2.S and three after mRNA vaccines (See et al., 2022). These case counts translated into reporting rates of 3.83 TTS cases per million doses of Ad26.COV2.S and 0.00855 TTS cases per million doses of mRNA vaccines. Reporting rates of TTS after Ad26.COV2.S were particularly pronounced among adults aged 18–49. No TTS events were reported for individuals under 18, although BNT162b2 was the only one authorized for use in the pediatric population during the study period (See et al., 2022).

Postmarketing reports of TTS after Ad26.COV2.S led to a pause in the use of the vaccine (April 13–23, 2021) and triggered an investigation by FDA and CDC (FDA, 2021c). In the most updated analyses, FDA reviewed TTS cases reported to VAERS through March 18, 2022, identifying 60 confirmed cases after Ad26.COV2.S, which translated into reporting rates of 3.23 cases per million doses (FDA, 2022a).

## From Evidence to Conclusions

The three observational studies (Andrews et al., 2022; Klein et al., 2021; Li et al., 2022) considered in the causality assessment failed to find an association between mRNA vaccinations and TTS. An analysis of cases of TTS reported to VAERS found only three after mRNA vaccination (See et al., 2022), translating into a reporting rate of 0.00855 per million doses, which the committee interpreted as likely representative of the background rate in the general population.

**Conclusion 5-1: The evidence favors rejection of a causal relationship between the BNT162b2 vaccine and thrombosis with thrombocytopenia syndrome.**

**Conclusion 5-2: The evidence favors rejection of a causal relationship between the mRNA-1273 vaccine and thrombosis with thrombocytopenia syndrome.**

The committee was not able to identify any data from comparative epidemiology studies on the association between Ad26.COV2.S and TTS. A study from VAERS estimated a reporting rate of 3.83 cases per 1 million doses of Ad26.COV2.S (See et al., 2022); these findings are consistent with the FDA evaluation of VAERS data (FDA, 2022b). The presence of anti-PF4 antibodies in individuals presenting with TTS after Ad26.COV2.S was deemed strong mechanistic evidence associating that vaccine with TTS, particularly when similar mechanistic data associating the ChAdOx1-S vaccine with TTS are taken into consideration. No evidence was available on a potential association with NVX-CoV2373.

**Conclusion 5-3: The evidence favors acceptance of a causal relationship between the Ad26.COV2.S vaccine and thrombosis with thrombocytopenia syndrome.**

**Conclusion 5-4: The evidence is inadequate to accept or reject a causal relationship between the NVX-CoV2373 vaccine and thrombosis with thrombocytopenia syndrome.**

## IMMUNE THROMBOCYTOPENIC PURPURA

---

**BOX 5-2**
**Conclusions for Immune Thrombocytopenic Purpura**

**Conclusion 5-5:** The evidence is inadequate to accept or reject a causal relationship between the BNT162b2 vaccine and immune thrombocytopenic purpura.

**Conclusion 5-6:** The evidence is inadequate to accept or reject a causal relationship between the mRNA-1273 vaccine and immune thrombocytopenic purpura.

**Conclusion 5-7:** The evidence is inadequate to accept or reject a causal relationship between the Ad26.COV2.S vaccine and immune thrombocytopenic purpura.

**Conclusion 5-8:** The evidence is inadequate to accept or reject a causal relationship between the NVX-CoV2373 vaccine and immune thrombocytopenic purpura.

---

### Background

ITP is an autoimmune disorder characterized primarily by a low platelet count, which can be associated with purpura and hemorrhagic episodes. It is often diagnosed through the exclusion of other causes of thrombocytopenia. IgG autoantibodies sensitize circulating platelets, leading to their accelerated removal by macrophages in the spleen and other components of the monocyte-macrophage system. Bone marrow responds by increasing platelet production. ITP is commonly observed in healthy children and young adults, often after a viral infection. The epidemiology varies; in children, spontaneous remission is common, whereas in adults, remission is rare, and patients are typically treated with a variety of therapies, including corticosteroids, rituximab, and thrombopoietin-mimetic agents.

The diagnosis of ITP is defined by a platelet count $<100 \times 10^9$ per L. Platelet counts of $100–150 \times 10^9$ per L are frequently encountered in apparently healthy individuals, and most individuals in this range are unlikely to develop more severe thrombocytopenia (Rodeghiero et al., 2009). The disease can be classified into different phases based on the duration postdiagnosis: newly diagnosed (within the first 3 months), persistent (3–12 months), chronic (over 12 months), and refractory (failure of splenectomy). ITP occurs with infections, such as HIV; malignancies, such as lymphoma; and autoimmune diseases, such as systemic lupus erythematosus. Drug-induced ITP is also notable, with several medications implicated in it.

Epidemiologically, the acute form of ITP affects children and adults, but in children, it is relatively benign, often resolving spontaneously within 3 months. Chronic ITP more frequently affects adults primarily aged 20–50 years, with a higher prevalence in women, and may present with prolonged bleeding episodes and fluctuating platelet counts.

### Mechanisms

ITP is highlighted by multiple immunological mechanisms, predominantly involving producing autoantibodies against platelet antigens. This autoimmune response is primarily driven by IgG autoantibodies targeting platelet membrane glycoproteins, such as GPIIb/IIIa and GPIb/IX (Kremer et al., 2022). Binding these autoantibodies to platelets tags them for destruction by the spleen's macrophages, leading to a precipitous decline in platelet count. This process is intricately associated with the adaptive immune system, where B-lymphocytes play a pivotal role in autoantibody production, and T-lymphocytes may contribute to the loss of tolerance to platelet antigens (Audia et al., 2021).

A particularly intriguing aspect of ITP is its association with vaccines, known as "vaccine-induced ITP." The exact immunological pathways are still being elucidated, but several hypotheses have been proposed. One suggests molecular mimicry, where vaccine antigens share structural similarities with platelet antigens, leading to cross-reactive immune responses (Segal and Shoenfeld, 2018). Another theory involves adjuvants, which can increase the immune response, potentially breaking the tolerance to self-antigens such as those found on platelets (McGonagle et al., 2021). Furthermore, the polyclonal activation of B cells by vaccines may inadvertently lead to producing autoantibodies against platelet antigens.

This ITP variant, although relatively rare, has been reported after various vaccinations, such as measles-mumps-rubella, varicella, and COVID-19 (Thomas et al., 2021). These cases are characterized by the rapid onset of thrombocytopenia, often within days to weeks. The immunological response to the vaccine's vector may trigger an autoimmune reaction in predisposed individuals, leading to platelet destruction. However, the absolute risk remains low, and it is rarely associated with significant bleeding.

Recurrent severe thrombocytopenia has been observed in 6.1 to 17 percent of patients with pre-existing ITP following vaccination against SARS-CoV-2 (Kuter, 2021; Lee et al., 2022; Mori et al., 2023). Most of these patients quickly recover with rescue therapy, usually consisting of corticosteroids with or without intravenous immunoglobulin, and major bleeding is uncommon. It is generally recommended that patients with pre-existing ITP still get vaccinated but that platelet counts should be monitored afterward. Recurrent ITP is not considered further in the text below.

## Epidemiological Evidence

Clinical trial results submitted to FDA for Emergency Use Authorization (EUA) and/or full approval do not indicate a signal regarding ITP and any of the vaccines under study (FDA, 2021d, 2023b,c,d). Table 5-2 presents seven studies that contributed to the causality assessment.

Shoaibi et al. (2023) followed an SCCS design to evaluate the risk of ITP after mRNA vaccines among Medicare beneficiaries aged 65+. Diagnosis codes from inpatient and outpatient claims were extracted; a medical review of health records of a random sample of cases was performed to validate the claims-based definition. From 91 cases of ITP identified in claims data and with health records available, only two were adjudicated as confirmed, one as probable, and six as possible. These statistics translated into a predictive positive value of 4 percent (1.37–11.11 percent), showing the high potential for misclassification based on diagnosis codes (Shoaibi et al., 2023). The limited validity of diagnosis codes in the detection of ITP was considered a major limitation of all studies that used them. As a result, the committee assigned limited weight to the epidemiology evidence in the causality conclusion. Shoaibi et al. (2023) found no association between the primary series of the BNT162b2 and mRNA-1273 and ITP; results were reported combining first and second doses under the primary series. No association was found between a booster dose of BNT162b2 and mRNA-1273 and the risk of ITP; however, the booster analysis was likely underpowered.

Two studies led by Simpson used National Health Service data from Scotland to evaluate the risk of ITP among other outcomes after administration of ChAdOx1-S and BNT162b2. The first study limited analyses to the first dose of each vaccine (Simpson et al., 2021), and the second evaluated risk after the second dose (Simpson et al., 2022). Both analyses constrained sampling to individuals aged 16+ and used read codes (equivalent to diagnosis codes) to define ITP. The assessment of the risk of ITP after first doses employed a matched case control nested within a cohort design; this analysis was complemented by a sensitivity analysis after an SCCS design (Simpson et al., 2021). The study evaluating risk of events after the second dose followed an SCCS design (Simpson et al., 2021). No significant association was found between the first dose of BNT162b2 and ITP (relative risk [RR] 0.54, 95% CI: 0.10–3.02) (Simpson et al., 2021). The risk of ITP did not significantly differ between days 0–27 after the second dose of BNT162b2 and the baseline period (Simpson et al., 2022). However, these findings are limited by a small number of ITP events (nine). Using Read codes is a major limitation of the analysis. The authors tried to overcome this limitation by the reporting of platelet counts for individuals with post-vaccination ITP; however, data were only available for a nonrepresentative share of cases.

**TABLE 5-2** Epidemiological Studies in the Immune Thrombocytopenic Purpura Evidence Review

| Author | Study Design and Control Group | Location | Data Source | Vaccine(s) | Age Range | N | Number of Events | Results (95% CI) |
|---|---|---|---|---|---|---|---|---|
| Burn et al. (2022a) | Cohort, historical comparator | United Kingdom | Electronic health records | BNT162b2 | 20+ | 5.6 million vaccinees | Dose 1: 21 Dose 2: 9 | Dose 1: SIR 1.28 (0.83–1.96)<br><br>Dose 2: SIR 0.79 (0.41–1.52) |
| Burn et al. (2022b) | Cohort, historical comparator | Spain | Electronic health records | BNT162b2 | 20+ | 4.5 million vaccinees | Dose 1: 97 Dose 2: 61 | Dose 1: SIR 1.03 (0.84–1.26)<br><br>Dose 2: SIR 0.69 (0.53–0.88) |
| Klein et al. (2021) | Cohort | United States | Vaccine Safety Datalink | BNT162b2 | 12+ | 6.8 million doses | BNT162b2 and mRNA-1273 combined: 48 | BNT162b2 and mRNA-1273 combined: RR 1.12 (0.65–1.97) |
|  |  |  |  | mRNA-1273 |  | 5.1 million doses |  |  |
| Shoaibi et al. (2023) | Self-controlled case series design | United States | Medicare claims | BNT162b2 | 65+ | Doses 1 and 2: 3.4 million vaccinees | Doses 1 and 2: 472<br><br>Booster dose: 24 | Doses 1 and 2: IRR 1.12 (0.94–1.33)<br><br>Booster dose: IRR 1.17 (0.66–2.04) |
|  |  |  |  | mRNA-1273 |  | Booster dose: 6.2 million vaccinees | Doses 1 and 2: 318<br><br>Booster dose: 22 | Doses 1 and 2: IRR 1.08 (0.86–1.37)<br><br>Booster dose: IRR 1.54 (0.82–2.91) |
| Simpson et al. (2021) | Matched case control nested within a cohort | Scotland | National Health Service data | BNT162b2 | 16+ | Dose 1: 2.5 million vaccinees | 45 | RR 0.54 (0.10–3.02) |
| Simpson et al. (2022) | Self-controlled case series | Scotland | National Health Service data | BNT162b2 | 16+ | Dose 2: 3.6 million vaccinees | 9 | IRR 1.68 (0.80–3.52) |
| Torabi et al. (2022) | Self-controlled case series | Wales | Electronic health records | BNT162b2 | 16+ | 2.1 million vaccinees | <10 for each risk period | Dose 1, days 0–7: IRR 2.80 (1.21–6.49)<br><br>Dose 2: IRR 0.47 (0.07–3.40)<br><br>Booster dose: IRR 0.89 (0.20–4.01) |

NOTES: BNT162b2 refers to the COVID-19 vaccine manufactured by Pfizer-BioNTech under the name Comirnaty®. mRNA-1273 refers to the COVID-19 vaccine manufactured by Moderna under the name Spikevax®. Shoaibi et al. (2023) combined the number of BNT162b2 and mRNA-1273 vaccinees. The primary series for mRNA vaccines is two doses. Number of events refers to events in vaccinees only. CI: confidence interval; IRR: incidence rate ratio; RR: relative risk; SIR: standardized incidence ratio.
SOURCES: Burn et al., 2022a,b; Klein et al., 2021; Shoaibi et al., 2023; Simpson et al., 2021, 2022; Torabi et al., 2022.

Two studies led by Burn compared the risk of ITP among other outcomes after ChAdOx1-S and BNT162b2 against historical rates. The first used UK electronic health record data for individuals aged 20+ (Burn et al., 2022a). ITP events were defined using diagnosis codes; however, the specific codes used were not reported. The risk of ITP in the 28 days after either the first or the second dose of ChAdOx1-S and BNT162b2 was compared against individuals in the database from January 2017 to December 2019. The committee noted that the use of historical background rates could have biased results, as the background incidence of ITP may have been lower during the COVID-19 pandemic compared to the pre-pandemic period (Sakurai et al., 2023). Individuals with a recorded diagnosis of ITP in the year before vaccination were excluded. ITP events after the first dose of ChAdOx1-S significantly exceeded the expectation based on historical rates (standardized incidence ratio [SIR] 1.79, 95% CI: 1.33–2.39) (Burn et al., 2022a). The number of ITP events after the second dose of ChAdOx1-S or the first or second dose of BNT162b2 was not significantly different from expectations. These results were limited by the lack of adjustment for potential differences in clinical characteristics between the historical comparators and the vaccinated people and the low validity of using diagnosis codes.

The second study by Burn et al. (2022b) used electronic health record data from Spain to compare the cases of ITP observed in the 21 days after the first dose of ChAdOx1-S or the first and second doses of BNT162b2 against historical rates from 2017. No definition was provided for how ITP was determined. Analyses were limited to individuals aged 20+, and those with ITP in the year before vaccination were excluded. No adjustment for potential differences in clinical characteristics between vaccinated subjects and historical comparators was conducted. ITP cases after the first dose of ChAdOx1-S ($n = 12$) were significantly lower than expected based on historical rates (SIR 0.48, 95% CI: 0.27–0.85) (Burn et al., 2022b). ITP cases after the first dose of BNT162b2 ($n = 97$) were not significantly different from expectations; however, those after the second dose of BNT162b2 ($n = 61$) were significantly lower than expected (SIR 0.69, 95% CI: 0.53–0.88) (Burn et al., 2022b). The association of the first dose of ChAdOx1-S and the second dose of BNT162b2 with a decreased risk of ITP may indicate residual confounding.

Klein et al. (2021) described under the TTS section, compared the risk of ITP after first and second doses of BNT162b2 and mRNA-1273 combined. ITP was defined using diagnosis codes from emergency department and inpatient and outpatient claims (Klein et al., 2021). No significant differences were observed in the risk of ITP in days 1–21 post-vaccination compared to days 22–42 (RR 1.12, 95% CI: 0.65–1.97).

Torabi et al. (2022) used electronic health record data from Wales and evaluated the risk of ITP after first and second doses of BNT162b2. ITP was defined using diagnosis codes. The study incorporated an SCCS method and compared the risk of events in the 28 days after vaccination against a 90-day prevaccination baseline period and a post-vaccination control period (median of 72 days). The study population included 2.1 million individuals aged 16+. They found an increased risk of ITP on days 0–7 after the first dose of BNT162b2 (incidence rate ratio [IRR] 2.80, 95% CI 1.21–6.49) but not on days 8–14, 15–21, or 22–28, nor was there an increased risk 0–7 days after dose 2 or a booster dose (Torabi et al., 2022). Their findings are limited by the number of events, which was fewer than 10 for each of the 7-day intervals (Torabi et al., 2022), and the high misclassification associated with diagnosis codes.

## Pharmacovigilance and Surveillance

In the briefing documents provided by the sponsor for the advisory committee convened to review the EUA amendment for the booster dose of Ad26.COV2.S, the manufacturer disclosed that ITP had been reported in the post-marketing setting (FDA, 2021b). The manufacturer reported analyzing a U.S.-based claims database and found an increased risk of ITP within 28, 42, and 90 days of vaccination, using both SCCS and comparative designs (RR estimates 1.86–2.22) (FDA, 2021b). This study was only briefly described by the manufacturer in the EUA addendum and not published; as a result, the committee was not able to evaluate the definition of ITP used and methodology employed. The manufacturer also conducted an analysis of ITP reports submitted to VAERS by July 31, 2021, and estimated an observed-to-expected ratio of 3.6 (95% CI: 3.0–4.1) for individuals 18–59 and 3.0 (95% CI: 2.4–3.8) for individuals 60+. In this evaluation, the manufacturer used a case definition of ITP that included reports with platelet counts below $100 \times 10^9$ per L (FDA, 2021b).

FDA conducted an independent investigation of ITP reports submitted to VAERS by September 30, 2021, and estimated an overall observed-to-expected ratio of 4.04 (95% CI: 3.42–4.72) in the 28 days after Ad26.COV2.S

(FDA, 2022a). This investigation, however, defined ITP as having a platelet count less than $150 \times 10^9$ per L or a diagnosis of thrombocytopenia without a documented platelet count. The committee considered this definition too imprecise, however, given the criteria for the diagnosis of ITP noted at the beginning of this section. An update using reports submitted to VAERS through December 2021 was published in the peer-reviewed literature (Woo and Dimova, 2022). In addition to the earlier definition of ITP, which was considered the base case, this FDA study also included a "narrow" definition, which only included cases with documented platelet counts below $100 \times 10^9$ per L; the observed-to-expected ratio decreased to 1.55 (95% CI: 1.20–1.98). The authors acknowledged multiple limitations, however, including the lack of adjudication of cases by hematologists. Several reports mentioned a "history of thrombocytopenia," and five had experienced "clinically significant thrombotic or thromboembolic events" without meeting the case definition of TTS, an atypical presentation for ITP. Given these methodologic concerns, the committee felt that the pharmacovigilance data were insufficient to support a causal relationship between Ad26.COV2.S and ITP.

FDA also reviewed pharmacovigilance data submitted to VAERS through February 4, 2021, looking at thrombocytopenia and ITP after mRNA vaccines (Welsh et al., 2021) and did not find an increased rate of reported cases.

### From Evidence to Conclusions

With the exception of Shoaibi et al. (2023), who performed a medical review of electronic health record data, the totality of the epidemiology evidence on the potential association of BNT162b2 and mRNA-1273 and ITP is based on diagnosis codes. Shoaibi et al. (2023) estimated that the use of diagnosis codes had a positive predictive value of 4.0 percent for case identification. As a result, the committee deemed the use of diagnosis codes in the ITP case definition a major limitation of the studies.

**Conclusion 5-5: The evidence is inadequate to accept or reject a causal relationship between the BNT162b2 vaccine and immune thrombocytopenic purpura.**

**Conclusion 5-6: The evidence is inadequate to accept or reject a causal relationship between the mRNA-1273 vaccine and immune thrombocytopenic purpura.**

No published comparative epidemiology assessments evaluated the potential association of Ad26.COV2.S with ITP. A manufacturer analysis (FDA, 2021b) of a U.S.-based claims database found an increased risk. As this study was not published, the committee was unable to assess the definition of ITP and methodological rigor. The manufacturer analysis of VAERS data through July 2021 and the initial FDA evaluation of reports through September were considered superseded by the FDA evaluation that included reports through December 2021. The narrow definition of ITP (platelet counts below $100 \times 10^9$ per L) yielded an observed-to-expected ratio of 1.55, considerably lower than that estimated with the definition that also included reports with platelet counts of 100–150 $\times 10^9$ per L. Additionally, there was a lack of evidence on a potential mechanism of action linking Ad26.COV2.S with ITP. No evidence was available on the association of NVX-CoV2373 with ITP.

**Conclusion 5-7: The evidence is inadequate to accept or reject a causal relationship between the Ad26.COV2.S vaccine and immune thrombocytopenic purpura.**

**Conclusion 5-8: The evidence is inadequate to accept or reject a causal relationship between the NVX-CoV2373 vaccine and immune thrombocytopenic purpura.**

## CAPILLARY LEAK SYNDROME

---

**BOX 5-3**
**Conclusions for Capillary Leak Syndrome**

**Conclusion 5-9:** The evidence is inadequate to accept or reject a causal relationship between the BNT162b2 vaccine and capillary leak syndrome.

**Conclusion 5-10:** The evidence is inadequate to accept or reject a causal relationship between the mRNA-1273 vaccine and capillary leak syndrome.

**Conclusion 5-11:** The evidence is inadequate to accept or reject a causal relationship between the Ad26.COV2.S vaccine and capillary leak syndrome.

**Conclusion 5-12:** The evidence is inadequate to accept or reject a causal relationship between the NVX-CoV2373 vaccine and capillary leak syndrome.

---

### Background

CLS, also known as "Clarkson disease," is a complex and potentially lethal condition characterized by an initial phase of nonspecific symptoms followed by the hallmark features of diffuse severe edema and hypovolemia, hemoconcentration, and hypoalbuminemia (Bichon et al., 2021). This condition is often triggered by factors such as drugs (including antitumor therapies), malignancy, infections (predominantly viral), and inflammatory diseases. Its pathophysiology involves severe, transient, and multifactorial endothelial disruption, the mechanisms of which remain unclear. Treatment is primarily empirical and symptomatic during the acute phase, with the addition of drugs that amplify cyclic adenosine monophosphate levels in severe cases. Prophylactic monthly polyvalent immunoglobulins are used to prevent relapses (Bichon et al., 2021; Siddall et al., 2017).

U.S. reports exist of fatal exacerbations of CLS in patients with mild-to-moderate COVID-19 symptoms (Bichon et al., 2021). In these cases, the clinical diagnostic triad for CLS (hypotension, hemoconcentration, hypoalbuminemia) was observed, indicating that individuals with known or suspected CLS may be at increased risk of a disease flare in the context of COVID-19 (Felten et al., 2021). The cytokine storm associated with COVID-19 is thought to potentially lead to a CLS flare; alternatively, the virus may directly affect endothelial cells (Mohseni Afshar et al., 2023). This highlights the need for increased vigilance in patients with CLS or related inflammatory diseases during the COVID-19 pandemic.

Diagnostically, CLS is identified clinically based on a symptomatic triad of hypotension, hemoconcentration, and hypoalbuminemia resulting from fluid extravasation. Blood tests are important for diagnosing CLS, looking for increased levels of hematocrit and hemoglobin, and low blood protein levels. The presence of abnormal monoclonal gammopathy (M protein) is also a diagnostic consideration (Kapoor et al., 2010).

Systemic CLS is a rare disorder, affecting fewer than 500 people worldwide. It predominantly occurs in middle-aged adults and is very rare in children (NORD, 2020). However, the actual incidence may be higher due to potential misdiagnosis (Kapoor et al., 2010).

### Mechanisms

CLS involves an increase in capillary permeability to proteins, leading to the loss of protein-rich fluid from the intravascular space to the interstitial space (Siddall et al., 2017). This phenomenon is most commonly associated with sepsis but can occur in a variety of other conditions, such as idiopathic systemic CLS, engraftment syndrome, differentiation syndrome, ovarian hyperstimulation syndrome, hemophagocytic lymph histiocytosis, viral hemorrhagic fevers, autoimmune diseases, snakebite, ricin poisoning, and adverse effects from certain drugs, such as some interleukins, monoclonal antibodies, and gemcitabine (Siddall et al., 2017). The diseases associated with CLS, including sepsis, often manifest with diffuse pitting edema, exudative serous cavity effusions, noncardiogenic pulmonary edema, hypotension, and sometimes hypovolemic shock with multiple-organ failure. Acute kidney injury is a common complication in these conditions, and cytokines are believed to play a significant role in acute kidney injury in CLS. Fluid management is critical in treating CLS, as both hypovolemia and hypotension can cause organ injury, and capillary leakage of administered fluid can worsen organ edema, leading to progressive organ injury (Ruggiero et al., 2022).

CLS is also strongly associated with cytokine activity states and an underrecognized early immune effect of checkpoint inhibitor treatment, which is more typically associated with cellular immune responses (Ruggiero et al., 2022). The interaction between checkpoint inhibitors, cellular immunity, cytokine action, and endothelial damage has been noted in individuals with CLS after checkpoint inhibitor treatment. This suggests that CLS may be an unusual effect of immunotherapy, resulting from complex interactions between cellular immunity and cytokine activation, and its expression likely depends on inherent immune variation (Wong So et al., 2023).

## Epidemiological Evidence

Clinical trial results submitted to FDA for EUA and/or full approval do not indicate a signal regarding CLS and any of the vaccines under study (FDA, 2021d, 2023b,c,d). The committee failed to identify any comparative epidemiology studies evaluating CLS after COVID-19 vaccination. A study from the European pharmacovigilance database EudraVigilance reported that CLS emerged as a new adverse event after immunization associated with COVID-19 vaccination. Between January 1, 2021, and January 14, 2022, there were 36 CLS case reports associated with BNT162b2, three with mRNA-1273, 36 with ChAdOx1-S, and nine with Ad26.COV2.S. A disproportionality analysis of these reports associated mRNA vaccines with a decreased CLS reporting probability compared to viral vaccines (rate of return 0.5, 95% CI: 0.3–0.7) (Ruggiero et al., 2022). This study evaluated the onset of CLS after COVID-19 mRNA vaccines compared to viral vector vaccines. Cytokine release after T cell activation could be involved in CLS, but a precise mechanism has not yet been identified (Ruggiero et al., 2022).

## From Evidence to Conclusions

No comparative epidemiology studies evaluated the risk of CLS with COVID-19 vaccinations. Pharmacovigilance data available were inconclusive. Despite plausible mechanistic hypotheses that link potential mechanisms for CLS with the COVID-19 vaccinations (e.g., cytokine activation, endothelial cell perturbation), no available mechanistic data clearly link vaccination with the clinical development of CLS.

**Conclusion 5-9: The evidence is inadequate to accept or reject a causal relationship between the BNT162b2 vaccine and capillary leak syndrome.**

**Conclusion 5-10: The evidence is inadequate to accept or reject a causal relationship between the mRNA-1273 vaccine and capillary leak syndrome.**

**Conclusion 5-11: The evidence is inadequate to accept or reject a causal relationship between the Ad26.COV2.S vaccine and capillary leak syndrome.**

**Conclusion 5-12: The evidence is inadequate to accept or reject a causal relationship between the NVX-CoV2373 vaccine and capillary leak syndrome.**

# REFERENCES

Andrews, N. J., J. Stowe, M. E. Ramsay, and E. Miller. 2022. Risk of venous thrombotic events and thrombocytopenia in sequential time periods after ChAdOx1 and BNT162b2 COVID-19 vaccines: A national cohort study in England. *Lancet Regional Health—Europe* 13:100260. https://doi.org/10.1016/j.lanepe.2021.100260.

Audia, S., M. Mahevas, M. Nivet, S. Ouandji, M. Ciudad, and B. Bonnotte. 2021. Immune thrombocytopenia: Recent advances in pathogenesis and treatments. *HemaSphere* 5(6):e574. https://doi.org/10.1097/HS9.0000000000000574.

Bichon, A., J. Bourenne, M. Gainnier, and J. Carvelli. 2021. Capillary leak syndrome: State of the art in 2021. *Journal of Internal Medicine* 42(11):789–796. https://doi.org/10.1016/j.revmed.2021.05.012.

Burn, E., X. Li, A. Delmestri, N. Jones, T. Duarte-Salles, C. Reyes, E. Martinez-Hernandez, E. Marti, K. M. C. Verhamme, P. R. Rijnbeek, V. Y. Strauss, and D. Prieto-Alhambra. 2022a. Thrombosis and thrombocytopenia after vaccination against and infection with SARS-CoV-2 in the United Kingdom. *Nature Communications* 13(1):7167. https://doi.org/10.1038/s41467-022-34668-w.

Burn, E., E. Roel, A. Pistillo, S. Fernández-Bertolín, M. Aragón, B. Raventós, C. Reyes, K. Verhamme, P. Rijnbeek, X. Li, V. Y. Strauss, D. Prieto-Alhambra, and T. Duarte-Salles. 2022b. Thrombosis and thrombocytopenia after vaccination against and infection with SARS-CoV-2 in Catalonia, Spain. *Nature Communications* 13(1):7169. https://doi.org/10.1038/s41467-022-34669-9.

Chen, R., and J. Buttery. 2021. *Updated Brighton Collaboration case definition of thrombosis with thrombocytopenia syndrome (TTS)*. https://brightoncollaboration.org/wp-content/uploads/2023/08/TTS-Updated-Brighton-Collaboration-Case-Defintion-Draft-Nov-11-2021.pdf (accessed December 12, 2023).

FDA (Food and Drug Administration). 2021a. *BLA clinical review memorandum—COMIRNATY*. https://www.fda.gov/media/152256/download (accessed December 5, 2023).

FDA. 2021b. *Vaccines and Related Biological Products Advisory Committee October 14–15, 2021 meeting announcement*. https://www.fda.gov/advisory-committees/advisory-committee-calendar/vaccines-and-related-biological-products-advisory-committee-october-14-15-2021-meeting-announcement (accessed December 12, 2023).

FDA. 2021c. *FDA and CDC lift recommended pause on Johnson & Johnson (Janssen) COVID-19 vaccine use following thorough safety review*. https://www.fda.gov/news-events/press-announcements/fda-and-cdc-lift-recommended-pause-johnson-johnson-janssen-covid-19-vaccine-use-following-thorough (accessed March 8, 2024).

FDA. 2021d. *Emergency use authorization (EUA) amendment for an unapproved product review memorandum*. https://www.fda.gov/media/153439/download (accessed May 3, 2023).

FDA. 2022a. CBER assessment of new safety information on immune thrombocytopenia (ITP) following administration of the Janssen COVID-19 vaccine. Center for Biologics Evaluation and Research.

FDA. 2022b. *BLA clinical review memorandum—SPIKEVAX*. https://www.fda.gov/media/156342/download (accessed December 5, 2023).

FDA. 2023a. *Coronavirus (COVID-19) update: FDA authorizes changes to simplify use of bivalent mRNA COVID-19 vaccines*. https://www.fda.gov/news-events/press-announcements/coronavirus-covid-19-update-fda-authorizes-changes-simplify-use-bivalent-mrna-covid-19-vaccines (accessed December 12, 2023).

FDA. 2023b. *BLA clinical review memorandum—COMIRNATY*. https://www.fda.gov/media/172333/download?attachment (accessed December 5, 2023).

FDA. 2023c. *BLA clinical review memorandum—SPIKEVAX*. https://www.fda.gov/media/172357/download?attachment (accessed December 5, 2023).

FDA. 2023d. *Emergency use authorization (EUA) for an unapproved product review memorandum*. https://www.fda.gov/media/168233/download?attachment (accessed December 5, 2023).

Felten, R., M. Scherlinger, A. Guffroy, V. Poindron, A. Meyer, M. Giannini, A. S. Korganow, C. Sordet, E. Chatelus, R. M. Javier, A. Meyer, L. Pijnenburg, J. F. Kleinmann, J. E. Gottenberg, J. Sibilia, T. Martin, and L. Arnaud. 2021. Incidence and predictors of COVID-19 and flares in patients with rare autoimmune diseases: A systematic survey and serological study at a national reference center in France. *Arthritis Research & Therapy* 23(1):188. https://doi.org/10.1186/s13075-021-02565-0.

Greinacher, A., T. Thiele, T. E. Warkentin, K. Weisser, P. A. Kyrle, and S. Eichinger. 2021. Thrombotic thrombocytopenia after ChAdOx1 nCoV-19 vaccination. *New England Journal of Medicine* 384(22):2092–2101. https://doi.org/10.1056/NEJMoa2104840.

Higgins, H., N. Andrews, J. Stowe, G. Amirthalingam, M. Ramsay, G. Bahra, A. Hackett, K. A. Breen, M. Desborough, D. Khan, H. Leary, C. Sweeney, E. Hutchinson, S. E. Shapiro, C. Lees, J. Dhanapal, P. K. MacCallum, S. Burke, V. McDonald, N. M. A. Entwistle, S. Booth, C. J. Atchison, and B. J. Hunt. 2022. Risk of thrombosis with thrombocytopenia syndrome after COVID-19 vaccination before the recognition of vaccine-induced thrombocytopenia and thrombosis: A self-controlled case series study in England. *Research and Practice in Thrombosis and Haemostasis* 6(3):e12698. https:// doi.org/10.1002/rth2.12698.

Huynh, A., D. M. Arnold, J. G. Kelton, J. W. Smith, P. Horsewood, R. Clare, A. Guarné, and I. Nazy. 2019. Characterization of platelet factor 4 amino acids that bind pathogenic antibodies in heparin-induced thrombocytopenia. *Journal of Thrombosis and Haemostasis* 17(2):389–399. https://doi.org/https://doi.org/10.1111/jth.14369.

Huynh, A., D. M. Arnold, N. Ivetic, R. Clare, M. Hadzi-Tosev, Y. Liu, J. W. Smith, A. L. Bissola, M. Daka, J. G. Kelton, and I. Nazy. 2023. Antibodies against platelet factor 4 and the risk of cerebral venous sinus thrombosis in patients with vaccine-induced immune thrombotic thrombocytopenia. *Journal of Thrombosis and Haemostasis* 21(10):2833–2843. https://doi.org/10.1016/j.jtha.2023.06.026.

Jay, R. M., and T. E. Warkentin. 2008. Fatal heparin-induced thrombocytopenia (HIT) during warfarin thromboprophylaxis after orthopedic surgery: Another example of "spontaneous" HIT? *Journal of Thrombosis and Haemostasis* 6(9):1598–1600. https://doi.org/10.1111/j.1538-7836.2008.03040.x.

Kanack, A. J., and A. Padmanabhan. 2022. Vaccine-induced immune thrombotic thrombocytopenia. *Best Practice & Research: Clinical Haematology* 35(3):101381. https://doi.org/10.1016/j.beha.2022.101381.

Kapoor, P., P. T. Greipp, E. W. Schaefer, S. J. Mandrekar, A. H. Kamal, N. C. Gonzalez-Paz, S. Kumar, and P. R. Greipp. 2010. Idiopathic systemic capillary leak syndrome (Clarkson's Disease): The Mayo Clinic experience. *Mayo Clinic Proceedings* 85(10):905–912. https://doi.org/10.4065/mcp.2010.0159.

Klein, N. P., N. Lewis, K. Goddard, B. Fireman, O. Zerbo, K. E. Hanson, J. G. Donahue, E. O. Kharbanda, A. Naleway, J. C. Nelson, S. Xu, W. K. Yih, J. M. Glanz, J. T. B. Williams, S. J. Hambidge, B. J. Lewin, T. T. Shimabukuro, F. DeStefano, and E. S. Weintraub. 2021. Surveillance for adverse events after COVID-19 mRNA vaccination. *JAMA* 326(14):1390–1399. https://doi.org/10.1001/jama.2021.15072.

Kremer, V., L. de Chaisemartin, and F. Jonsson. 2022. The role of neutrophils in antibody-driven autoimmune cytopenias. *International Journal of Biochemistry and Cell Biology* 147:106231. https://doi.org/10.1016/j.biocel.2022.106231.

Kuter, D. J. 2021. Exacerbation of immune thrombocytopenia following COVID-19 vaccination. *British Journal of Haematology* 195(3):365–370. https://doi.org/10.1111/bjh.17645.

Lee, E. J., M. Beltrami-Moreira, H. Al-Samkari, A. Cuker, J. DiRaimo, T. Gernsheimer, A. Kruse, C. Kessler, C. Kruse, A. D. Leavitt, A. I. Lee, H. A. Liebman, A. C. Newland, A. E. Ray, M. D. Tarantino, J. Thachil, D. J. Kuter, D. B. Cines, and J. B. Bussel. 2022. SARS-CoV-2 vaccination and ITP in patients with de novo or preexisting ITP. *Blood* 139(10):1564–1574. https://doi.org/10.1182/blood.2021013411.

Leung, H. H. L., J. Perdomo, Z. Ahmadi, S. S. Zheng, F. N. Rashid, A. Enjeti, S. B. Ting, J. J. H. Chong, and B. H. Chong. 2022. Netosis and thrombosis in vaccine-induced immune thrombotic thrombocytopenia. *Nature Communications* 13(1):5206. https://doi.org/10.1038/s41467-022-32946-1.

Li, X., E. Burn, T. Duarte-Salles, C. Yin, C. Reich, A. Delmestri, K. Verhamme, P. Rijnbeek, M. A. Suchard, K. Li, M. Mosseveld, L. H. John, M. A. Mayer, J. M. Ramirez-Anguita, C. Cohet, V. Strauss, and D. Prieto-Alhambra. 2022. Comparative risk of thrombosis with thrombocytopenia syndrome or thromboembolic events associated with different COVID-19 vaccines: International network cohort study from five European countries and the U.S. *British Journal of Medicine* 379:e071594. https://doi.org/10.1136/bmj-2022-071594.

McGonagle, D., G. De Marco, and C. Bridgewood. 2021. Mechanisms of immunothrombosis in vaccine-induced thrombotic thrombocytopenia (VITT) compared to natural SARS-CoV-2 infection. *Journal of Autoimmunity* 121:102662. https:// doi.org/10.1016/j.jaut.2021.102662.

Mohseni Afshar, Z., M. Barary, A. Babazadeh, A. Tavakoli Pirzaman, R. Hosseinzadeh, A. Alijanpour, A. Allahgholipour, S. R. Miri, T. T. Sio, M. J. M. Sullman, K. Carson-Chahhoud, and S. Ebrahimpour. 2023. The role of cytokines and their antagonists in the treatment of COVID-19 patients. *Reviews in Medical Virology* 33(1):e2372. https://doi.org/10.1002/ rmv.2372.

Mori, A., M. Onozawa, M. Kobayashi, S. Tsukamoto, H. Senjo, T. Ishio, E. Yokoyama, K. Izumiyama, M. Saito, H. Muraki, M. Morioka, T. Teshima, and T. Kondo. 2023. Humoral response to mRNA-based COVID-19 vaccine in patients with immune thrombocytopenia. *British Journal of Haematology* 200(6):717–721. https://doi.org/10.1111/bjh.18578.

NORD (National Organization for Rare Disorders). 2020. Systemic capillary leak syndrome. https://rarediseases.org/rare-diseases/systemic-capillary-leak-syndrome (accessed February 22, 2024).

Pavord, S., M. Scully, B. J. Hunt, W. Lester, C. Bagot, B. Craven, A. Rampotas, G. Ambler, and M. Makris. 2021. Clinical features of vaccine-induced immune thrombocytopenia and thrombosis. *New England Journal of Medicine* 385(18):1680–1689. https://doi.org/10.1056/NEJMoa2109908.

Rodeghiero, F., R. Stasi, T. Gernsheimer, M. Michel, D. Provan, D. M. Arnold, J. B. Bussel, D. B. Cines, B. H. Chong, N. Cooper, B. Godeau, K. Lechner, M. G. Mazzucconi, R. McMillan, M. A. Sanz, P. Imbach, V. Blanchette, T. Kuhne, M. Ruggeri, and J. N. George. 2009. Standardization of terminology, definitions and outcome criteria in immune thrombocytopenic purpura of adults and children: Report from an international working group. *Blood* 113(11):2386–2393. https://doi.org/10.1182/blood-2008-07-162503.

Ruggiero, R., N. Balzano, R. Di Napoli, A. Mascolo, P. M. Berrino, C. Rafaniello, L. Sportiello, F. Rossi, and A. Capuano. 2022. Capillary leak syndrome following COVID-19 vaccination: Data from the European pharmacovigilance database EudraVigilance. *Frontiers in Immunology* 13:956825. https://doi.org/10.3389/fimmu.2022.956825.

Sakurai, M., Y. Kogure, K. Mizuno, E. Matsuki, and K. Kataoka. 2023. Long-term reduction in the incidence of aplastic anemia and immune thrombocytopenia during the COVID-19 pandemic. *Haematologica* 108(9):2546–2550. https://doi.org/10.3324/haematol.2022.282351.

Schultz, N. H., I. H. Sørvoll, A. E. Michelsen, L. A. Munthe, F. Lund-Johansen, M. T. Ahlen, M. Wiedmann, A.-H. Aamodt, T. H. Skattør, and G. E. Tjønnfjord. 2021. Thrombosis and thrombocytopenia after ChAdOx1 NCOV-19 vaccination. *New England Journal of Medicine* 384(22):2124–2130.

Scully, M., D. Singh, R. Lown, A. Poles, T. Solomon, M. Levi, D. Goldblatt, P. Kotoucek, W. Thomas, and W. Lester. 2021. Pathologic antibodies to platelet factor 4 after ChAdOx1 NCOV-19 vaccination. *New England Journal of Medicine* 384(23):2202–2211. https://doi.org/10.1056/NEJMoa2105385.

See, I., J. R. Su, A. Lale, E. J. Woo, A. Y. Guh, T. T. Shimabukuro, M. B. Streiff, A. K. Rao, A. P. Wheeler, S. F. Beavers, A. P. Durbin, K. Edwards, E. Miller, T. A. Harrington, A. Mba-Jonas, N. Nair, D. T. Nguyen, K. R. Talaat, V. C. Urrutia, S. C. Walker, C. B. Creech, T. A. Clark, F. DeStefano, and K. R. Broder. 2021. U.S. case reports of cerebral venous sinus thrombosis with thrombocytopenia after Ad26.COV2.S vaccination, March 2 to April 21, 2021. *JAMA* 325(24):2448–2456. https://doi.org/10.1001/jama.2021.7517.

See, I., A. Lale, P. Marquez, M. B. Streiff, A. P. Wheeler, N. K. Tepper, E. J. Woo, K. R. Broder, K. M. Edwards, R. Gallego, A. I. Geller, K. A. Jackson, S. Sharma, K. R. Talaat, E. B. Walter, I. J. Akpan, T. L. Ortel, V. C. Urrutia, S. C. Walker, J. C. Yui, T. T. Shimabukuro, A. Mba-Jonas, J. R. Su, and D. K. Shay. 2022. Case series of thrombosis with thrombocytopenia syndrome after COVID-19 vaccination—United States, December 2020 to August 2021. *Annals of Internal Medicine* 175(4):513–522. https://doi.org/10.7326/m21-4502.

Segal, Y., and Y. Shoenfeld. 2018. Vaccine-induced autoimmunity: The role of molecular mimicry and immune crossreaction. *Cellular & Molecular Immunology* 15(6):586–594. https://doi.org/10.1038/cmi.2017.151.

Shoaibi, A., P. C. Lloyd, H. L. Wong, T. C. Clarke, Y. Chillarige, R. Do, M. Hu, Y. Jiao, A. Kwist, A. Lindaas, K. Matuska, R. McEvoy, M. Ondari, S. Parulekar, X. Shi, J. Wang, Y. Lu, J. Obidi, C. K. Zhou, J. A. Kelman, R. A. Forshee, and S. A. Anderson. 2023. Evaluation of potential adverse events following COVID-19 mRNA vaccination among adults aged 65 years and older: Two self-controlled studies in the U.S. *Vaccine* 41(32):4666–4678. https://doi.org/10.1016/j.vaccine.2023.06.014.

Siddall, E., M. Khatri, and J. Radhakrishnan. 2017. Capillary leak syndrome: Etiologies, pathophysiology, and management. *Kidney International* 92(1):37–46. https://doi.org/10.1016/j.kint.2016.11.029.

Simpson, C. R., T. Shi, E. Vasileiou, S. V. Katikireddi, S. Kerr, E. Moore, C. McCowan, U. Agrawal, S. A. Shah, L. D. Ritchie, J. Murray, J. Pan, D. T. Bradley, S. J. Stock, R. Wood, A. Chuter, J. Beggs, H. R. Stagg, M. Joy, R. S. M. Tsang, S. de Lusignan, R. Hobbs, R. A. Lyons, F. Torabi, S. Bedston, M. O'Leary, A. Akbari, J. McMenamin, C. Robertson, and A. Sheikh. 2021. First-dose ChAdOx1 and BNT162b2 COVID-19 vaccines and thrombocytopenic, thromboembolic and hemorrhagic events in Scotland. *Nature Medicine* 27(7):1290–1297. https://doi.org/10.1038/s41591-021-01408-4.

Simpson, C. R., S. Kerr, S. V. Katikireddi, C. McCowan, L. D. Ritchie, J. Pan, S. J. Stock, I. Rudan, R. S. M. Tsang, S. de Lusignan, F. D. R. Hobbs, A. Akbari, R. A. Lyons, C. Robertson, and A. Sheikh. 2022. Second-dose ChAdOx1 and BNT162b2 COVID-19 vaccines and thrombocytopenic, thromboembolic and hemorrhagic events in Scotland. *Nature Communications* 13(1):4800. https://doi.org/10.1038/s41467-022-32264-6.

Singh, A., F. Toma, G. Uzun, T. R. Wagner, L. Pelzl, J. Zlamal, V. Freytag, K. Weich, S. Nowak-Harnau, U. Rothbauer, K. Althaus, and T. Bakchoul. 2022. The interaction between anti-PF4 antibodies and anticoagulants in vaccine-induced thrombotic thrombocytopenia. *Blood* 139(23):3430–3438. https://doi.org/10.1182/blood.2021013839.

Thomas, W., A. Albano, D. Kirkel, N. Rouhizad, and F. Arinze. 2021. Immune thrombocytopenic purpura following administration of mRNA-based SARS-CoV-2 and MMR vaccinations: A cautionary tale. *Case Reports in Infectious Diseases* 2021:2704249. https://doi.org/10.1155/2021/2704249.

Torabi, F., S. Bedston, E. Lowthian, A. Akbari, R. K. Owen, D. T. Bradley, U. Agrawal, P. Collins, R. Fry, L. J. Griffiths, J. Beggs, G. Davies, J. Hollinghurst, J. Lyons, H. Abbasizanjani, S. Cottrell, M. Perry, R. Roberts, A. Azcoaga-Lorenzo, A. F. Fagbamigbe, T. Shi, R. S. M. Tsang, C. Robertson, F. D. R. Hobbs, S. de Lusignan, C. McCowan, M. Gravenor, C. R. Simpson, A. Sheikh, and R. A. Lyons. 2022. Risk of thrombocytopenic, haemorrhagic and thromboembolic disorders following COVID-19 vaccination and positive test: A self-controlled case series analysis in Wales. *Scientific Reports* 12(1):16406. https://doi.org/10.1038/s41598-022-20118-6.

Warkentin, T. E. 2022. Platelet-activating anti-PF4 disorders: An overview. *Seminars in Hematology* 59(2):59–71. https://doi.org/10.1053/j.seminhematol.2022.02.005.

Warkentin, T. E., A. Greinacher, A. Koster, and A. M. Lincoff. 2008. Treatment and prevention of heparin-induced thrombocytopenia: American College of Chest Physicians evidence-based clinical practice guidelines (8th edition). *Chest* 133(6 Suppl):340s–380s. https://doi.org/10.1378/chest.08-0677.

Welsh, K. J., J. Baumblatt, W. Chege, R. Goud, and N. Nair. 2021. Thrombocytopenia including immune thrombocytopenia after receipt of mRNA COVID-19 vaccines reported to the Vaccine Adverse Event Reporting System (VAERS). *Vaccine* 39(25):3329–3332. https://doi.org/10.1016/j.vaccine.2021.04.054.

Wong So, J., F. Bouibede, A. P. Jonville-Bera, F. Maillot, F. Barbier, and B. Largeau. 2023. Immune checkpoint inhibitor-associated capillary leak syndrome: A systematic review and a worldwide pharmacovigilance study. *Journal of Internal Medicine* 294(1):58–68. https://doi.org/10.1111/joim.13641.

Woo, E. J., and R. B. Dimova. 2022. Thrombocytopenia after Ad.26.COV2.S COVID-19 vaccine: Reports to the Vaccine Adverse Event Reporting System. *Vaccine* 40(31):4116–4120. https://doi.org/10.1016/j.vaccine.2022.05.078.

# 6

# Vascular Conditions and COVID-19 Vaccines: Myocardial Infarction, Stroke, Pulmonary Embolism, Deep Vein Thrombosis, and Venous Thromboembolism

This chapter describes the potential relationship between COVID-19 vaccines and potential vascular-related harms: myocardial infarction (MI), ischemic stroke, hemorrhagic stroke (HS), deep vein thrombosis (DVT), pulmonary embolism (PE), and the composite venous thromboembolism (VTE).

Each outcome is addressed in a separate section in this chapter. Twelve scientific reports were selected for evaluation of the six clinical outcomes considered; these are summarized and referenced in Table 6-1. Many of these reports addressed more than one clinical outcome and more than one vaccine. Additionally, some of these reports included outcomes and vaccines that were addressed in other chapters of this report. The 12 reports in Table 6-1 generally represented large populations, with only one study from the United States, conducted on the Medicare populations (persons 65+); multiple studies from the United Kingdom and Scandinavia; two from the French National Health Data System (covering different age groups); and individual studies from Israel, Hong Kong, Japan, Spain, and Malaysia. These studies may in some sense represent broad global coverage, but many countries, cultures, and health systems were not covered, including most low- and middle-income countries. Although these studies applied standard epidemiological methods and analytical techniques overall, they did not appear to have followed a common or harmonized protocol. For example, they varied in how age groups were presented and in the post-vaccination exposure interval, although many centered on approximately 28 days. One study examined outcomes for weeks 1 and 2 separately, resulting in smaller sample sizes. None of the reports emphasized vaccine outcomes in children, which is unsurprising given the emphasis on the chronic vascular conditions of older persons. Only a minority of the studies adjusted their analytic models for a history of comorbid conditions. Several studies used patient self-controls, with a few employing case-control or cohort designs, including non-immunized comparator groups (Grosso et al., 2011). Further information can be found on the studies as part of the descriptions of the vaccine–disease outcomes in the respective sections of this chapter.

Some other general methodological issues of potential import to the reports were discussed sparingly or not at all, such as the potential health impact of multiple vaccines at the same time of administration (e.g., COVID-19 and influenza). A particularly interesting and difficult issue is possible exposure to severe acute respiratory syndrome coronavirus-2 (SARS-CoV-2) simultaneously with vaccination, although some reports provided separate comparator groups of patients with documented SARS-CoV-2 infection, possibly making it more difficult to distinguish harms caused by vaccination from those caused by COVID-19 infection. The studies also varied in whether sources of patient data included both inpatient and ambulatory care, although all studies reported information on

**TABLE 6-1** Epidemiological Studies in the Vascular Conditions Evidence Review

| Author | Study Design and Comparison Group | Location | Data Source | Vaccine(s) | Age Range | Total Sample Size |
|---|---|---|---|---|---|---|
| Ab Rahman et al. (2022) | Self-controlled case series | Malaysia | Malaysia Vaccine Administration System (myVAS) | BNT162b2 | 18–60+ years | 20 million |
| Barda et al. (2021) | Cohort, unvaccinated individuals | Israel | Clalit Health Services | BNT162b2 | 16+ years | 1.7 million |
| Botton et al. (2022) | Self-controlled case series | France | French National Health Data System | BNT162b2, mRNA-1273, Ad26.COV2.S | 18–74 years | 46.5 million |
| Burn et al. (2022a) | Cohort, historical comparator | UK | Electronic health records | BNT162b2 | 20+ years | 5.6 million |
| Burn et al. (2022b) | Cohort, historical comparator | Spain | Electronic health records | BNT162b2 | 20+ years | 4.6 million |
| Chui et al. (2022) | Self-controlled case series | China | Electronic health records | BNT162b2 | 16+ years | 2.9 million (BNT162b2 vaccinees) |
| Hippisley-Cox et al. (2021) | Self-controlled | England | National Immunization Management System data | BNT162b2 | 16+ years | 29 million |
| Hviid et al. (2022) | Nationwide exploratory retrospective cohort, unvaccinated comparison group | Denmark | Danish Civil Registration System | BNT162b2 | 16–64 years | 355,209 |
| Jabagi et al. (2022) | Self-controlled case series | France | French National Health Data System | BNT162b2 | 75+ years | 3.9 million |
| Patone et al. (2021) | Self-controlled case series | Scotland | English National Immunisation (NIMS) Database | BNT162b2 | 16–90+ years | 12.1 million |
| Shoaibi et al. (2023) | Self-controlled case series | US | Medicare claims | BNT162b2, mRNA-1273 | 65+ years | 3.3 million (Doses 1 and 2) |
| Whiteley et al. (2022) | Cohort | England | English NHS, General Practice Extraction Service Data for Pandemic Planning and Research | BNT162b2 | ≥18 years | 46 million |

NOTES: BNT162b2 refers to the COVID-19 vaccine manufactured by Pfizer-BioNTech under the name Comirnaty®. mRNA-1273 refers to the COVID-19 vaccine manufactured by Moderna under the name Spikevax®. Ad26.COV2.S refers to the COVID-19 vaccine manufactured by Janssen.
SOURCES: Ab Rahman et al., 2022; Barda et al., 2021; Botton et al., 2022; Burn et al., 2022a,b; Chui et al., 2022; Hippisley-Cox et al., 2021; Hviid et al., 2022; Jabagi et al., 2022; Patone et al., 2021; Shoaibi et al., 2023; Whiteley et al., 2022.

hospitalized patients. These and other issues should be the topic of more intensive research to better refine the evaluation of vaccine safety.

The committee attempted to focus on the six thromboembolic outcomes from the first and/or second dose of the primary series. No studies of adverse outcomes from bivalent or monovalent updated booster vaccines were considered here, in part because few such studies were available, and a variety of important selective forces likely affected who received subsequent doses, such as variation in individual clinical circumstances.

The studies had generally modest variations in analysis and presentation, such as differences in the post-vaccination analytical intervals, age groups of the vaccinees, and clinical history of COVID-19 infection (see Table 6-1).

All studies used in this chapter applied general administrative disease coding according to the International Classification of Diseases (ICD-10) nosology. Importantly, some studies only included hospitalized patients, likely deterring identification of diseases and conditions that might be identified largely in ambulatory settings.

Due to expected variation in cross-national medical care and coding practices, harmonization across disease rubrics and nosology could not be assured. Some studies reported diagnoses that could have been placed in alternative disease categories or classification codes. For example, "subarachnoid hemorrhage" may or may not be the same as "hemorrhagic stroke." This was not unexpected, but it challenges the validity of disease classification. This is explained further in the subsections of this chapter. Studies were only included if the disease reports used identical terms to those requested in the Statement of Task. Only Shoaibi et al. (2023) provided a supplemental validation study of disease coding accuracy, using medical charts as the standard. For both MI and PE, the majority of diagnoses were consistent with this manual evaluation. No study reported an evaluation of the accuracy of population immunization registries used to link vaccine receipt data to the respective medical care systems. See Boxes 6-1 through 6-4 for all conclusions in this chapter.

The following is a brief synopsis of the 12 studies contained in Table 6-1, in order to orient the reader to study characteristics and interpretation. They are presented in alphabetical order, as they appear also in Table 6-1. Vaccines analyzed are identified throughout the table headings and in this chapter's subheadings. Clinical trial results submitted to FDA for Emergency Use Authorization and/or full approval do not indicate a signal regarding any of the outcomes reviewed in this chapter and any of the vaccines under study (FDA, 2021, 2023a,b,c).

Ab Rahman et al. (2022) explored adverse events of special interest among patients admitted to major urban hospitals in Malaysia, during February through September 2021. The basic analyses were conducted using a self-controlled case series, and outcomes were represented as incidence rate ratios. Three vaccine platforms were evaluated, although as noted elsewhere in this report only those vaccines used in the United States were presented in our evaluations. Several but not all adverse events of special interest were analyzed relevant to this chapter, but only those occurring within 21 days after immunization were included. More than one vaccine dose may have been administered during the study window.

Barda et al. (2021) conducted an analysis of adverse events after the first dose of the BNT162b2 vaccine, in the setting of the largest health care organization in Israel, starting among persons with no medical history of any of the adverse events of interest. One person with a history of vaccine receipt was matched with another with no vaccine history, and with adjustment for various sociodemographic variables. Adverse everts in both groups were monitored using medical records and were followed for an observation interval of 42 days using system medical records. Study participants' ages were 16 years of age and above. Other inclusion and exclusion criteria were applied. In addition to the analysis of adverse events, a second, similarly matched analytical cohort was created using those with a history of COVID-19 infection, matched to similar persons with no history of infection at the same time; then, the clinical outcomes were followed in both groups to separately assess the role of general infection on these outcomes as a comparator. Other studies used in this chapter and in other chapters used similar methodology to contrast rates of adverse events following vaccination with similar rates of adverse events following infection.

Botton et al. (2022) explored three adverse vascular effects, MI, stroke, and PE, for three vaccines used in the United States: BNT162b2, mRNA-1273, and Ad26.COV2.S, among persons ages 18–74 years. The study population included over 46 million adults using the French National Health Data System, using a self-controlled case series method adapted to the event-dependent exposure and overall high rate of general mortality characteristic of this large population size. The relative incidence (RI) of each clinical outcome of interest was determined for 3 separately reported weeks after the recorded date of vaccine receipt, derived from separate population vaccine use files. Study data were separately reported for the first and second doses of the primary series for each of the vaccines. Of note, the same overall study methods were used for persons 75 years or older in the same geographic region but are reported separately by Jabagi et al. (2022).

Burn et al. (2022a) conducted a series of cohort studies from September 2020 through May 2021 in the United Kingdom, using a series of national clinical databases that included clinical characteristics of patients as well as vaccine receipt. Clinical outcomes included both vascular and hematological conditions, which also served to better understand prevaccination health status for a variety of comorbid conditions. Only data on the BNT162b2 were relevant to this chapter, and both first and second doses were considered, encompassing over 3 million doses distributed to vaccinees who were 20 years of age and older. Additionally, a separate cohort of patients who sustained the COVID-19 infection was analyzed to use as a comparator to the vaccine receipt cohorts with regard to clinical outcomes. Adverse events were counted in the 28 days after vaccine receipt. Of note, this study used some of the same clinical data resources as another study by Hippisley-Cox et al. (2021), but this was not deemed an important problem.

Burn et al. (2022b) analyzed hospital and primary care data from the region of Catalonia, Spain, including the first and second doses of BNT162b2. Another vaccine was studied but not used in the United States. Over 3 million persons were reported to have used at least one dose of this vaccine and were available for study. The outcomes assessed relevant to this chapter were VTE, MI, and ischemic stroke, with results among vaccinated persons compared to a historical comparator group. However, several other comorbid conditions were studied as "pre-morbid" risk factors, or as potential harms assessed in other chapters of this report (e.g., immune thrombocytopenia). As in other reports utilized in this chapter and others, a separate cohort of persons with the viral COVID-19 infection was identified as a separate comparator for outcome events relative to those receiving the study vaccines.

Chui et al. (2022) conducted a series of studies on the potential harms of the BNT162b2 vaccine in 2.9 million vaccinees in the period between February and September 2021. Data were obtained from Hong Kong's (China) territory-wide electronic health and vaccination records. The basic analytical design was a "modified" self-controlled case series using a variety of preselected vascular and thromboembolic events and HS. The period of adverse event risk assessment was 27 days after vaccination, and first and second doses of the vaccine were considered separately. An additional cohort of patients acquiring COVID-19 infection was also analyzed as a separate comparator. Of note, this was one of the first studies to concede that citizens had the right to change the scheduling of the first and second primary series doses.

Hippisley-Cox et al. (2021) conducted self-controlled case series analyses of thromboembolism and thrombocytopenia in over 9.5 million persons receiving the BNT162b2 vaccine in England, United Kingdom, between December 2020 and April 2021 who were 16 years of age or older. All information was derived from national databases of mortality, hospitalization, and vaccinations. Only clinical outcomes after the first dose were considered by the authors. Important to this chapter, MI, ischemic stroke, and VTE outcomes were available and were assessed in the 28 days after vaccination. Additionally, a separate cohort was analyzed using patients who were noted to be infected with the COVID-19 virus, as a comparator for relevant clinical outcomes. As noted above, there may be a small amount of database overlap between this study and that of Burn et al. (2022a).

Hviid et al. (2022) conducted a cohort study in Denmark of "frontline workers," who were among the first priority groups to receive COVID-19 vaccines when available in that country. These workers, born after 1957, were the only study group of its type to be evaluated in this chapter (the remainder were all from the general community). They were largely health care and institutional workers ($n \sim 101{,}000$) although some others were not further classified occupationally. Analytical information was obtained from national health and immunization registers. Only the BNT162b2 vaccine was assessed in this chapter, and the most important outcomes here were PE and DVT. The study sample size was more modest than most of the other studies considered in this chapter, limiting the statistical power of the analysis. The window of observation extended from December 2020 to April 2021.

Jabagi et al. (2022) conducted a self-controlled case series analysis of persons from the French National Health Data System linked to the national COVID-19 vaccination database, which can be considered an "extension" of the report by Botton et al. (2022) (see above), except that it included persons 75 years and older. The paper by Botton et al. (2022) only considered persons only up to 74 years of age. The separate reporting emphasis was deemed useful because older persons were priority vaccinees in many global communities. Main outcomes included in this paper were MI, stroke, and PE. In this paper over 3.9 million persons were included and only the BNT162b2 vaccine findings were reported, perhaps in part because of the limited sample availability for other vaccines during the study interval. Data on first and second doses were reported separately, but only a 2-week post vaccination interval was reported.

Patone et al. (2021) conducted a study in England, United Kingdom, that was mostly devoted to identifying potential neurological harms of two COVID-19 vaccines; only BNT162b2 was considered in this chapter because of relevance to U.S. vaccine exposures, as noted above, and over 12 million persons received this vaccine between December 2020 and May 2021. The study was considered for assessment in this chapter because HS was one of the prespecified safety outcomes. The study analysis was a self-controlled case series, and 811 HS events were detected among those who received the BNT162b2 vaccine. The follow-up interval was weekly for 28 days after immunization, and only the first dose of vaccine and the first detected adverse event were considered in the analysis. Additional cohorts were developed among patients from Scottish data to serve as validation of the findings from England, and among those who were found to have a positive COVID-19 test for infection, to be used as a comparator for the core findings.

Shoaibi et al. (2023) studied two messenger ribonucleic acid (mRNA) vaccines (BNT162b2 and mRNA-1273); this study differed in certain important ways from the other studies in this chapter. It was the only study reviewed in this section conducted on a U.S. population (the "Medicare" population consisting of nearly all Americans 65 years and older). Vascular, coagulation, and certain neurological outcomes were evaluated, but only those related to this chapter (see Background Information section of this chapter) were included. The study design was also different from some of the others. The two mRNA vaccines were considered separately and assessed using self-controlled case series methods. However, after a prevaccination data collection period, where demographic and general clinical information on the study cohorts were collected, the selected outcomes were assessed in both ambulatory and hospital settings for 90 days after the vaccines became available. Thus, it was not possible to separate out first and second dose effects of the individual vaccines. Shoaibi et al. also conducted secondary and exploratory analyses, including a validation study of outcome codes using medical case record reviews. These findings strengthened the understanding and challenges of medical record data, even if the findings may not be similar in other reports reviewed in this chapter.

Whiteley et al. (2022) examined the adult population of England, United Kingdom, using hospitalization and primary care data, comprising a total population of approximately 46 million persons observed between December 2020 and March 2021. Extensive clinical and demographic information were noted in the pre-vaccine period; a 28-day period of observation was used following the first immunization, and only the first dose was considered in the authors' analysis. Additionally, only the findings from the BNT162b2 vaccine were utilized in this chapter, as it was the only vaccine used in the United States. The clinical outcomes data in this report are specifically categorized in two groups—those 69 years or younger and those 70 years and older. The authors noted two main limitations of their analyses: reliance on the accuracy of coded electronic health records and residual confounding within the adjusted models.

## MYOCARDIAL INFARCTION

---

**BOX 6-1**
**Conclusions for Myocardial Infarction**

**Conclusion 6-1:** The evidence favors rejection of a causal relationship between the BNT162b2 vaccine and myocardial infarction.

**Conclusion 6-2:** The evidence favors rejection of a causal relationship between the mRNA-1273 vaccine and myocardial infarction.

**Conclusion 6-3:** The evidence is inadequate to accept or reject a causal relationship between the Ad26.COV2.S vaccine and myocardial infarction.

**Conclusion 6-4:** The evidence is inadequate to accept or reject a causal relationship between the NVX-CoV2373 vaccine and myocardial infarction.

---

## Background

A heart attack (MI) usually occurs when a blood clot blocks blood flow to the heart. Tissues, particularly heart muscle, lose oxygen and may die. Symptoms include tightness or pain in the chest, neck, back, or arms; fatigue; lightheadedness; abnormal heartbeat; and anxiety (Thygesen et al., 2018). MI is important and common; with other cardiovascular diseases, it is the leading cause of death in many developed countries. MI rates will vary among regional and national populations because of differences in risk factor levels and their management, in medical treatment, or in access to and use of health care resources and vary worldwide in part because of these differences in populations and communities. Sometimes a definitive diagnosis is difficult to make because of timing of clinical events, variation in symptom rates, premature death, or therapeutic interventions; this is likely to be a worldwide finding. The global epidemiology and occurrence have been reasonably well characterized (Salari et al., 2023).

SARS-CoV-2 is believed to cause both MI and other vascular conditions (Siddiqi et al., 2021), due to a variety of mechanisms, including infection and inflammation of atherosclerotic plaques and coagulation abnormalities. In the studies evaluated in this section, MI was substantially more common among COVID-19-infected persons than those who were uninfected but received any COVID-19 vaccine. Concordant exposure to both vaccine and infection during the pandemic can make it difficult to attribute MI to either potential cause.

## Mechanisms

MI is primarily defined as the sudden ischemic death of myocardial tissue. This often occurs due to thrombotic blockage of a coronary vessel after a plaque ruptures. The lack of blood flow triggers significant metabolic and ionic disturbances in the myocardium, leading to rapid deterioration of systolic function (Prabhu and Frangogiannis, 2016). Prolonged lack of blood flow activates a "wavefront" of cardiomyocyte death, which progresses from the subendocardium to the subepicardium. This process involves mitochondrial changes that are central to apoptosis and necrosis of cardiomyocytes (Davidson et al., 2020). Given the limited regenerative capacity of the adult mammalian heart, healing primarily occurs through scar formation. The immune system plays a significant role in both the homeostatic and perturbed conditions of the heart. Immune cells infiltrate the heart during gestation and persist in the myocardium throughout life, participating in essential housekeeping functions. After MI or in response to infection, large numbers of immune cells are recruited to the heart to remove dying tissue, scavenge pathogens, and promote healing (Prabhu and Frangogiannis, 2016). However, in some cases, these immune cells can cause irreversible damage, contributing to heart failure.

Reports exist of vaccine-related MI cases, particularly after ChAdOx1-S, which were mostly characterized by ST-segment elevation and occurred after the first dose. However, no definitive mechanistic link is established in the literature between COVID-19 vaccination and MI. Furthermore, most cases occurred after the first dose, which suggests that the immune response elicited by the vaccine may play a minimal role in MI (Hana et al., 2022; Zafar et al., 2022); an overactive immune response would presumably lead to a higher incidence of MI after booster dose. The immune response to vaccination does not correlate with a single inflammatory biomarker associated with MI but shows a range of markers, including IL-6 (interleukin-6), C-reactive protein, and components of the interferon signaling pathway (Hervé et al., 2019).

## Epidemiological Evidence

*BNT162b2 and MI*

Table 6-2 presents eight studies that contributed to the causality assessment.

All studies have varying designs; the majority were self-controlled, and the remainder were cohort studies, except for a case-control study (Whiteley et al., 2022). The number of MI events after BNT162b2[1] was higher than the background rate, except for the Israeli study ($n = 59$) (Barda et al., 2021).

Shoaibi et al. (2023) used the two-dose primary series as the "exposure," without presenting the separate

---

[1] The COVID-19 vaccine manufactured by Pfizer-BioNTech under the name Comirnaty®.

**TABLE 6-2** Epidemiological Studies in the BNT162b2–Myocardial Infarction Evidence Review

| Author | N | Number of Events | Results (95% CI) |
|---|---|---|---|
| Ab Rahman et al. (2022) | Dose 1: 8.7 million vaccinees | 409 | IRR 0.97 (0.87–1.08) |
| | Dose 2: 6.7 million vaccinees | 387 | IRR 1.08 (0.97–1.21) |
| Barda et al. (2021) | Dose 1: 884,828 vaccinees | 59 | RR 1.07 (0.74–1.60) |
| Botton et al. (2022) | Dose 1: 16,728 vaccinees | Week 1: 543 | RI 0.91 (0.83–1.00) |
| | | Week 2: 492 | RI 0.86 (0.78–0.94) |
| | Dose 2: 14,004 vaccinees | Week 1: 408 | RI 0.89 (0.80–1.00) |
| | | Week 2: 404 | RI 0.95 (0.85–1.06) |
| Burn et al. (2022a) | Dose 1: 1.8 million vaccinees | 442 | SIR 0.88 (0.80–0.97) |
| | Dose 2: 1.3 million vaccinees | 283 | SIR 0.80 (0.71–0.89) |
| Burn et al. (2022b) | Dose 1: 2.0 million vaccinees | 280 | SIR 1.05 (0.93–1.18) |
| | Dose 2: 1.3 million vaccinees | 272 | SIR 1.10 (0.98–1.24) |
| Jabagi et al. (2022) | Dose 1: 3.9 million vaccinees | 6,510 | RI 0.97 (0.88–1.06) |
| | Dose 2: 3.2 million vaccinees | 4,843 | RI 1.04 (0.93–1.16) |
| Shoaibi et al. (2023) | Doses 1 and 2: 3.4 million vaccinees | 2,783 | IRR 1.04 (0.91–1.18) |
| Whiteley et al. (2022) | Dose 1: 8.7 million vaccinees | 3,722 | Age <70: HR 0.88 (0.83–0.94) |
| | | | Age >70: HR 0.76 (0.71–0.81) |

NOTES: BNT162b2 refers to the COVID-19 vaccine manufactured by Pfizer-BioNTech under the name Comirnaty®. Shoaibi et al. (2023) combined the number of BNT162b2 and mRNA-1273 vaccinees. The primary series for BNT162b2 is two doses. Number of events refers to events in vaccinees only. CI: confidence interval; HR: hazard ratio; IRR: incidence rate ratio; RI: relative incidence; RR: risk ratio; SIR: standardized incidence ratio.
SOURCES: Ab Rahman et al., 2022; Barda et al., 2021; Botton et al., 2022; Burn et al., 2022a,b; Jabagi et al., 2022; Shoaibi et al., 2023; Whiteley et al., 2022.

outcomes. This study was retained in the report, in part because it was the only U.S. study. The two studies from France are respectively the younger and older cohorts of patients from the same national health system (Botton et al., 2022; Jabagi et al., 2022); they reported MI outcomes only from a 2-week interval post-vaccination. Whiteley et al. (2022) from England also presented data separately for two age categories (younger and older than 70). All the studies used a post-vaccination analysis interval of 1 month or less, except Shoaibi et al. (2023), which used 90 days with appropriate adjustments.

The findings were generally uniform across all eight studies. Seven of them showed no statistically significant increases in the risk of MI associated with BNT162b2. Shoaibi et al. (2023), in partially adjusted analyses, showed a modest increased risk: 1.17 (95% confidence interval [CI]: 1.08–1.28). However, these investigators included additional adjustments: current history of COVID-19 infection and seasonality. These factors were considered important; the latter was not explored in any other study contained in this chapter. After adjusting for these additional variables, the MI–BNT162b2 association was no longer significant: 1.04 (95% CI: 0.91–1.18). Shoaibi et al. (2023) also demonstrated that ICD codes for MI in their dataset were generally valid using medical chart reviews, with a positive predictive value (PPV) of 80 percent. In summary, all the studies in Table 6-2 showed no significant association between vaccination with BNT162b2 and MI.

*mRNA-1273 and MI*

Table 6-3 presents two studies that contributed to the causality assessment.

**TABLE 6-3** Epidemiological Studies in the mRNA-1273–Myocardial Infarction Evidence Review

| Author | N | | Number of Events | Results (95% CI) |
|---|---|---|---|---|
| Botton et al. (2022) | Dose 1: 2,435 vaccinees | | Week 1: 58 | RI 0.78 (0.59–1.03) |
| | | | Week 2: 78 | RI 1.06 (0.83–1.37) |
| | Dose 2: 1,831 vaccinees | | Week 1: 46 | RI 0.85 (0.61–1.18) |
| | | | Week 2: 61 | RI 1.21 (0.90–1.62) |
| Shoaibi et al. (2023) | Doses 1 and 2: 3.4 million vaccinees | | 302 | IRR 1.01 (0.82–1.26) |

NOTES: mRNA-1273 refers to the COVID-19 vaccine manufactured by Moderna under the name Spikevax®. Shoaibi et al. (2023) combined the number of BNT162b2 and mRNA-1273 vaccinees. The primary series for mRNA-1273 is two doses. Number of events refers to events in vaccinees only. CI: confidence interval; IRR: incidence rate ratio; RI: relative incidence.
SOURCES: Botton et al., 2022; Shoaibi et al., 2023.

Two studies evaluated the association between mRNA-1273[2] and MI, one using data from the French National Health Data System (Botton et al., 2022) and one using data from the U.S. Medicare system (Shoaibi et al., 2023) (see Tables 6-1 and 6-3.) Botton et al. (2022) covered adults under 75, and the vaccine was one of four evaluated in this report. Botton et al. (2022) used standard epidemiological methods but reported only on outcomes over a 2-week post-vaccination interval, and each week was reported separately. Shoaibi et al. (2023) used a 90-day post-vaccination interval to study MI risk of the two-dose primary series.

Botton et al. (2022) found no increase in risk of MI with mRNA-1273 in the first (RI 0.78, 95% CI: 0.59–1.03) or second (RI 1.06, 95% CI: 0.83–1.37) outcome week (Botton et al., 2022). Shoaibi et al. (2023) showed no increased risk of MI: incidence rate ratio (IRR) 1.01 (95% CI: 0.82–1.26), after full adjustment for selected study variables.

*Ad26.COV2.S and MI*

Table 6-4 summarizes one study that contributed to the causality assessment.

As noted, this study from the French National Health Data System, covering adults 18–74 years, evaluated four vaccines (see Table 6-1). Ad26.COV2.S[3] was received by about 30,000 persons overall, and of those receiving the first dose, 282 MIs were identified. Data were presented separately for the first and second post-vaccination weeks only. Outcomes were RI 1.57 (95% CI: 1.02–2.44) for the first week and RI 1.75 (95% CI: 1.16–2.62) for the second week.

---

[2] Refers to the COVID-19 vaccine manufactured by Moderna under the name Spikevax®.
[3] The COVID-19 vaccine manufactured by Janssen.

**TABLE 6-4** Epidemiological Study in the Ad26.COV2.S–Myocardial Infarction Evidence Review

| Author | N | Number of Events | Results (95% CI) |
|---|---|---|---|
| Botton et al. (2022) | Dose 1: 282 vaccinees | Week 1: 33 | RI 1.57 (1.02–2.44) |
| | | Week 2: 34 | RI 1.75 (1.16–2.62) |

NOTES: Ad26.COV2.S refers to the COVID-19 vaccine manufactured by Janssen. The primary series for Ad26.COV2.S is one dose. Number of events refers to events in vaccinees only. CI: confidence interval; RI: relative incidence.
SOURCE: Botton et al., 2022.

### From Evidence to Conclusions

Eight studies assessed the relationship between BNT162b2 and MI across different demographic groups and national populations on three continents. Despite some variation in the types of observational epidemiological study designs, all of these studies showed no important overall statistical evidence of increased risk of MI associated with either dose of BNT162b2 (Ab Rahman et al., 2022; Barda et al., 2021; Botton et al., 2022; Burn et al., 2022a,b; Jabagi et al., 2022; Shoaibi et al., 2023; Whiteley et al., 2022).

**Conclusion 6-1: The evidence favors rejection of a causal relationship between the BNT162b2 vaccine and myocardial infarction.**

Only two studies evaluated the association between mRNA-1273 and MI; neither showed evidence of increased risk (Botton et al., 2022; Shoaibi et al., 2023), but the findings aligned with those for BNT162b2.

**Conclusion 6-2: The evidence favors rejection of a causal relationship between the mRNA-1273 vaccine and myocardial infarction.**

Only one study evaluated the relation between Ad26.COV2.S and MI, and the number of MI events was modest (Botton et al., 2022).

**Conclusion 6-3: The evidence is inadequate to accept or reject a causal relationship between the Ad26.COV2.S vaccine and myocardial infarction.**

No studies examined the relationship between NVX-CoV2373[4] and MI.

**Conclusion 6-4: The evidence is inadequate to accept or reject a causal relationship between the NVX-CoV2373 vaccine and myocardial infarction.**

---

[4] The COVID-19 vaccine manufactured by Novavax.

## ISCHEMIC STROKE

---

**BOX 6-2**
**Conclusions for Ischemic Stroke**

**Conclusion 6-5: The evidence favors rejection of a causal relationship between the BNT162b2 vaccine and ischemic stroke.**

**Conclusion 6-6: The evidence is inadequate to accept or reject a causal relationship between the mRNA-1273 vaccine and ischemic stroke.**

**Conclusion 6-7: The evidence is inadequate to accept or reject a causal relationship between the Ad26.COV2.S vaccine and ischemic stroke.**

**Conclusion 6-8: The evidence is inadequate to accept or reject a causal relationship between the NVX-CoV2373 vaccine and ischemic stroke.**

---

### Background

A stroke may occur due to either a blockage in blood flow to the brain or sudden bleeding within the brain. The primary form is known as an ischemic stroke, where the brain is deprived of necessary oxygen and nutrients due to a blockage in blood flow, leading to rapid cell death. The secondary type is termed an HS, characterized by blood leakage that applies pressure on brain cells, causing damage (NHLBI, 2023). HSs are discussed and evaluated in the next section.

Ischemic strokes are usually caused by either atherosclerotic lesions in cerebral arteries or emboli, often blood clots, from the heart or other parts of the vascular tree. However, several other mechanisms are possible. Strokes can occur at any age but are most common in older people. In the United States, strokes are overall the fifth leading cause of death. Typically, strokes are acute and relatively sudden, often within hours or less, even though the lesions themselves may take a long time to develop. Sometimes, neurological manifestations occur intermittently and incompletely; these clinical events may be diagnosed as a "transient ischemic attack," which is often considered diagnostically separate from "completed" strokes, which can be important in studies that assess stroke outcomes. The clinical presentation may also be modified by various medical interventions, leading to other diagnostic challenges. Stroke diagnoses may also vary by relative access to technology, such as imaging procedures, which can differ by country and within-country region. All of these factors can possibly affect apparent incidence rates across studies. To complicate matters further, persons with cardiovascular diseases are two to four times more likely to have a stroke (Robinson et al., 2023), raising issues of the underlying causes. These complex diagnostic challenges apply to all the thromboembolic outcomes assessed in this chapter, as discussed. However, in a comprehensive global review of ICD coding validity study, McCormick et al. (2015) found that the PPV was 82 and over 93 percent for ischemic and ICD-9 HS codes.

For diagnosis, ischemic stroke is identified by the abrupt onset of focal neurologic deficits, with speech disturbance and weakness on one-half of the body being the most common symptoms. Diagnostic studies are crucial to differentiate it from other conditions, such as intracerebral hemorrhage, or entities mimicking it, such as seizures or hypoglycemia. Neuroimaging, particularly noncontrast computed tomography (CT) or magnetic resonance imaging (MRI), plays a vital role in this differentiation. Noncontrast CT is sensitive for detecting mass lesions and acute hemorrhage but less effective in detecting strokes within 3 hours of the event and has even lower sensitivity for small or posterior fossa strokes. In contrast, MRI, especially diffusion-weighted imaging, offers better resolution and greater sensitivity for detecting acute ischemic stroke and is as sensitive as noncontrast CT for intracerebral HS (Vymazal et al., 2012).

## Mechanisms

A key aspect of ischemic stroke pathophysiology involves the immune system. In the acute phase, innate immune cells invade the brain and meninges, contributing to damage but also potentially offering protection. This phase is characterized by the damaged brain cells releasing danger signals, such as damage-associated molecular patterns, into the circulation, activating systemic immunity. In the chronic phase, antigen presentation triggers an adaptive immune response targeted at the brain, possibly underlying the neuropsychiatric sequelae that significantly contribute to morbidity (Chamorro et al., 2012; Nakamura and Shichita, 2019).

A mechanism of ischemic stroke as a result of COVID-19 vaccination remains to be established. However, it can be hypothesized that temporary inflammation of the arterial wall could be a contributing factor in cerebral hemorrhage (de Mélo Silva and Lopes, 2021). The proposed immune response could also trigger a systemic prothrombotic state, characterized by endothelial dysfunction and activation, complement and platelet activation, and infiltration of inflammatory cells into atherosclerotic plaques. These processes lead to amplified inflammatory responses and potential thrombosis within these plaques (Bonaventura et al., 2021). This is in line with the concept that inflammatory conditions, especially in atherosclerosis, are precursors to thrombotic events, including cerebrovascular ones (Assiri et al., 2022).

Some argue that COVID-19 vaccination could induce an inflammatory cascade similar to that in COVID-19 infection, leading to disseminated intravascular coagulation, vascular endothelial dysfunction, and large-vessel cerebral infarctions. Following mRNA vaccination, the introduction of mRNA sequences coding for the SARS-CoV-2 spike protein into host cells leads to its synthesis and release, stimulating an inflammatory immune response (Assiri et al., 2022; Famularo, 2022).

## Epidemiological Evidence

### BNT162b2 and Ischemic Stroke

Table 6-5 presents six studies that contributed to the causality assessment.

The two papers from France report on one study, addressing adults younger than and over 75, respectively (Botton et al., 2022; Jabagi et al., 2022). This study, as noted, reported only 2 separate weeks of post-vaccination outcomes. Botton et al. (2022) showed no increased risk of stroke after either week (Botton et al., 2022), and Jabagi et al. (2022) studied the oldest population (over 75) and found similar results. The UK study (Burn et al., 2022a) and the Catalonia, Spain, study (Burn et al., 2022b) also found no increased stroke risk with this vaccine. The Malaysian study, with a different design, had the same findings (Ab Rahman et al., 2022). Whiteley et al. (2022) from England had one of the largest immunized populations, over 8 million, but presented findings separately for those over and under 70. Hazard ratios were reported for two separate age groups: younger than 70 and 70+. All studies showed no increased risk of ischemic stroke with the BNT162b2 vaccine in all major analytical groups.

### mRNA-1273 and Ischemic Stroke

Table 6-6 summarizes one study that contributed to the causality assessment.

Only one relevant scientific report attempted to link mRNA-1273 with ischemic stroke risk. As seen in other sections, Botton et al. (2022), covering adults 18–74 years, reported ischemic stroke risk in the 2 weeks after immunization. Some weaknesses included the inability to fully assess the risk association on the day of immunization; the reporting of each outcome week risk separately; and that, as in many of the other reports, outpatient-only clinical events were not surveyed. The risk was not significantly increased in either post-vaccination week. The companion paper (Jabagi et al., 2022) on persons 75+ in this study did not include this vaccine.

### Ad26.COV2.S and Ischemic Stroke

Table 6-7 summarizes one study that contributed to the causality assessment.

**TABLE 6-5** Epidemiological Studies in the BNT162b2–Ischemic Stroke Evidence Review

| Author | N | Number of Events | Results (95% CI) |
|---|---|---|---|
| Ab Rahman et al. (2022) | Dose 1: 8.7 million vaccinees | Dose 1: 535 | IRR 1.05 (0.95–1.15) |
| | Dose 2: 6.7 million vaccinees | Dose 2: 471 | IRR 1.11 (1.00–1.23) |
| Botton et al. (2022) | Dose 1: 11,282 vaccinees | Week 1: 329 | RI 0.84 (0.74–0.94) |
| | | Week 2: 366 | RI 0.95 (0.85–1.06) |
| | Dose 2: 9,344 vaccinees | Week 1: 279 | RI 0.93 (0.81–1.06) |
| | | Week 2: 307 | RI 1.09 (0.96–1.23) |
| Burn et al. (2022a) | Dose 1: 1.8 million vaccinees | 146 | SIR 1.10 (0.93–1.29) |
| | Dose 2: 1.3 million vaccinees | 68 | SIR 0.68 (0.54–0.86) |
| Burn et al. (2022b) | Dose 1: 2.0 million vaccinees | 521 | SIR 0.98 (0.90–1.07) |
| | Dose 2: 1.3 million vaccinees | 515 | SIR 1.01 (0.92–1.10) |
| Jabagi et al. (2022) | Dose 1: 3.9 million vaccinees | 9,162 | RI 0.90 (0.84–0.98) |
| | Dose 2: 3.2 million vaccinees | 6,531 | RI 1.04 (0.93–1.16) |
| Whiteley et al. (2022) | Dose 1: 8.7 million vaccinees | 4,143 | <70 years: HR 0.90 (0.83–0.97) |
| | | | >70 years: HR 0.71 (0.68–0.75) |

NOTES: BNT162b2 refers to the COVID-19 vaccine manufactured by Pfizer-BioNTech under the name Comirnaty®. Number of events refers to events in vaccinees only. CI: confidence interval; HR: hazard ratio; IRR: incidence rate ratio; RI: relative incidence; SIR: standardized incidence ratio.
SOURCES: Ab Rahman et al., 2022; Botton et al., 2022; Burn et al., 2022a,b; Jabagi et al., 2022; Whiteley et al., 2022.

**TABLE 6-6** Epidemiological Study in the mRNA-1273–Ischemic Stroke Evidence Review

| Author | N | Number of Events | Results (95% CI) |
|---|---|---|---|
| Botton et al. (2022) | Dose 1: 1,491 vaccinees | Week 1: 42 | RI 0.76 (0.55–1.07) |
| | | Week 2: 40 | RI 0.76 (0.54–1.07) |
| | Dose 2: 1,200 vaccinees | Week 1: 45 | RI 1.15 (0.82–1.62) |
| | | Week 2: 41 | RI 1.12 (0.77–1.62) |

NOTES: mRNA-1273 refers to the COVID-19 vaccine manufactured by Moderna under the name Spikevax®. Number of events refers to events in vaccinees only. CI: confidence interval; RI: relative incidence.
SOURCE: Botton et al., 2022.

**TABLE 6-7** Epidemiological Study in the Ad26.COV2.S–Ischemic Stroke Evidence Review

| Author | N | Number of Events | Results (95% CI) |
|---|---|---|---|
| Botton et al. (2022) | Dose 1: 196 vaccinees | Week 1: 14 | RI 0.78 (0.43–1.41) |
| | | Week 2: 19 | RI 1.09 (0.66–1.81) |

NOTES: Ad26.COV2.S refers to the COVID-19 vaccine manufactured by Janssen.
The primary series of Ad26.COV2.S is one dose. CI: confidence interval; RI: relative incidence.
SOURCE: Botton et al., 2022.

Botton et al. (2022), as mentioned in the discussion on BNT162b2 and mRNA-1273, was the only available report on the association of Ad26.COV2.S with ischemic stroke. Its strengths and limitations are similar. One additional limitation for this vaccine is that the number of outcome events was modest, which should be considered in statistical evaluation of the findings. However, within these limitations, no significantly increased risk of ischemic stroke was found.

## From Evidence to Conclusions

All six studies that assessed the association between BNT162b2 and ischemic stroke, comprising five robust studies from multiple countries and exploring younger and older adults, found no evidence of increased risk, despite modest difference in the study designs (Ab Rahman et al., 2022; Botton et al., 2022; Burn et al., 2022a,b; Jabagi et al., 2022; Whiteley et al., 2022).

**Conclusion 6-5: The evidence favors rejection of a causal relationship between the BNT162b2 vaccine and ischemic stroke.**

A single study assessed the relationship between mRNA-1273 and Ad26.COV2.S and ischemic stroke (Botton et al., 2022). Although it was generally well designed, it had limitations: a lack of representation of older persons (over 75), separate presentation of outcome rates for each post-vaccination week, a group with high ischemic stroke risk, and a modest number of stroke outcomes. No studies evaluated the relationship between NVX-CoV2373 and ischemic stroke.

**Conclusion 6-6: The evidence is inadequate to accept or reject a causal relationship between the mRNA-1273 vaccine and ischemic stroke.**

**Conclusion 6-7: The evidence is inadequate to accept or reject a causal relationship between the Ad26.COV2.S vaccine and ischemic stroke.**

**Conclusion 6-8: The evidence is inadequate to accept or reject a causal relationship between the NVX-CoV2373 vaccine and ischemic stroke.**

## HEMORRHAGIC STROKE

---

**BOX 6-3**
**Conclusions for Hemorrhagic Stroke**

**Conclusion 6-9: The evidence is inadequate to accept or reject a causal relationship between the BNT162b2 vaccine and hemorrhagic stroke.**

**Conclusion 6-10: The evidence is inadequate to accept or reject a causal relationship between the mRNA-1273 vaccine and hemorrhagic stroke.**

**Conclusion 6-11: The evidence is inadequate to accept or reject a causal relationship between the Ad26.COV2.S vaccine and hemorrhagic stroke.**

**Conclusion 6-12: The evidence is inadequate to accept or reject a causal relationship between the NVX-CoV2373 vaccine and hemorrhagic stroke.**

---

## Background

As with other strokes, HS is usually an acute event that occurs after bleeding within the cerebrum or more specifically within the brain, usually caused by a ruptured blood vessel. It has been estimated that about 750,000 persons in the United States die of stroke each year. About 20 percent of incident strokes are due to hemorrhage. Often, the bleeding that comes with HS can damage the brain and impair neurological function by many mechanisms, such as due to physical pressure or inflammation. HS has many causes, such as ruptured aneurysms, head trauma, vascular malformations, and anticoagulants (Caplan, 2023). Some of the risk factors are similar to those of other important vascular conditions, such as MI or ischemic stroke (e.g., smoking, hypertension, diabetes), so prevention is an important part of the management of this condition.

HS may occur in several areas of the brain, such as epidural, intraparenchymal, subdural, and subarachnoid locations. The extent of diagnostic specificity depends, as with other vascular conditions, on regional and national diagnostic and therapeutic practices and health care resources, such as advanced imaging and other neuro-radiological techniques. This is particularly important because in studies of vaccine use and clinical outcomes, the latter will depend on these resources and diagnostic nomenclature. For example, an HS may be primarily called a "ruptured aneurysm" or a "subarachnoid hemorrhage," which may have causal implications. As COVID-19 infection may be a cause of HS, this complicates assessing vaccine causation due to interacting comorbid conditions and treatments (Wang et al., 2020). Research has advanced the use of artificial intelligence to help identify anatomic locations of hemorrhage and its classification (Neves et al., 2023), but how this is being applied to causal studies, such as those related to vaccines, is uncertain. Yet, as noted, validation studies of ICD coding of HS have been positive and useful (Kirkman et al., 2009).

## Mechanisms

HS occurs when a blood vessel within the brain ruptures, leading to bleeding in or around the brain, and can result from various etiologies, including hypertension, aneurysms, and arteriovenous malformations. Chronic hypertension may lead to Charcot-Bouchard microaneurysms in small penetrating arterioles, which are prone to rupture under sustained high pressure. Subarachnoid hemorrhage is often due to the rupture of a saccular aneurysm, and arteriovenous malformations, which are tangles of blood vessels with abnormal connections between arteries and veins, can also rupture (Montano et al., 2021; Smith and Eskey, 2011).

The secondary injury mechanisms include the mass effect and increased intracranial pressure, where blood accumulation causes compression of brain tissue, leading to blocked blood flow and the toxic effects of blood breakdown products (Serrone et al., 2015). Hemoglobin degradation products can be toxic to brain tissue and contribute to vasospasm, particularly in subarachnoid hemorrhage (Gross et al., 2019).

An immune response after hemorrhage is characterized by the activation of microglia and infiltration of macrophages and lymphocytes, which can exacerbate neuronal damage. Proinflammatory cytokines, such as TNF-α, IL-1β, and IL-6, are elevated, contributing to secondary injury and brain edema (Li and Chen, 2023).

Some vaccines, notably those associated with a risk of thrombocytopenia, could theoretically lead to HS, although this is exceedingly rare; an autoimmune response leading to platelet destruction and severe thrombocytopenia might predispose individuals to hemorrhage. The proposed mechanism of HS is similar to that of ischemic stroke, as mentioned.

## Epidemiological Evidence

*BNT162b2 and HS*

Table 6-8 presents six studies that contributed to the causality assessment.

Six reports represent five studies addressing the association of HS with this vaccine, and several reports were used in other sections of this chapter. One was a cohort study; the remainder were self-controlled designs. The committee examined the data on the first dose of the primary series. All but Patone et al. (2021) and Chui et al. (2022) have been discussed.

Patone et al. (2021) was conducted using the English National Immunisation (NIMS) Database, using a self-controlled design. Only first-dose outcomes and hospitalized patients were evaluated. The study showed a modestly increased risk (RI 1.24, 95% CI: 1.07–1.43). However, this group also conducted a validation study using similar methods on Scottish data and found no increased risk of HS, using a somewhat smaller sample size. An important issue with this report is that subarachnoid hemorrhage was considered as a separate outcome from HS; as discussed

**TABLE 6-8** Epidemiological Studies in the BNT162b2–Hemorrhagic Stroke Evidence Review

| Author | N | Number of Events | Results (95% CI) |
|---|---|---|---|
| Ab Rahman et al. (2022) | Dose 1: 8.7 million vaccinees | 119 | IRR 1.29 (1.05–1.59) |
| | Dose 2: 6.7 million vaccinees | 80 | IRR 1.05 (0.82–1.34) |
| Botton et al. (2022) | Dose 1: 3,141 vaccinees | Week 1: 112 | RI 0.97 (0.80–1.19) |
| | | Week 2: 119 | RI 1.07 (0.88–1.30) |
| | Dose 2: 2,372 vaccinees | Week 1: 86 | RI 0.98 (0.77–1.25) |
| | | Week 2: 71 | RI 0.86 (0.67–1.11) |
| Chui et al. (2022) | Dose 1: 2.9 million vaccinees | 31 | IRR 1.67 (1.04–2.69) |
| | Dose 2: 2.7 million vaccinees | 26 | IRR 1.68 (0.99–2.84) |
| Jabagi et al. (2022) | Dose 1: 3.9 million vaccinees | 2,050 | RI 0.90 (0.78–1.04) |
| | Dose 2: 3.2 million vaccinees | 1,366 | RI 0.97 (0.81–1.15) |
| Patone et al. (2021) | Dose 1: 12.1 million vaccinees | 151 | RI 1.24 (1.07–1.43) |
| Whiteley et al. (2022) | Dose 1: 8.7 million vaccinees | 440 | <70 years: HR 0.77 0.62–0.96) |
| | | | >70 years: HR 0.65 (0.57–0.74) |

NOTES: BNT162b2 refers to the COVID-19 vaccine manufactured by Pfizer-BioNTech under the name Comirnaty®. Number of events refers to events in vaccinees only. CI: confidence interval; HR: hazard ratio; IRR: incidence rate ratio; RI: relative incidence.
SOURCES: Ab Rahman et al., 2022; Botton et al., 2022; Chui et al., 2022; Jabagi et al., 2022; Patone et al., 2021; Whiteley et al., 2022.

in the background of this section, these two diseases may have some amount of overlap and/or misclassification, although no further information was offered.

Chui et al. (2022) conducted a study in Hong Kong, China, using geography-wide medical care and immunization databases, a "modified" self-control design with seasonal adjustment, and a 28-day post-vaccination outcomes interval. They found an increased risk of HS associated with BNT162b2 (IRR 1.67, 95% CI: 1.04–2.69).

In addition, Ab Rahman et al. (2022) from Malaysia showed a marginally increased risk of HS (IRR 1.29, 95% CI: 1.05–1.59).

The remaining studies showed no increased risk, including two analyses that separated the findings into older and younger adults (Botton et al., 2022; Jabagi et al., 2022).

*mRNA-1273 and HS*

Table 6-9 summarizes the one study that contributed to the causality assessment.

**TABLE 6-9** Epidemiological Study in the mRNA-1273–Hemorrhagic Stroke Evidence Review

| Author | N | Number of Events | Results (95% CI) |
|---|---|---|---|
| Botton et al. (2022) | Dose 1: 414 vaccinees | Week 1: 12 | RI 0.73 (0.39–1.37) |
| | | Week 2: 14 | RI 0.91 (0.51–1.61) |
| | Dose 2: 299 vaccinees | Week 1: 10 | RI 1.06 (0.56–2.00) |
| | | Week 2: 4 | RI 0.45 (0.16–1.23) |

NOTES: mRNA-1273 refers to the COVID-19 vaccine manufactured by Moderna under the name Spikevax®. Number of events refers to events in vaccinees only. CI: confidence interval; RI: relative incidence.
SOURCE: Botton et al., 2022.

**TABLE 6-10** Epidemiological Study in the Ad26.COV2.S–Hemorrhagic Stroke Evidence Review

| Author | N | Number of Events | Results (95% CI) |
|---|---|---|---|
| Botton et al. (2022) | Dose 1: 38 vaccinees | Week 1: 6 | RI 1.28 (0.46–3.61) |
| | | Week 2: 6 | RI 1.59 (0.60–4.21) |

NOTES: Ad26.COV2.S refers to the COVID-19 vaccine manufactured by Janssen. The primary series for Ad26.COV2.S is one dose. Number of events refers to events in vaccinees only. CI: confidence interval; RI: relative incidence.
SOURCE: Botton et al., 2022.

Botton et al. (2022) used the French National Health Data System to explore the association between mRNA-1273 and HS. This was a study of HS outcomes after the first dose of the primary series. As in the other applications of this study, only 2 weeks of the post-vaccination interval were presented, and the risks for each week were presented separately. This study included adults up to 74, but the number of HS case outcomes in the first 2 weeks was only 26. The portion of the study describing outcomes in persons 75+ showed no findings on mRNA-1273 and HS (Jabagi et al., 2022), likely because of an inadequate number of case outcomes.

*Ad26.COV2.S and HS*

Table 6-10 summarizes one study that contributed to the causality assessment.

As with mRNA-1273, only one study evaluated Ad26.COV2.S for adults aged 18–74 (Botton et al., 2022). The same limitations apply here, and only 12 HS cases occurred in the 2-week post-vaccination interval. The outcomes for the older patient set (75+ years) were not available (Jabagi et al., 2022).

**From Evidence to Conclusions**

The findings from the studies evaluating BNT162b2 and HS were mixed, with some finding an increased risk. Additionally, evidence of possible disease misclassification of HS with other sources of intracranial hemorrhage could not be resolved, as suggested by the general medical literature. Only two of the five studies showed an increased signal of HS risk, and an additional study showed a marginally increased risk (Ab Rahman et al., 2022; Chui et al., 2022; Patone et al., 2021).

**Conclusion 6-9: The evidence is inadequate to accept or reject a causal relationship between the BNT162b2 vaccine and hemorrhagic stroke.**

Only one study evaluated the relationship between mRNA-1273 and HS; it had only 2 weeks of post-vaccination follow-up (Botton et al., 2022). Only 26 HS cases occurred in those who received mRNA-1273.

**Conclusion 6-10: The evidence is inadequate to accept or reject a causal relationship between the mRNA-1273 vaccine and hemorrhagic stroke.**

Only one study evaluated the relationship between Ad26.COV2.S and HS, which showed no evidence of increased risk; it had only 2 weeks of post-vaccination follow-up with only 12 cases (Botton et al., 2022). No studies evaluated the association between NVX-CoV2373 and HS.

**Conclusion 6-11: The evidence is inadequate to accept or reject a causal relationship between the Ad26.COV2.S vaccine and hemorrhagic stroke.**

**Conclusion 6-12: The evidence is inadequate to accept or reject a causal relationship between the NVX-CoV2373 vaccine and hemorrhagic stroke.**

## DEEP VEIN THROMBOSIS, PULMONARY EMBOLISM, AND VENOUS THROMBOEMBOLISM

---

**BOX 6-4**
**Conclusions for Deep Vein Thrombosis,**
**Pulmonary Embolism, and Venous Thromboembolism**

**Conclusion 6-13:** The evidence is inadequate to accept or reject a causal relationship between the BNT162b2 vaccine and deep vein thrombosis, pulmonary embolism, and venous thromboembolism.

**Conclusion 6-14:** The evidence is inadequate to accept or reject a causal relationship between the mRNA-1273 vaccine and deep vein thrombosis, pulmonary embolism, and venous thromboembolism.

**Conclusion 6-15:** The evidence is inadequate to accept or reject a causal relationship between the Ad26.COV2.S vaccine and deep vein thrombosis, pulmonary embolism, and venous thromboembolism.

**Conclusion 6-16:** The evidence is inadequate to accept or reject a causal relationship between the NVX-CoV2373 vaccine and deep vein thrombosis, pulmonary embolism, and venous thromboembolism.

---

### Background

DVT, PE, and VTE are related conditions, often with common risk factors, clinical manifestations, pathogenetic mechanisms, treatments, and preventive interventions. "VTE" mostly or entirely may represent a category including PE and DVT. Occurrence rates can depend on the chronicity, comorbidity, and prevalent risk factors. The mortality risk among adults ≥65 with VTE is 3.1 percent at 30 days and 19.6 percent at 1 year (Giorgio et al., 2023). Other vascular and related immunologic outcomes, such as immune thrombotic purpura and immune thrombocytopenic purpura, are considered separately in Chapter 5. The evidence regarding association of each of the three conditions with COVID-19 vaccines will be discussed separately, but conclusions and the relevant justifications appear together at the end of this section.

DVT, PE, and VTE, in part because of these overlapping characteristics, present a dilemma in research and clinical outcome studies because regional and national variation in diagnostic practices and medical terminology may lead to misclassification, which can be substantial. For example, in an important report cited in this chapter (Shoaibi et al., 2023), a medical chart review of PE from the U.S. Medicare system found that the PPV for accuracy of 101 cases was only 45 percent. Other similar validation studies show varying results. In a study of over 4,000 VTE cases, also from the United States, Fang et al. (2017) found a PPV of 64.6 percent in patients who were hospitalized or seen in an emergency department but only 30.9 percent for outpatients. On the other hand, Tamariz et al. (2012) found the highest PPV values among ICD-9 codes for combined PE and DVT to range from 65–95 percent accuracy, with the highest among those at greatest risk of VTE. These studies overall found important variation in accuracy according to patient risk, location seen in the health care system, whether the diagnosis was primary or secondary, and anatomic site.

### Pathophysiology

The pathophysiology of DVT is often explained by Virchow's triad: venous stasis, endothelial injury, and hypercoagulability. PE involves not only the mechanical obstruction of the pulmonary artery but also the release of vasoactive substances that cause pulmonary vasoconstriction, leading to an increase in pulmonary vascular resistance and right ventricular strain. Immune responses, particularly those involving inflammatory mediators, can exacerbate this by increasing vascular permeability and promoting further thrombosis.

VTE occurs at higher frequency in the context of inflammation, such as during infections, in autoimmune conditions, and postoperatively. In an immune-mediated context, inflammation plays a critical role. Proinflammatory cytokines can alter the coagulation cascade, leading to a prothrombotic state. For instance, elevated levels of IL-6 have been implicated in increased thrombin generation (Tang et al., 2015). COVID-19 vaccines have been shown to increase IL-6 production both in situ (Zhu et al., 2023) and ex vivo (Langgartner et al., 2023). Other ways that the immune system can lead to a hypercoagulable state include monocytes and neutrophil release of tissue factor, a potent activator of the coagulation cascade, and the formation of neutrophil extracellular traps, which can provide a scaffold for thrombus formation.

## Deep Vein Thrombosis

DVT occurs when blood clots develop and persist in a larger vein, such as in the thighs, pelvis, arms, splanchnic vasculature, and cerebrum. Most of these clots, however, form in the legs, with varying signs and symptoms, altered persistence, and uncertain clinical consequences (Mithoowani, 2022). Signs and symptoms may include edema, redness, pain, and disability. The diagnosis can be challenging, made by a combination of clinical signs and symptoms, biomarkers, imaging studies, and physiological measures. DVT may occur acutely or chronically, the latter supporting the importance of having a history of DVT. This is important because prior DVT and its underlying conditions may be central to understanding the pathogenetic underpinnings during acute exposures, such as vaccines. Various studies, some reviewed here, may or may not have included prior comorbidity occurrence in DVT risk models. DVT (and VTE in general) may have different rates across countries and global regions.

*Epidemiological Evidence*

**BNT162b2 and DVT** Table 6-11 lists five studies that contributed to the causality assessment.

Five scientific reports from Europe and Israel explored the association of relevant COVID-19 vaccines to DVT. Of the four vaccines that are the focus of the committee's review, only BNT162b2 was included in these analyses. The five studies included three cohort designs and one each with a self-controlled design and a matched case-control design. The sample sizes were generally robust, except for the Danish study (Hviid et al., 2022), where these were more modest. This study was also the only one that presented its outcome statistics as risk differences. Whiteley et al. (2022) presented their findings separately for persons under and over 70. Burn et al. (2022a) from the United Kingdom included VTE and DVT outcomes. Hviid et al. (2022) had many fewer cases, and the CI was wide but not significant in this relative difference analysis. All the studies showed no significantly increased risk.

**TABLE 6-11** Epidemiological Studies in the BNT162b2–Deep Vein Thrombosis Evidence Review

| Author | N | Number of Events | Results (95% CI) |
|---|---|---|---|
| Barda et al. (2021) | Dose 1: 884,828 vaccinees | 39 | RR 0.87 (0.55–1.40) |
| Burn et al. (2022a) | Dose 1: 1.8 million vaccinees | 303 | SIR 1.00 (0.89–1.12) |
| | Dose 2: 1.3 million vaccinees | 182 | SIR 0.85 (0.74 to 0.99) |
| Burn et al. (2022b) | Dose 1: 2.0 million vaccinees | 182 | SIR 1.03 (0.89–1.19) |
| | Dose 2: 1.3 million vaccinees | 130 | SIR 0.80 (0.67–0.95) |
| Hviid et al. (2022) | Dose 1: 101,212 vaccinees | 13 | RD 2.05 (−2.49–6.59) |
| Whiteley et al. (2022) | Dose 1: 8.7 million vaccinees | 555 | Age <70: HR 0.82 (0.71–0.95) |
| | | | Age >70: HR 0.61 (0.53–0.70) |

NOTES: BNT162b2 refers to the COVID-19 vaccine manufactured by Pfizer-BioNTech under the name Comirnaty®. Number of events refers to events in vaccinees only. CI: confidence interval; HR: hazard ratio; RD: risk difference; RR: risk ratio; SIR: standardized incidence ratio.
SOURCES: Barda et al., 2021; Burn et al., 2022a,b; Hviid et al., 2022; Whiteley et al., 2022.

## Pulmonary Embolism

PE is the obstruction of a pulmonary artery by a physical entity, the embolus, that travels to the heart, lodging in the lungs. This "obstruction" may often be from blood clots forming elsewhere, usually due to some form of DVT, but it could be a tumor, air, or fat globule. This could be quite traumatic and acute or chronic, and it may be fatal, depending on the extent and cause of the embolus. According to the American Lung Association, about 900,000 people have a PE each year (ALA, 2023). Because these may be symptomatic or asymptomatic and have varying degrees of clinical severity, difficulties may arise in making a definitive diagnosis. Due to the challenges and variations in PE diagnostic practices and technology and in coding and classification systems, apparent PE rates may vary across populations and countries, and this variation may lead to variations in community and regional study findings and in identifying risk factors and outcomes, as is the case for DVT (see above).

As is with DVT, the nomenclature for diagnostic coding varies, leading to some of these thromboembolic events being designated under different rubrics, such as DVT, PE, or VTE. This complicates the interpretation of vaccine-related population studies, and only a few of them address these issues in detail or with validation studies.

*Epidemiological Evidence*

**BNT162b2 and PE** Table 6-12 presents eight studies that contributed to the causality assessment.

PE outcomes were explored in nine scientific reports, including eight separate studies and three vaccines (BNT162b2, mRNA-1273, and Ad26.COV2.S). Eight represented findings from the first dose of the primary COVID-19 vaccination series; Shoaibi et al. (2023) reflected the combined effects of doses 1 and 2. The eight studies represented countries in Europe, and one was in the United States. Two studies in three reports presented older and younger vaccinees separately (see Table 6-1 for more detail) (Botton et al., 2022; Jabagi et al., 2022; Whiteley et al., 2022). All the outcomes shown were listed only as derived from the outcome rubric "PE."

**TABLE 6-12** Epidemiological Studies in the BNT162b2–Pulmonary Embolism Evidence Review

| Author | N | | Number of Events | Results (95% CI) |
|---|---|---|---|---|
| Barda et al. (2021) | Dose 1: 884,828 vaccinees | | 10 | RR 0.56 (0.21–1.15) |
| Botton et al. (2022) | Dose 1: 7,242 vaccinees | | Week 1: 203 | RI 0.81 (0.70–0.94) |
| | | | Week 2: 200 | RI 0.83 (0.71–0.96) |
| | Dose 2: 5,665 vaccinees | | Week 1: 156 | RI 0.83 (0.70–0.99) |
| | | | Week 2: 178 | RI 1.00 (0.85–1.17) |
| Burn et al. (2022a) | Dose 1: 1.8 million vaccinees | | 324 | SIR 1.25 (1.12–1.40) |
| | Dose 2: 1.3 million vaccinees | | 153 | SIR 0.84 (0.71–0.98) |
| Burn et al. (2022b) | Dose 1: 2.0 million vaccinees | | 154 | SIR 1.25 (1.07–1.46) |
| | Dose 2: 1.3 million vaccinees | | 116 | SIR 1.00 (0.84–1.20) |
| Hviid et al. (2022) | Dose 1: 101,212 vaccinees | | 8 | RD 1.32 (−2.55–5.19) |
| Jabagi et al. (2022) | Dose 1: 3.9 million vaccinees | | 3,993 | RI 0.85 (0.75–0.96) |
| | Dose 2: 3.2 million vaccinees | | 2,889 | RI 1.10 (0.95–1.26) |
| Shoaibi et al. (2023) | Doses 1 and 2: 3.4 million vaccinees | | 1,684 | IRR 1.19 (1.03–1.38) |
| Whiteley et al. (2022) | Dose 1: 8.7 million vaccinees | | 928 | Age <70: HR 0.78 (0.69–0.88) |
| | | | | Age >70: HR 0.54 (0.49–0.69) |

NOTES: BNT162b2 refers to the COVID-19 vaccine manufactured by Pfizer-BioNTech under the name Comirnaty®. Shoaibi et al. (2023) combined the number of BNT162b2 and mRNA-1273 vaccinees. The primary series for BNT162b2 is two doses. Number of events refers to events in vaccinees only. CI: confidence interval; HR: hazard ratio; IRR: incidence rate ratio; RD: risk difference; RI: relative incidence; RR: risk ratio; SIR: standardized incidence ratio.
SOURCES: Barda et al., 2021; Botton et al., 2022; Burn et al., 2022a,b; Hviid et al., 2022; Jabagi et al., 2022; Shoaibi et al., 2023; Whiteley et al., 2022.

As described for certain reports, some of the statistical models were adjusted for demographic characteristics, length of post-vaccination follow-up interval, prevalent comorbidity at baseline, and other features, such as season. Study designs included self-controls, cohort studies and matched case-control, all noted in Table 6-1. Hviid et al. (2022) from Denmark had the smallest number of follow-up patients.

Six reports from five studies showed no evidence of increased risk of PE, but three studies showed increased risk (Burn et al., 2022a,b; Shoaibi et al., 2023). Hviid et al. (2022), despite not showing an increased risk, had a very wide CI of the estimate, likely due to a smaller sample size in the base population and number of cases (RD 1.32, 95% CI: −2.55–5.19).

**mRNA-1273 and PE** Table 6-13 presents two studies that contributed to the causality assessment.

The mRNA-1273 association with PE was explored in two reports (Botton et al., 2022; Shoaibi et al., 2023). These studies are summarized in this section and Tables 6-1 and 6-13. The findings from Botton et al. (2022), representing persons 18–74 years of age, showed no increased risk of PE, but only 44 cases were noted. Shoaibi et al. (2023) also showed no increased risk. However, uniquely among all the reports assessed in this chapter, Shoaibi et al. (2023) conducted a medical record review of PE validated against the ICD codes. For the 101 cases identified by code, over half of the diagnoses were inaccurate or could not be determined. This suggests that case misclassification could be an important problem.

**TABLE 6-13** Epidemiological Studies in the mRNA-1273–Pulmonary Embolism Evidence Review

| Author | N | | Number of Events | Results (95% CI) |
|---|---|---|---|---|
| Botton et al. (2022) | Dose 1: 1,003 vaccinees | | Week 1: 18 | RI 0.43 (0.26–0.71) |
| | | | Week 2: 26 | RI 0.72 (0.48–1.09) |
| | Dose 2: 769 vaccinees | | Week 1: 36 | RI 1.31 (0.90–1.91) |
| | | | Week 2: 23 | RI 0.88 (0.56–1.40) |
| Shoaibi et al. (2023) | Doses 1 and 2: 3.4 million vaccinees | | 786 | IRR 1.15 (0.94–1.41) |

NOTES: Shoaibi et al. (2023) combined the number of BNT162b2 and mRNA-1273 vaccinees. The primary series for mRNA-1273 is two doses. Number of events refers to events in vaccinees only. CI: confidence interval; IRR: incidence rate ratio; RI: relative incidence.
SOURCES: Botton et al., 2022; Shoaibi et al., 2023.

**TABLE 6-14** Epidemiological Study in the Ad26.COV2.S–Pulmonary Embolism Evidence Review

| Author | N | Number of Events | Results (95% CI) |
|---|---|---|---|
| Botton et al. (2022) | Dose 1: 77 vaccinees | Week 1: 7 | RI 0.94 (0.40–2.21) |
| | | Week 2: 3 | RI 0.42 (0.13–1.32) |

NOTES: Ad26.COV2.S refers to the COVID-19 vaccine manufactured by Janssen. The primary series for Ad26.COV2.S is one dose. Number of events refers to events in vaccinees only. CI: confidence interval; RI: relative incidence.
SOURCE: Botton et al., 2022.

**Ad26.COV2.S and PE** Table 6-14 summarizes one study that contributed to the causality assessment.

Only one scientific report related Ad26.COV2.S to PE: Botton et al. (2022), an assessment from the French National Health Data System, covering persons aged 18–74. The findings showed no increased association of this vaccine with PE, but only 10 cases of PE recorded in the 2 post-vaccination weeks were available for analysis.

## Venous Thromboembolism

Although VTE is used throughout the literature on vascular and coagulation-related diseases, it appears to be used differently in different literature reports, as noted. For example, it often appears to include both thrombotic conditions (deep and superficial) in various anatomic sites and for embolic phenomena. A few studies have been done on validation of the rubric as used in ICD coding. One study of VTE using ICD-9 coding concluded that it was not an effective code for determining underlying conditions (Fang et al., 2017). Another study of VTE coding in the emergency department setting concluded that the ICD-10 code was only moderately effective in identifying DVT and PE (Al-Ani et al., 2015). Shoaibi et al. (2023) found validation problems with these entities, and this calls into question the potential validity of VTE outcomes in certain population studies that apply institutional coding systems, where validation studies have not been performed.

*Epidemiological Evidence*

**BNT162b2 and VTE** Table 6-15 presents four studies that contributed to the causality assessment.

Despite issues of outcome identification and the possibility of case misclassification, the committee assessed the three studies that used the VTE outcome rubric. The four reports presented VTE outcomes, available for BNT162b2 only. Hippisley-Cox et al. (2021) presented VTE outcomes for four separate 1-week post-vaccination

**TABLE 6-15** Epidemiological Studies in the BNT162b2–Venous Thromboembolism Evidence Review

| Author | N | Number of Events | Results (95% CI) |
|---|---|---|---|
| Ab Rahman et al. (2022) | Dose 1: 8.7 million vaccinees | 103 | IRR 1.34 (1.07–1.26) |
| | Dose 2: 6.7 million vaccinees | 63 | IRR 1.09 (0.83–1.44) |
| Burn et al. (2022a) | Dose 1: 1.8 million vaccinees | 595 | SIR 1.12 (1.03–1.21) |
| | Dose 2: 1.3 million vaccinees | 324 | SIR 0.86 (0.77–0.96) |
| Burn et al. (2022b) | Dose 1: 2.0 million vaccinees | 313 | SIR 1.18 (1.06–1.32) |
| | Dose 2: 1.3 million vaccinees | 227 | SIR 0.92 (0.81–1.05) |
| Hippisley-Cox et al. (2021) | Dose 1: 9.5 million vaccinees | Total: 2,054 Days 8–14: 555 | Days 8–14: IRR 0.99 (0.90–1.08) |

NOTES: BNT162b2 refers to the COVID-19 vaccine manufactured by Pfizer-BioNTech under the name Comirnaty®. Number of events refers to events in vaccinees only. CI: confidence interval; IRR: incidence rate ratio; SIR: standardized incidence ratio.
SOURCES: Ab Rahman et al., 2022; Burn et al., 2022a,b; Hippisley-Cox et al., 2021.

outcomes, without any further summarization; the week with the highest risk outcome (days 8–14) is included in Table 6-15. Burn et al. (2022a,b) showed a very slight increased risk after dose 1. Given the limitations noted, three of the four studies showed an increased risk of VTE associated with this vaccine, albeit modest increases.

### From Evidence to Conclusions

Five population studies from Europe and Israel evaluated the association between BNT162b2 and the risk of DVT. None showed any significant increased risk. However, Hviid et al. (2022) had a much smaller number of patient outcomes and a wide CI. The dilemma for these five studies is that some had other clinical rubrics or outcome categories denoting coagulation disorders or "VTE." This and the general problem of uncertainty in disease classification raised the issue that some of these patients may not have had DVT, leading to some possible loss of sample size and disease misclassification.

Eight reports from seven studies addressed the association between BNT162b2 and risk of PE (Barda et al., 2021; Botton et al., 2022; Burn et al., 2022a,b; Hviid et al., 2022; Jabagi et al., 2022; Shoaibi et al., 2023; Whiteley et al., 2022). All studies were informative for the committee's analysis, but they varied to some extent in epidemiological design. All but one study had suitably robust sample sizes. Some concern arose based on a validation study whether all diagnoses of PE could be confirmed on further review. Four studies showed no evidence of increased risk of PE, but three found a statistically significant increased risk.

The number of studies addressing VTE was limited (four) and addressed only BNT162b2; three pointed in the direction of increased risk, albeit modest (Ab Rahman et al., 2022; Burn et al., 2022a,b; Hippisley-Cox et al., 2021). A composite outcome, VTE could have been analyzed in the other studies that reported only PE and DVT as the outcomes, so the results might be at greater risk of reporting bias compared with other outcomes. The remaining issue is potential validation problems for VTE, and its constituent DVT and PE diagnoses, based on some of the quality assessment literature consulted.

**Conclusion 6-13: The evidence is inadequate to accept or reject a causal relationship between the BNT162b2 vaccine and deep vein thrombosis, pulmonary embolism, and venous thromboembolism.**

No studies evaluated the relationship between mRNA-1273 and DVT or VTE. Only two studies provided evidence for PE outcomes (Botton et al., 2022; Shoaibi et al., 2023); both showed no evidence of increased risk. The sample sizes were generally more modest than with BNT162b2. The results are complicated by the problem noted with diagnostic validation.

**Conclusion 6-14: The evidence is inadequate to accept or reject a causal relationship between the mRNA-1273 vaccine and deep vein thrombosis, pulmonary embolism, and venous thromboembolism.**

Only one study was available to assess the evidence between Ad26.COV2.S and PE (Botton et al., 2022). The number of cases was very small in the 2-week post-vaccination follow-up period, although no increased risk was found. The committee notes the case validation issue. No studies evaluated the relationship between NVX-CoV2373 and DVT, PE, or VTE.

**Conclusion 6-15: The evidence is inadequate to accept or reject a causal relationship between the Ad26.COV2.S vaccine and deep vein thrombosis, pulmonary embolism, and venous thromboembolism.**

**Conclusion 6-16: The evidence is inadequate to accept or reject a causal relationship between the NVX-CoV2373 vaccine and deep vein thrombosis, pulmonary embolism, and venous thromboembolism.**

# REFERENCES

Ab Rahman, N., M. T. Lim, F. Y. Lee, S. C. Lee, A. Ramli, S. N. Saharudin, T. L. King, E. B. Anak Jam, N. A. Ayub, R. K. Sevalingam, R. Bahari, N. N. Ibrahim, F. Mahmud, S. Sivasampu, and K. M. Peariasamy. 2022. Risk of serious adverse events after the BNT162b2, CoronaVac, and ChAdOx1 vaccines in Malaysia: A self-controlled case series study. *Vaccine* 40(32):4394–4402. https://doi.org/10.1016/j.vaccine.2022.05.075.

ALA (American Lung Association). 2023. Learn about pulmonary embolism. https://www.lung.org/lung-health-diseases/lung-disease-lookup/pulmonary-embolism/learn-about-pulmonary-embolism (accessed December 12, 2023).

Al-Ani, F., S. Shariff, L. Siqueira, A. Seyam, and A. Lazo-Langner. 2015. Identifying venous thromboembolism and major bleeding in emergency room discharges using administrative data. *Thrombosis Research* 136(6):1195–1198. https://doi.org/10.1016/j.thromres.2015.10.035.

Assiri, S. A., R. M. M. Althaqafi, K. Alswat, A. A. Alghamdi, N. E. Alomairi, D. M. Nemenqani, Z. S. Ibrahim, and A. Elkady. 2022. Post COVID-19 vaccination-associated neurological complications. *Neuropsychiatric Disease and Treatment* 18:137–154. https://doi.org/10.2147/ndt.S343438.

Barda, N., N. Dagan, Y. Ben-Shlomo, E. Kepten, J. Waxman, R. Ohana, M. A. Hernán, M. Lipsitch, I. Kohane, D. Netzer, B. Y. Reis, and R. D. Balicer. 2021. Safety of the BNT162b2 mRNA COVID-19 vaccine in a nationwide setting. *New England Journal of Medicine* 385(12):1078–1090. https://doi.org/10.1056/NEJMoa2110475.

Bonaventura, A., A. Vecchié, L. Dagna, K. Martinod, D. L. Dixon, B. W. Van Tassell, F. Dentali, F. Montecucco, S. Massberg, M. Levi, and A. Abbate. 2021. Endothelial dysfunction and immunothrombosis as key pathogenic mechanisms in COVID-19. *Nature Reviews: Immunology* 21(5):319–329. https://doi.org/10.1038/s41577-021-00536-9.

Botton, J., M. J. Jabagi, M. Bertrand, B. Baricault, J. Drouin, S. Le Vu, A. Weill, P. Farrington, M. Zureik, and R. Dray-Spira. 2022. Risk for myocardial infarction, stroke, and pulmonary embolism following COVID-19 vaccines in adults younger than 75 years in France. *Annals of Internal Medicine* 175(9):1250–1257. https://doi.org/10.7326/m22-0988.

Burn, E., X. Li, A. Delmestri, N. Jones, T. Duarte-Salles, C. Reyes, E. Martinez-Hernandez, E. Marti, K. M. C. Verhamme, P. R. Rijnbeek, V. Y. Strauss, and D. Prieto-Alhambra. 2022a. Thrombosis and thrombocytopenia after vaccination against and infection with SARS-CoV-2 in the United Kingdom. *Nature Communications* 13(1):7167. https://doi.org/10.1038/s41467-022-34668-w.

Burn, E., E. Roel, A. Pistillo, S. Fernández-Bertolín, M. Aragón, B. Raventós, C. Reyes, K. Verhamme, P. Rijnbeek, X. Li, V. Y. Strauss, D. Prieto-Alhambra, and T. Duarte-Salles. 2022b. Thrombosis and thrombocytopenia after vaccination against and infection with SARS-CoV-2 in Catalonia, Spain. *Nature Communications* 13(1):7169. https://doi.org/10.1038/s41467-022-34669-9.

Caplan, L. R. 2023. *Patient education: Hemorrhagic stroke treatment (beyond the basics)*. https://www.uptodate.com/contents/hemorrhagic-stroke-treatment-beyond-the-basics (accessed November 6, 2023).

Chamorro, A., A. Meisel, A. M. Planas, X. Urra, D. van de Beek, and R. Veltkamp. 2012. The immunology of acute stroke. *Nature Reviews: Neurology* 8(7):401–410. https://doi.org/10.1038/nrneurol.2012.98.

Chui, C. S. L., M. Fan, E. Y. F. Wan, M. T. Y. Leung, E. Cheung, V. K. C. Yan, L. Gao, Y. Ghebremichael-Weldeselassie, K. K. C. Man, K. K. Lau, I. C. H. Lam, F. T. T. Lai, X. Li, C. K. H. Wong, E. W. Chan, C. L. Cheung, C. W. Sing, C. K. Lee, I. F. N. Hung, C. S. Lau, J. Y. S. Chan, M. K. Lee, V. C. T. Mok, C. W. Siu, L. S. T. Chan, T. Cheung, F. L. F. Chan, A. Y. Leung, B. J. Cowling, G. M. Leung, and I. C. K. Wong. 2022. Thromboembolic events and hemorrhagic stroke after mRNA (BNT162b2) and inactivated (CoronaVac) COVID-19 vaccination: A self-controlled case series study. *EClinicalMedicine* 50:101504. https://doi.org/10.1016/j.eclinm.2022.101504.

Davidson, S. M., A. Adameova, L. Barile, H. A. Cabrera-Fuentes, A. Lazou, P. Pagliaro, K. O. Stenslokken, D. Garcia-Dorado, and E.-C. C. Action. 2020. Mitochondrial and mitochondrial-independent pathways of myocardial cell death during ischaemia and reperfusion injury. *Journal of Cellular and Molecular Medicine* 24(7):3795–3806. https://doi.org/10.1111/jcmm.15127.

de Mélo Silva, M. L., Jr., and D. P. Lopes. 2021. Large hemorrhagic stroke after ChAdOx1 NCOV-19 vaccination: A case report. *Acta Neurologica Scandinavica* 144(6):717–718. https://doi.org/10.1111/ane.13505.

Famularo, G. 2022. Stroke after COVID-19 vaccination. *Acta Neurologica Scandinavica* 145(6):787–788. https://doi.org/10.1111/ane.13608.

Fang, M. C., D. Fan, S. H. Sung, D. M. Witt, J. R. Schmelzer, S. R. Steinhubl, S. H. Yale, and A. S. Go. 2017. Validity of using inpatient and outpatient administrative codes to identify acute venous thromboembolism: The CVRN VTE study. *Medical Care* 55(12):e137–e143. https://doi.org/10.1097/MLR.0000000000000524.

FDA (Food and Drug Administration). 2021. *Emergency use authorization (EUA) amendment for an unapproved product review memorandum*. Food and Drug Administration. https://www.fda.gov/media/153439/download (accessed May 3, 2023).

FDA. 2023a. *BLA clinical review memorandum—COMIRNATY*. Food and Drug Administration. https://www.fda.gov/media/172333/download?attachment (accessed December 5, 2023).

FDA. 2023b. *BLA clinical review memorandum—SPIKEVAX*. Food and Drug Administration. https://www.fda.gov/media/172357/download?attachment (accessed December 5, 2023).

FDA. 2023c. *Emergency use authorization (EUA) for an unapproved product review memorandum*. Food and Drug Administration. https://www.fda.gov/media/168233/download?attachment (accessed December 5, 2023).

Giorgio, K., R. F. Walker, R. F. MacLehose, D. Adrianzen-Herrera, W. Wang, A. Alonso, N. A. Zakai, and P. L. Lutsey. 2023. Venous thromboembolism mortality and trends in older U.S. adults, 2011–2019. *American Journal of Hematology* 98(9):1364–1373. https://doi.org/10.1002/ajh.26996.

Gross, B. A., B. T. Jankowitz, and R. M. Friedlander. 2019. Cerebral intraparenchymal hemorrhage: A review. *JAMA* 321(13):1295–1303. https://doi.org/10.1001/jama.2019.2413.

Grosso, A., I. Douglas, R. MacAllister, I. Petersen, L. Smeeth, and A. D. Hingorani. 2011. Use of the self-controlled case series method in drug safety assessment. *Expert Opinion on Drug Safety* 10(3):337–340. https://doi.org/10.1517/14740338.2011.562187.

Hana, D., K. Patel, S. Roman, B. Gattas, and S. Sofka. 2022. Clinical cardiovascular adverse events reported post-COVID-19 vaccination: Are they a real risk? *Current Problems in Cardiology* 47(3):101077. https://doi.org/10.1016/j.cpcardiol.2021.101077.

Hervé, C., B. Laupèze, G. Del Giudice, A. M. Didierlaurent, and F. Tavares Da Silva. 2019. The how's and what's of vaccine reactogenicity. *NPJ Vaccines* 4:39. https://doi.org/10.1038/s41541-019-0132-6.

Hippisley-Cox, J., M. Patone, X. W. Mei, D. Saatci, S. Dixon, K. Khunti, F. Zaccardi, P. Watkinson, M. Shankar-Hari, J. Doidge, D. A. Harrison, S. J. Griffin, A. Sheikh, and C. A. C. Coupland. 2021. Risk of thrombocytopenia and thromboembolism after COVID-19 vaccination and SARS-CoV-2 positive testing: Self-controlled case series study. *British Journal of Medicine* 374:n1931. https://doi.org/10.1136/bmj.n1931.

Hviid, A., J. V. Hansen, E. M. Thiesson, and J. Wohlfahrt. 2022. Association of AZD1222 and BNT162b2 COVID-19 vaccination with thromboembolic and thrombocytopenic events in frontline personnel: A retrospective cohort study. *Annals of Internal Medicine* 175(4):541–546. https://doi.org/10.7326/m21-2452.

Jabagi, M. J., J. Botton, M. Bertrand, A. Weill, P. Farrington, M. Zureik, and R. Dray-Spira. 2022. Myocardial infarction, stroke, and pulmonary embolism after BNT162b2 mRNA COVID-19 vaccine in people aged 75 years or older. *JAMA* 327(1):80–82. https://doi.org/10.1001/jama.2021.21699.

Kirkman, M. A., W. Mahattanakul, B. A. Gregson, and A. D. Mendelow. 2009. The accuracy of hospital discharge coding for hemorrhagic stroke. *Acta Neurologica Belgica* 109(2):114–119.

Langgartner, D., R. Winkler, J. Brunner-Weisser, N. Rohleder, M. N. Jarczok, H. Gündel, K. Weimer, and S. O. Reber. 2023. COVID-19 vaccination exacerbates ex vivo IL-6 release from isolated PBMCS. *Scientific Reports* 13(1):9496. https://doi.org/10.1038/s41598-023-35731-2.

Li, X., and G. Chen. 2023. CNS-peripheral immune interactions in hemorrhagic stroke. *Journal of Cerebral Blood Flow and Metabolism* 43(2):185–197. https://doi.org/10.1177/0271678x221145089.

McCormick, N., V. Bhole, D. Lacaille, and J. A. Avina-Zubieta. 2015. Validity of diagnostic codes for acute stroke in administrative databases: A systematic review. *PLoS One* 10(8):e0135834. https://doi.org/10.1371/journal.pone.0135834.

Mithoowani, S. 2022. *Deep vein thrombosis (DVT) (beyond the basics)*. www.uptodate.com/contents/deep-vein-thrombosis-dvt-beyond-the-basics (accessed November 16, 2023).

Montano, A., D. F. Hanley, and J. C. Hemphill, III. 2021. Hemorrhagic stroke. *Handbook of Clinical Neurology* 176:229–248. https://doi.org/10.1016/B978-0-444-64034-5.00019-5.

Nakamura, K., and T. Shichita. 2019. Cellular and molecular mechanisms of sterile inflammation in ischaemic stroke. *Journal of Biochemistry* 165(6):459–464. https://doi.org/10.1093/jb/mvz017.

Neves, G., P. I. Warman, A. Warman, R. Warman, T. Bueso, J. D. Vadhan, and T. Windisch. 2023. External validation of an artificial intelligence device for intracranial hemorrhage detection. *World Neurosurgery* 173:e800–e807. https://doi.org/10.1016/j.wneu.2023.03.019.

NHLBI (National Heart, Lung, and Blood Institute). 2023. *What is a stroke?* https://www.nhlbi.nih.gov/health/stroke (accessed November 16, 2023).

Patone, M., L. Handunnetthi, D. Saatci, J. Pan, S. V. Katikireddi, S. Razvi, D. Hunt, X. W. Mei, S. Dixon, F. Zaccardi, K. Khunti, P. Watkinson, C. A. C. Coupland, J. Doidge, D. A. Harrison, R. Ravanan, A. Sheikh, C. Robertson, and J. Hippisley-Cox. 2021. Neurological complications after first dose of COVID-19 vaccines and SARS-CoV-2 infection. *Nature Medicine* 27(12):2144–2153. https://doi.org/10.1038/s41591-021-01556-7.

Prabhu, S. D., and N. G. Frangogiannis. 2016. The biological basis for cardiac repair after myocardial infarction: From inflammation to fibrosis. *Circulation Research* 119(1):91–112. https://doi.org/10.1161/CIRCRESAHA.116.303577.

Robinson, K., J. M. Katzenellenbogen, T. J. Kleinig, J. Kim, C. A. Budgeon, A. G. Thrift, and L. Nedkoff. 2023. Large burden of stroke incidence in people with cardiac disease: A linked data cohort study. *Clinical Epidemiology* 15:203–211. https://doi.org/10.2147/CLEP.S390146.

Salari, N., F. Morddarvanjoghi, A. Abdolmaleki, S. Rasoulpoor, A. A. Khaleghi, L. A. Hezarkhani, S. Shohaimi, and M. Mohammadi. 2023. The global prevalence of myocardial infarction: A systematic review and meta-analysis. *BMC Cardiovascular Disorders* 23(1):206. https://doi.org/10.1186/s12872-023-03231-w.

Serrone, J. C., H. Maekawa, M. Tjahjadi, and J. Hernesniemi. 2015. Aneurysmal subarachnoid hemorrhage: Pathobiology, current treatment and future directions. *Expert Review of Neurotherapeutics* 15(4):367–380. https://doi.org/10.1586/14737175.2015.1018892.

Shoaibi, A., P. C. Lloyd, H. L. Wong, T. C. Clarke, Y. Chillarige, R. Do, M. Hu, Y. Jiao, A. Kwist, A. Lindaas, K. Matuska, R. McEvoy, S. Ondari, S. Parulekar, X. Shi, J. Wang, Y. Lu, J. Obidi, C. K. Zhou, J. A. Kelman, R. A. Forshee, and S. A. Anderson. 2023. Evaluation of potential adverse events following COVID-19 mRNA vaccination among adults aged 65 years and older: Two self-controlled studies in the U.S. *Vaccine* 41(32):4666–4678. https://doi.org/10.1016/j.vaccine.2023.06.014.

Siddiqi, H. K., P. Libby, and P. M. Ridker. 2021. COVID-19 - a vascular disease. *Trends in Cardiovascular Medicine* 31(1):1–5. https://doi.org/10.1016/j.tcm.2020.10.005.

Smith, S. D., and C. J. Eskey. 2011. Hemorrhagic stroke. *Radiologic Clinics of North America* 49(1):27–45. https://doi.org/10.1016/j.rcl.2010.07.011.

Tamariz, L., T. Harkins, and V. Nair. 2012. A systematic review of validated methods for identifying venous thromboembolism using administrative and claims data. *Pharmacoepidemiology and Drug Safety* 21(Suppl 1):154–162. https://doi.org/10.1002/pds.2341.

Tang, Y. H., S. Vital, J. Russell, H. Seifert, and D. N. Granger. 2015. Interleukin-6 mediates enhanced thrombus development in cerebral arterioles following a brief period of focal brain ischemia. *Experimental Neurology* 271:351–357. https://doi.org/10.1016/j.expneurol.2015.06.004.

Thygesen, K., J. S. Alpert, A. S. Jaffe, B. R. Chaitman, J. J. Bax, D. A. Morrow, and H. D. White. 2018. Fourth universal definition of myocardial infarction (2018). *Journal of the American College of Cardiology* 72(18):2231–2264. https://doi.org/doi:10.1016/j.jacc.2018.08.1038.

Vymazal, J., A. M. Rulseh, J. Keller, and L. Janouskova. 2012. Comparison of CT and MR imaging in ischemic stroke. *Insights Imaging* 3(6):619–627. https://doi.org/10.1007/s13244-012-0185-9.

Wang, H., X. Tang, H. Fan, Y. Luo, Y. Song, Y. Xu, and Y. Chen. 2020. Potential mechanisms of hemorrhagic stroke in elderly COVID-19 patients. *Aging* 12(11):10022–10034. https://doi.org/10.18632/aging.103335.

Whiteley, W. N., S. Ip, J. A. Cooper, T. Bolton, S. Keene, V. Walker, R. Denholm, A. Akbari, E. Omigie, S. Hollings, E. Di Angelantonio, S. Denaxas, A. Wood, J. A. C. Sterne, and C. Sudlow. 2022. Association of COVID-19 vaccines ChAdOx1 and BNT162b2 with major venous, arterial, or thrombocytopenic events: A population-based cohort study of 46 million adults in England. *PLoS Medicine* 19(2):e1003926. https://doi.org/10.1371/journal.pmed.1003926.

Zafar, U., H. Zafar, M. S. Ahmed, and M. Khattak. 2022. Link between COVID-19 vaccines and myocardial infarction. *World Journal of Clinical Cases* 10(28):10109–10119. https://doi.org/10.12998/wjcc.v10.i28.10109.

Zhu, X., K. A. Gebo, A. G. Abraham, F. Habtehyimer, E. U. Patel, O. Laeyendecker, T. J. Gniadek, R. E. Fernandez, O. R. Baker, M. Ram, E. R. Cachay, J. S. Currier, Y. Fukuta, J. M. Gerber, S. L. Heath, B. Meisenberg, M. A. Huaman, A. C. Levine, A. Shenoy, S. Anjan, J. E. Blair, D. Cruser, D. N. Forthal, L. L. Hammitt, S. Kassaye, G. S. Mosnaim, B. Patel, J. H. Paxton, J. S. Raval, C. G. Sutcliffe, M. Abinante, P. Broderick, V. Cluzet, M. E. Cordisco, B. Greenblatt, J. Petrini, W. Rausch, D. Shade, K. Lane, A. L. Gawad, S. L. Klein, A. Pekosz, S. Shoham, A. Casadevall, E. M. Bloch, D. Hanley, D. J. Sullivan, and A. A. R. Tobian. 2023. Dynamics of inflammatory responses after SARS-CoV-2 infection by vaccination status in the USA: A prospective cohort study. *The Lancet Microbe* 4(9):e692–e703. https://doi.org/https://doi.org/10.1016/S2666-5247(23)00171-4.

# 7

# Myocarditis, Pericarditis, and COVID-19 Vaccines

This chapter describes the potential relationship between COVID-19 vaccines and myocarditis and pericarditis (see Box 7-1 for all conclusions in this chapter).

---

**BOX 7-1**
**Conclusions for Myocarditis and Pericarditis**

**Conclusion 7-1: The evidence establishes a causal relationship between the BNT162b2 vaccine and myocarditis.**

**Conclusion 7-2: The evidence establishes a causal relationship between the mRNA-1273 vaccine and myocarditis.**

**Conclusion 7-3: The evidence is inadequate to accept or reject a causal relationship between the Ad26.COV2.S vaccine and myocarditis.**

**Conclusion 7-4: The evidence is inadequate to accept or reject a causal relationship between the NVX-CoV2373 vaccine and myocarditis.**

**Conclusion 7-5: The evidence is inadequate to accept or reject a causal relationship between the BNT162b2 vaccine and pericarditis without myocarditis.**

**Conclusion 7-6: The evidence is inadequate to accept or reject a causal relationship between the mRNA-1273 vaccine and pericarditis without myocarditis.**

**Conclusion 7-7: The evidence is inadequate to accept or reject a causal relationship between the Ad26.COV2.S vaccine and pericarditis without myocarditis.**

**Conclusion 7-8: The evidence is inadequate to accept or reject a causal relationship between the NVX-CoV2373 vaccine and pericarditis without myocarditis.**

---

## BACKGROUND

### Myocarditis

Myocarditis is defined as inflammation of the myocardium with or without necrosis (Cooper, 2009), and the gold standard for diagnosis is based on endomyocardial biopsy and established histologic, immunologic, and immuno-histochemical criteria (Caforio et al., 2013; Matsumori, 2003) based on the position statement of the Working Group on Myocardial and Pericardial Diseases of the European Society of Cardiology (Van Linthout and Tschöpe, 2018). For cases where a biopsy is not obtained, which is typical in the United States, the diagnosis can be made based on cardiac magnetic resonance imaging (MRI) (Ferreira et al., 2018). Cardiac MRI provides strong evidence for myocarditis based on a combination of T2- and T1-based markers that indicate cardiac edema as a sign of myocardial inflammation (Ferreira et al., 2018) in patients with the classical clinical findings associated with otherwise unexplained troponin elevation. No approved imaging modalities directly detect cardiac inflammation. A clinical definition of severe acute respiratory syndrome coronavirus-2 (SARS-CoV-2) severe acute respiratory syndrome coronavirus-2 (SARS-CoV-2)–induced myocarditis has been proposed that includes new or worsening clinical symptoms and one or more of the following: arrhythmias on electrocardiogram, cardiac dysfunction using echocardiography, or cardiac MRI indicative of myocarditis after infection (Heidecker et al., 2022; Tschöpe et al., 2021).

Most individuals develop acute myocarditis symptoms within a few days to 2 weeks after a viral infection (Cooper, 2009), and lymphocytic myocarditis is the most common form of myocarditis in the post-viral settings. Myocarditis has a variable presentation, ranging from subclinical disease to fatigue, chest pain, new-onset heart failure, cardiogenic shock, and sudden death (Cooper, 2009), and it is a common cause of sudden cardiac death in young adults. In cases of myocarditis following COVID-19 vaccination, signs and symptoms have been similar to those associated with other forms of myocarditis (Heidecker et al., 2022). However, the prognosis for myocarditis after COVID-19 vaccination appears to be much less severe. In a study of nearly 4 million residents of Hong Kong, only one death occurred (1 percent) among 104 cases of post-vaccination myocarditis, compared with 84 deaths (11 percent) among 762 cases of viral infection-related myocarditis (hazard ratio 0.08, 95% confidence interval [CI] 0.01–0.57) (Lai et al., 2022). In a surveillance study of cases of myocarditis related to COVID-19 vaccination in the United States reported to the Vaccine Adverse Event Reporting System (VAERS), among 484 hospitalizations there were no deaths, and evidence of ongoing myocarditis at follow-up cardiac MRI was uncommon (13 percent) (Kracalik et al., 2022).

Myocarditis is classified based on histological findings, including lymphocytic (the most common form in Europe and the United States), fulminant, eosinophilic, and giant cell (Caforio et al., 2013). Myocarditis can also be described by presumed causes, including viral, autoimmune, or other causes (Ball et al., 2019). Most patients with lymphocytic myocarditis recover fully, but some may develop dilated cardiomyopathy (DCM) several weeks to months later and progress to chronic heart failure that may need a heart transplant (McNamara et al., 2011; Schultheiss et al., 2019; Tschöpe et al., 2021). Fulminant, eosinophilic, and giant cell myocarditis are rare, result in a more severe clinical course, and have a greater risk of sudden death (Abston et al., 2012a; Ammirati et al., 2019; Cooper et al., 1997; Maleszewski et al., 2015). Pediatric myocarditis tends to be more fulminant (Law et al., 2021).

### Pericarditis

Pericarditis is defined as inflammation of the pericardium, the fibroelastic sac that surrounds the heart, according to the World Health Organization classification (Adler et al., 2015). The major clinical manifestations and diagnostic criteria include chest pain, which is typically sharp and pleuritic; pericardial friction rub; electrocardiogram changes; and pericardial effusion (Chiabrando et al., 2020; Imazio et al., 2015). The diagnosis is typically made based on clinical signs and symptoms, which in many cases can be challenging.

Acute myocarditis and pericarditis frequently co-occur in clinical practice and animal models of viral or auto-immune myocarditis and are often referred to as "myopericarditis" (primary myocarditis phenotype) or "perimyo-carditis" (primarily pericarditis phenotype) depending on the primary clinical symptoms. The etiology is similar for both myocarditis and perimyocarditis, with viral infections being the predominant causative agent, including coxsackieviruses, influenza, and SARS-CoV-2 (Aljohani et al., 2022; Fairweather et al., 2023a). Because of the challenges in distinguishing myocarditis alone from myocarditis with features of pericarditis, and because of the clinical and prognostic importance of myocarditis, we included both in our review of the evidence for myocarditis related to COVID-19 vaccines. Separately, we reviewed evidence for the potential effect of COVID-19 vaccines on acute pericarditis alone (i.e., pericarditis without myocarditis). In this chapter, the term pericarditis and our conclusions about pericarditis refer only to pericarditis without myocarditis.

## EPIDEMIOLOGY OF MYOCARDITIS AND PERICARDITIS

The latest Global Burden of Disease report estimates the worldwide age-standardized morbidity and mortality of myocarditis combined with all types of cardiomyopathy in men versus women prior to the COVID-19 pandemic to be 6.5 per 100,000 years lived with disability (YLDs) (95% uncertainty interval [UI]: 4.3–9.3 per 100,000 YLDs) and 4.2 per 100,000 YLDs (95% UI: 2.8 –6.0 per 100,000 YLDs), respectively, and 148.9 per 100,000 years of life lost (YLLs) (95% UI: 120.2–168.7 per 100,000 YLLs) and 71.4 per 100,000 YLLs (95% UI: 61.0–79.9 per 100,000 YLLs), respectively. After adjustment for a 7-day risk period, estimated background or expected rates of myocarditis and pericarditis after COVID-19 vaccination in the United States are 0.2 and 1.4 per 1 million people, respectively (Pillay et al., 2022). Similar to myocarditis, men aged 16–65 have a greater risk of acute pericarditis than women (Fairweather et al., 2023a; Kytö et al., 2014). Prevalence refers to the frequency of a condition at a given point in time, which cannot be used to estimate a background rate of an event during a unit of time (e.g., incidence). For myocarditis only, the prevalence of myocarditis in individuals 35–39 years of age is 6.1 per 100,000 (95% UI: 4.2–8.7 per 100,000) in men and 4.4 per 100,000 (95% UI: 3.0–6.3 per 100,000) in women.

## MECHANISMS

### Myocarditis and Pericarditis

Most of the understanding of the pathogenesis or mechanisms of myocarditis and myopericarditis comes from animal models, where pericarditis always occurs with myocarditis. Myocarditis can be caused by many infectious and noninfectious agents, such as viruses, bacteria, parasites (*Trypanasoma cruzi* leading to Chagas disease), and toxins, including anthracyclines, ethanol, arsenic, cocaine, and heavy metals (Jain et al., 2022). Myocarditis is often considered to result from direct damage by infections or toxins, but it may also involve autoimmune mechanisms, perhaps triggered by infections/toxins (Fairweather et al., 2001; Root-Bernstein and Fairweather, 2014; Root-Bernstein et al., 2023). The primary mouse models of myocarditis are viral, autoimmune, or both (Ciháková et al., 2004; Fairweather et al., 2012; Poli et al., 2020), and most use male mice. Regardless of the animal model, common immune mechanisms have been identified in all models that increase the severity of the condition (myocardial inflammation), particularly in males (Fairweather et al., 2023a). All models in male mice have shown that the inflammatory infiltrate during peak acute myocarditis consists of a mixed infiltrate of predominantly macrophages, with fewer T and B cells and small numbers of natural killer cells, dendritic cells, mast cells, and other cell types (Ciháková et al., 2008; Frisancho-Kiss et al., 2007; Huber and Job, 1983; Liu et al., 2013). In contrast, female mice have far less cardiac inflammation (Fairweather et al., 2023a; Frisancho-Kiss et al., 2007; Huber and Job, 1983). In animal models of myocarditis, male mice have more mast cells and macrophages than females (Frisancho-Kiss et al., 2006a, 2007, 2009). Similar histologic findings are also observed in biopsies from patients with myocarditis (Baumeier et al., 2022; Fairweather et al., 2014, 2023b; Heidecker et al., 2022; Lüscher and Akhtar, 2022). Mechanisms that drive sex differences in young male white-genetic-background mice (i.e., BALB/c, A/J) have been well described (Fairweather et al., 2013, 2023b; Huber and Job, 1983). Increased viral myocarditis in male mice is associated with elevated numbers of mast cells and macrophages in the heart that express complement receptors (CR3, also called "CD11b," and C3aR and C5aR) and Toll-like receptor 4 (TLR4)/ inflammasome (Cooper et al., 2010; Fairweather et al., 2003; Frisancho-Kiss et al., 2007). Only white-background mice are susceptible to autoimmune myocarditis/perimyocarditis and progressing to DCM (Fairweather et al.,

2001; Neu et al., 1987). This is due to higher levels of mast cells in the peritoneum, spleen, and heart that drive the immune response toward a proinflammatory and profibrotic immune response after infection or in response to self-antigens (Fairweather et al., 2004a).

Evidence of the importance of the complement and TLR4/inflammasome pathways in the pathogenesis of myocarditis was recently illustrated when microRNA (in extracellular vesicles [EVs]) targeting these specific pathways was able to prevent myocardial inflammation in a viral animal model (Beetler et al., 2023). EVs, with their receptors and content, can be proinflammatory or immunoregulatory (Beetler et al., 2023), which is important when discussing potential vaccine mechanisms, particularly messenger ribonucleic acid (mRNA) vaccines that consist of mRNA packaged in a lipid nanoparticle (LNP). Activation of the innate immune response is critical for the induction and progression of viral and autoimmune myocarditis. Key innate pathways include complement pathways, and TLR4/ inflammasome pathways are known to play a role in animal models and human myocarditis (Cooper et al., 2010; Fairweather et al., 2003, 2006; Frisancho-Kiss et al., 2007; Roberts et al., 2013; Tschöpe et al., 2017). The majority of immune cells in the hearts of male mice and humans during acute myocarditis are CR3 positive activated mast cells and macrophages (Fairweather et al., 2014; Frisancho-Kiss et al., 2007). TLR4 signaling works through the inflammasome (NLRP3) to produce the cytokines interleukin (IL)-1β and IL-18 during myocarditis in males (Fairweather et al., 2003; Tschöpe et al., 2017). IL-1β increases inflammation and remodeling, leading to cardiac fibrosis and then DCM in susceptible strains of mice (Coronado et al., 2012; Fairweather et al., 2004b). IL-18 strongly induces interferon (IFN) γ responses that drive M1 macrophages and T helper (Th)1-type immune responses in male mice with viral myocarditis and are needed to control viral replication (Frisancho-Kiss et al., 2006b; Toldo and Abbate, 2023). TLR2 has also been found to be important in mouse models of myocarditis; TLR2 signaling can be activated by cardiac myosin antigens and promote autoimmune T helper 17 (Th17)-type immune responses that contribute to remodeling and progression to DCM in male mice (Baldeviano et al., 2010; Myers et al., 2016; Roberts et al., 2013).

Susceptibility to myocarditis in animal models is associated with mast cells, which are abundantly present in allergy-prone white-background mouse strains, that promote inflammation, pericarditis, and fibrosis, leading to DCM (Abston et al., 2012b, 2013; Afanasyeva et al., 2001; Coronado et al., 2012; Fairweather et al., 2004a). Mouse strains with very few mast cells, such as C57BL/6 (B6) or B10, do not develop autoimmune myocarditis or progress to DCM after acute myocarditis (Abston et al., 2012a, 2013; Afanasyeva et al., 2001; Fairweather et al., 2004a). Mast cells are the first antigen-presenting cells to respond to virus in the autoimmune coxsackievirus B3 (CVB3) model of myocarditis in BALB/c mice, where they upregulate CD11b/CR3 and TLR4 (Frisancho-Kiss et al., 2006b, 2007). Mast cells are critical in driving macrophages to an alternatively activated M2 phenotype during acute myocarditis, where they work together to increase cardiac inflammation and remodeling/fibrosis in males (Coronado et al., 2012). Mast cell degranulation is associated with pericarditis/perimyocarditis in mice (Bruno et al., 2019, 2021; Fairweather et al., 2004a, 2006).

Almost no research has examined mechanisms underlying pericarditis in the absence of myocarditis because in these animal models the two are always present together. The efficacy of colchicine in treating patients with pericarditis (Imazio et al., 2005a,b, 2011, 2013, 2014) points to an important role for the NLRP3 inflammasome in its pathogenesis. The NLRP3 inflammasome cleaves caspase-1, leading to the production of IL-1β and IL-18 (Martinon et al., 2006). TLR4 produces proIL-1β and proIL-18 that caspase-1 cleaves, leading to active IL-1β and IL-18 that promote soluble ST2 and IL-6 levels, which are serum biomarkers for all forms of heart failure, including myocarditis (Coronado et al., 2019; Potere et al., 2023). Colchicine also impairs neutrophil adhesion to vascular endothelium, increases leukocytic cyclic adenosine monophosphate levels, and inhibits IL-1β and TNF (tumor necrosis factor) production from macrophages (Potere et al., 2023).

## SARS-CoV-2-Associated Myocarditis and Pericarditis

SARS-CoV-2 infection dramatically increased the reported incidence of myocarditis and pericarditis. The overall U.S. incidence of myocarditis from SARS-CoV-2 infection has been estimated in a study by the Centers for Disease Control and Prevention (CDC) at around 150 cases per 100,000 versus 9 cases per 100,000 in non-COVID-19 cases during the same time period (Boehmer et al., 2021). A separate study in the United States and Europe estimated 240 and 410 cases per 100,000 of definite/probable or possible myocarditis, respectively (Ammirati et al., 2022). These data indicate more than a 15-fold increased risk of developing myocarditis from SARS-CoV-2 infection compared to pre-COVID-19 rates.

The signs and symptoms of COVID-19-associated myocarditis are very similar to other forms. Much like in other causes of myocarditis, immunohistochemistry performed on biopsies found a predominant infiltrate of CD68+ macrophages (CD11b is not typically assessed in clinical biopsies) with fewer T cells—the same as animal models of myocarditis (Basso et al., 2020; Heidecker et al., 2022; Lovell et al., 2022). Thus, COVID-19-associated myocarditis is histologically similar to other forms of myocarditis.

SARS-CoV-2 infection causes an immune response (and sex differences in the immune response) that is very similar to that which has been found to drive myocarditis/perimyocarditis in animal models. For example, most studies of COVID-19 reported more male than female patients and higher numbers of circulating neutrophils and macrophages; female patients had more T cells (Lau et al., 2021; Takahashi et al., 2020). Male patients with COVID-19 were also reported to have higher circulating levels of ferritin, C-reactive protein, IL-6, IL-8, and IL-18 (Lau et al., 2021; Takahashi et al., 2020). COVID-19 has been documented to strongly complement and activate other innate immune pathways, such as TLR4 and the inflammasome, which leads to increased IL-1β and IL-18 levels (Amin et al., 2022; Carvelli et al., 2020; Huber et al., 2021; Toldo et al., 2021). TLR4 signaling is key in driving proinflammatory responses associated with COVID-19 and contributes to an increased Th1-type immune response because IL-18 (and IL-1β) strongly induces IFNs (Cai et al., 2000; Frisancho-Kiss et al., 2006a). T cell immuno-globulin mucin (Tim-3) is a receptor that is upregulated on mast cells and macrophages in female patients during viral myocarditis that inhibits T cell responses and is associated with increased IL-10 release from alternatively activated M2 macrophages, conferring protection (Frisancho-Kiss et al., 2007, 2009). Tim-3 and IL-10 upregulation are also observed in COVID-19 and thought to contribute to the immunosuppressive state (Shahbazi et al., 2021).

Angiotensin-converting enzyme 2 (ACE2) had been identified as the receptor for SARS-CoV-2 (Lan et al., 2020). The spike protein binds ACE2 and is cleaved by type II transmembrane serine protease 2 (TMPRSS2), facilitating viral entry into the cytosol, and is also required for entry into cells (Hoffmann et al., 2020); this process is detailed in Chapter 2. A number of cell types in the heart and immune cells express ACE2, including cardiomyocytes, pericytes (located around vessels in the heart), fibroblasts, endothelial cells, and macrophages and mast cells (Chen et al., 2020; Hikmet et al., 2020; Theoharides, 2021). Other accessory proteins (i.e., neuropilin-1 receptor/NRP1, CD147, integrin α5β1, and cathepsin B/L) are also needed for SARS-CoV-2 infection and found on mast cells (Theoharides, 2021). As described earlier, mast cells and macrophages are found in much higher levels in males than females. Thus, the spike protein activating mast cells by ACE2 is a potential mechanism that contributes to the development of myocarditis following COVID-19 in males (Fairweather et al., 2023b).

## COVID-19 Vaccine–Associated Myocarditis/Pericarditis

Similar to other forms of myocarditis (Halsell et al., 2003; Roth et al., 2020), myocarditis after COVID-19 vaccination has been reported to occur most frequently in White male patients aged 16–30 and primarily in individuals under 50 (Straus et al., 2023), with few reports past age 50. The findings of a similar sex, age, and race/ethnicity for myocarditis of all types, including vaccine-associated cases, suggest similar mechanisms are at play.

Most vaccine-associated cases of myocarditis were reported after vaccination with mRNA platform vaccines, specifically after the second dose. The second dose was already known from healthy volunteers to promote a robust humoural, cell-mediated, and innate immune response (Arunachalam et al., 2021). These vaccines contain modified mRNA that encodes the spike protein encapsulated by LNPs that are similar in structure and composition to EVs. The mRNA vaccines do not contain live or heat-inactivated virus. Cases of myocarditis were also reported after adenoviral vector SARS-CoV-2 vaccines (Husby et al., 2021), but by far most cases were associated with mRNA platforms (Diaz et al., 2021).

When biopsies were obtained from patients with myocarditis after COVID-19 vaccination, the immune infiltrate was found to resemble classic lymphocytic myocarditis, with macrophages and T and B cell infiltrates (Baumeier et al., 2022; Fairweather et al., 2023b; Heidecker et al., 2022; Lüscher and Akhtar, 2022). The authors of case reports and small case series often identified the vaccine as the probable cause because people developed myocarditis shortly after receiving it (Baumeier et al., 2022). Some studies also carefully tested for viral infections to eliminate that as a cause (Baumeier et al., 2022). That similar infiltrates occur in vaccine-associated cases of myocarditis as in those from other causes and animal models suggests a common mechanism. Evidence that mRNA vaccine components may increase complement and TLR4/inflammasome/IL-1β immune responses and activate mast cells comes from a number of studies. LNPs have been used in mRNA vaccine platforms to prevent mRNA degradation, facilitate mRNA delivery, and stimulate the immune response but have also been linked with complement activation-related mast cell hypersensitivity reactions and TLR-mediated release of proinflammatory cytokines (Halamoda-Kenzaoui and Bremer-Hoffmann, 2018; Kauffman et al., 2016; Lamerton et al., 2022; Power et al., 2022; Samaridou et al., 2020; Seneff et al., 2022). A number of components in the mRNA LNPs, including polyethylene glycol, cholesterol, and saponin, are well known to activate mast cells and a primary reason individuals develop allergic responses (Hou et al., 2021; Tsilingiris et al., 2022). Ndeupen et al. (2021) found that the mRNA platform's LNP component was highly inflammatory. They observed significant upregulation of gene transcripts associated with activating the TLR4/inflammasome, such as NLRP3, IL-1β, and IL-6, and confirmed increased IL-1β and IL-6 levels in mice. Overall, these findings indicate that mRNA vaccines have contents that can activate the precise pathways known to drive myocarditis in mice in a sex- and background-specific manner (elevated in males and white-background mice with many mast cells), including complement and TLR4/inflammasome/IL-1β.

Regardless of vaccine platform, all COVID-19 vaccines include or lead to the production of the spike protein, which binds ACE2. As noted previously, ACE2 is expressed on antigen-presenting cells such as mast cells and macrophages, and binding may activate an innate immune response (Fairweather et al., 2023b). However, Yonker et al. (2023) found that in patients with vaccine-associated myocarditis, levels of circulating spike protein remained elevated in the blood for at least 3 weeks after vaccination, instead of the protein being quickly cleared. No healthy controls had detectable free spike protein in their serum at any time after vaccination. The patients with vaccine-associated myocarditis also had elevated serum levels of IL-1β, IL-6, and other cytokines, suggesting a persistent innate proinflammatory response (Yonker et al., 2023). Thus, it is possible that persistent free spike protein may activate mast cells not only at the site of vaccination but also at other sites, including the heart, where mast cells are located at their highest levels at vessels and along the pericardium. Spike protein has been found in biopsies from the hearts of patients with myocarditis after vaccination, indicating that it can reach, and deposit in, the heart (Baumeier et al., 2022).

Additionally, several studies have reported that exosomes (a type of EV) leave cells after vaccination, enter the circulation, and express the spike protein on their surface (Bansal et al., 2021; Chaudhary et al., 2021; Seneff et al., 2022). They also found that circulating spike protein–expressing exosomes increased by a factor of 12 after the second vaccination. These exosomes may activate ACE2 on mast cells and macrophages contributing to the increased incidence of myocarditis reported after the second mRNA vaccination.

Animal models of many autoimmune diseases require two injections to initiate diseases (Cihákova et al., 2004). One factor that may contribute to the much higher incidence of vaccine-associated myocarditis after the second vaccination is "trained immunity," which is used to explain how innate immune cells mount a much higher response the second time they are exposed to an antigen, as long as the second exposure is not too long after the first. It has been revealed that the TLR4/inflammasome/IL-1β pathway is critical to developing this innate immunological memory (Moorlag et al., 2018). These findings provide a potential mechanism for how COVID-19 vaccines that use spike protein to induce an immune response may activate the precise immune pathways that are known to drive myocarditis. The risk may be increased by adding the lipid layer in mRNA vaccine platforms that has additional elements that may further activate these pathways. In support of this idea, patients with myocarditis after COVID-19 vaccination with mRNA in LNP have been found to have immune responses associated with activation of the TLR4/inflammasome/IL-1β/IL-18 pathway. TLR4 expression on mast cells and macrophages could drive this response, and it is well established in animal models of viral and autoimmune myocarditis that inhibiting this pathway using therapies, such as mesenchymal stem cells or EVs, or drugs, such as colchicine, reduce myocardial and pericardial inflammation (Beetler et al., 2023; Fairweather et al., 2003; Miteva et al., 2018; Pappritz et al., 2022). A case series by Frustaci et al. (2022) reported three cases of severe eosinophilic myocarditis after mRNA vaccination (eosinophils are activated by mast cells) in individuals who had experienced hypersensitivity/allergic reactions to mRNA vaccines. Another case report described a patient with Still's disease and myocarditis after an mRNA vaccine (Hugues et al., 2022). Still's disease is associated with elevated levels of IL-1β and IL-18, and treatment with IL-1β and IL-6 inhibitors was effective (Hugues et al., 2022). Another case report examined the immune response of a patient with myocarditis after mRNA vaccination and found elevated circulating levels of IL-18 (Won et al., 2022). Another case study of vaccine-associated myocarditis cases found antibodies against IL-1R antagonist (IL-1RA) in the serum of patients with myocarditis after mRNA vaccination, indicating activation/regulation of the IL-1β receptor pathway (Thurner et al., 2022). Overall, these several reports found consistent associations with inflammasome activation.

Last, one animal study reported that the COVID-19 mRNA vaccine was able to induce myopericarditis in BALB/c mice (Li et al., 2022), though these animals did not demonstrate myocardial inflammation typical of myocarditis animal models. Mast cells are most concentrated in BALB/c mice along the pericardium, where they could be activated by the spike protein, leading to pericardial inflammation. Unfortunately, these investigators did not examine mast cell numbers or activation. However, pericardial mast cell activation is well known as a major driver of myocarditis/perimyocarditis in viral animal models, as described. Evidence of activation of this pathway was observed in male BALB/c mice given mRNA vaccines that had higher levels of IL-1β, indicating TLR4/inflammasome activation (Li et al., 2022).

Overall, these findings provide a possible mechanism for how mRNA vaccines (and, to a lesser extent, other platforms) may activate complement and TLR4/inflammasome pathways on mast cells and macrophages to induce myocardial and pericardial inflammation. The potential role of mast cells in effects from COVID-19 vaccines has been reviewed in Fairweather et al. (2023b) and Theoharides (2021).

## COVID-19 VACCINES: CLINICAL AND EPIDEMIOLOGICAL EVIDENCE

The committee considered randomized controlled trials (RCTs) and observational studies to determine the relationship between COVID-19 vaccines and myocarditis and pericarditis.

## BNT162b2

*RCTs, BNT162b2*

A Cochrane Systematic Review of 41 RCTs of COVID-19 vaccines did not report findings for myocarditis or pericarditis (Graña et al., 2022). A Brighton Collaboration systematic review of serious adverse events after mRNA vaccination (Fraiman et al., 2022) reported on myocarditis/pericarditis in two large Phase 3 placebo-controlled RCTs of BNT162b2[1] and mRNA-1273[2] but with no imbalance in the number of events, and no inference about causality or association was attempted (Fraiman et al., 2022). The number of events in the Brighton Collaboration review does not align with the more detailed review of the trial results described from Food and Drug Administration (FDA) source materials.

Next, the committee reviewed myocarditis/pericarditis events from published and unpublished reports of individual RCTs of BNT162b2. The primary unpublished data sources include the FDA advisory committee, emergency use authorization (EUA), and biologic license application materials, which reported individual counts of events in each arm of each trial and details about them. These counts sometimes changed with additional follow-up and clinical review, so counts from the most recent FDA review documents were used when possible.

In the Phase 2/3 RCT C4591001, among individuals aged 16+ (*n* = 22,030), no myocarditis or pericarditis events were observed that were considered at least possibly related (FDA, 2020a,b, 2021a). In the same RCT, among individuals aged 12–15 (*n* = 1,131), one myocarditis event and no pericarditis events were observed (FDA, 2021b,c). In this trial, one 15-year-old boy in the placebo arm crossed over to receive open-label BNT162b2 at age 16, and 3 days later, he developed myocarditis; the FDA reviewer noted a "reasonable possibility that the myopericarditis was related to the vaccine administration due to the plausible temporal relationship" (FDA, 2021c).

[1] Refers to the COVID-19 vaccine manufactured by Pfizer-BioNTech under the name Comirnaty®.
[2] Refers to the COVID-19 vaccine manufactured by Moderna under the name Spikevax®.

In the Phase 2/3 RCT C4591007, among children aged 5–11 ($n$ = 3,109), no myocarditis or pericarditis events were observed that were at least possibly related (FDA, 2021c). In that same RCT, among children 6 months to 4 years ($n$ = 3,013), no myocarditis or pericarditis events were observed (FDA, 2022a).

The count of myocarditis and pericarditis events in these trials was so low (one myocarditis event across all trial populations) that no statistical inference could be made. The lack of a clear signal for myocarditis or pericarditis in these trials effectively excludes a large average increase in risk in broad populations studied but not the possibility of a causal effect that results in one case per tens of thousands of vaccine exposures.

*Observational Studies, BNT162b2*

Because of the large number of observational studies on myocarditis and pericarditis after mRNA vaccines, the committee next reviewed findings from systematic reviews or meta-analyses of observational studies. Many of the systematic reviews had serious methodological limitations, including a failure to account for different study designs and especially differences in outcome surveillance and ascertainment methods, which can vary substantially by country and across health care systems and surveillance systems *within* a country.

Rates of myocarditis tended to be lower in passive surveillance studies (i.e., spontaneous adverse event reporting) than in those that relied on diagnosis codes from health care encounters. Although passive surveillance (i.e., pharmacovigilance) studies suffer from reporting bias and are typically considered a weaker design than epidemiological studies with a well-enumerated population base and outcome identification through health care encounters, the likelihood of nondifferential misclassification of outcomes by exposure status is also high in studies nested within health care systems, given the high level of public awareness about myocarditis as a potential harm of some COVID-19 vaccines. Some pharmacovigilance studies used the most rigorous methods to identify outcomes, such as verifying cases by reviewing medical records and applying CDC clinical criteria for myocarditis (Oster et al., 2022). Confounding by age and sex was also a serious limitation in many studies. Because of the substantial evidence of effect modification of vaccine-related myocarditis risk by sex and age and possible confounding by these factors, the committee prioritized analyses that carefully accounted for both.

The most comprehensive review of epidemiologic studies of myocarditis and pericarditis related to COVID-19 mRNA vaccines was A Living Evidence Synthesis by Canada's Strategy for Patient-Oriented Research (SPOR), which provided detailed results stratified by age and sex for each mRNA vaccine from a protocolized review of the literature. Results from an interim review of the evidence were published in 2022 (Pillay et al., 2022), and more recent updates have been posted on the SPOR website (Update #4 on March 29, 2023) (Gaudet et al., 2023). This review reported incidences by age groups consistent with the age eligibility criteria in the registration clinical trials of the mRNA vaccines. The main findings from SPOR (Gaudet et al., 2023) are summarized in Table 7-1.

The key findings from the SPOR review were that BNT162b2 and mRNA-1273 likely increased the risk of myocarditis in male adolescents (12–17) and young adults (18–39) (Gaudet et al., 2023). Absolute risk estimates varied across studies by an order of magnitude, but even the highest reflect a low absolute risk. Nonetheless, the absolute risk estimates in certain male age groups appear to be orders of magnitude greater than the estimated background rate in the general population, making confounding or reporting bias an unlikely explanation. The risk in women, young children, and older adults may also be elevated, but the magnitude of the risk and the certainty of this finding are lower. The evidence reflected moderate to higher certainty that the risk of myocarditis is greater with mRNA-1273 compared with BNT162b2 in the older age groups, but risk associated with BNT162b2 remained elevated. The results from this review are consistent with results from several other systematic reviews.

The evidence from the SPOR review on pericarditis without myocarditis was sparse (Gaudet et al., 2023). For example, no studies in children aged 0–4 were identified, and only a single study included those aged 5–11. With just two studies, the certainty was low for boys and girls aged 12–17, women aged 18–24, and men aged 25–39, with an estimated absolute risk of <20 cases per million in those age–sex groups.

In addition to the SPOR review, Tables 7-2 and 7-3 summarize findings from some of the most informative individual epidemiological studies, prioritizing studies that had large numbers of vaccine-related myocarditis and pericarditis cases, respectively used an appropriate control group, attempted to address confounding by factors that may be associated with the vaccine, and reported risk estimates stratified by sex and age. These studies

**TABLE 7-1** Findings from Canada's Strategy for Patient-Oriented Research

| | Myocarditis | | | | | |
|---|---|---|---|---|---|---|
| | Male | | | Female | | |
| Age Group | Cases/million | Certainty | Studies | Cases/million | Certainty | Studies |
| 6m–4y | <20 | Low | 1 | <20 | Low | 1 |
| 5–11y | <20 | Moderate | 6 | <20 | Low | 7 |
| 12–17y | 13–390 | Moderate | 16 | 1–50 | Very low | 16 |
| 18–29y | 29–157 | Moderate | 14 | 2–37 | Very low | 12 |
| 18–39y | 8–104 | Moderate | 12 | <20 | Low | 9 |
| | mRNA-1273 Risk Compared to BNT162b2 | | | | | |
| Age Group | RR | Certainty | Studies | RR | Certainty | Studies |
| 6m–4y | Same | Low | 1 | Same | Low | 1 |
| 5–11y | — | — | 0 | Uncertain | Very low | 0 |
| 12–17y | Higher | Low | 1 | Uncertain | Uncertain | 1 |
| 18–29y | 2–3× | Moderate | 6 | 2–3× | Moderate | 5 |
| 30–39y | Higher | High | 5 | Higher | Low | 5 |
| | Pericarditis | | | | | |
| Age Group | Cases/million | Certainty | Studies | Cases/million | Certainty | Studies |
| 6m–4y | — | — | 0 | — | — | 0 |
| 5–11y | Uncertain | Very low | 1 | Uncertain | Very low | 1 |
| 12–17y | <20 | Low | 2 | <20 | Low | 2 |
| 18–24y | Uncertain | Very low | 2 | <20 | Low | 2 |
| 25–39y | <20 | Low | 2 | Uncertain | Uncertain | 2 |

NOTES: Certainty refers to certainty of the risk estimates using Grading of Recommendations, Assessment, Development, and Evaluations (GRADE) (Siemieniuk and Guyatt, 2024). Rates are *excess* incidence compared to background rate. Estimated background rate after vaccination is 0.2/million for myocarditis and 1.4/million for pericarditis. <20 per million reported when incidence rates from all studies reported as low. BNT162b2 refers to the COVID-19 vaccine manufactured by Pfizer-BioNTech under the name Comirnaty®. mRNA-1273 refers to the COVID-19 vaccine manufactured by Moderna under the name Spikevax®. m: month; RR: risk ratio; y: years.
SOURCE: Gaudet et al., 2023.

ascertained myocarditis events (Table 7-2) and pericarditis events (Table 7-3) after the first or second dose of the vaccine. All but one study relied on administrative data (diagnosis codes from health care encounters) to identify cases (Goddard et al., 2022a,b). Validation studies have reported that the positive predictive value of myocarditis International Classification of Diseases–10 diagnosis codes for validated events is approximately 70 percent (Wu et al., 2023). Therefore, bias due to outcome misclassification, which may be differential, is a potential limitation of nearly all of these population-based studies. Collectively, these studies strongly suggested an increased risk of myocarditis associated with BNT162b2, although it is likely to be lower than with mRNA-1273.

In contrast with myocarditis, few high-quality epidemiological studies of pericarditis without myocarditis were identified. Three found no increased risk, and two found an increased risk for BNT162b2. The relative risk estimates for pericarditis in the positive studies were much lower than the corresponding relative risk estimates for myocarditis.

Evidence from passive surveillance studies of potential harms was also considered. An analysis of cases of myocarditis related to mRNA vaccines in VAERS corroborated the findings from the epidemiological studies and was considered just as informative for the causality assessment (Oster et al., 2022). Notably, the myocarditis cases in VAERS were validated by medical record review and the application of CDC clinical criteria, and the observed

**TABLE 7-2** Selected Epidemiological Studies of Risk of Myocarditis Associated with BNT162b2

| Author | Age | Setting | Design | Confounding | Outcome | Interval | N | Vaccinated Cases | Results (95% CI) |
|---|---|---|---|---|---|---|---|---|---|
| Bots et al. (2022) | 5+ | Europe (4 countries) | Self-controlled | Self-controlled | ICD codes | 28d | 12.4 million | 72 | Myocarditis only<br><br>All ages: RR 3.18 (1.65–6.12)<br><br>Men: RR 2.78 (1.53–5.07)<br><br>Aged 12–29: RR 7.78 (2.58–23.5) |
| Goddard et al. (2022a) | 5–39 | VSD | Vaccinated only | None | Record review | 7d | 2.6 million | 101 | Myocarditis/pericarditis<br><br>Higher risk for males, second dose, and 12–15 and 16–17 age groups |
| Goddard et al. (2022b) | 18–39 | VSD | Self-controlled | Self-controlled | Record review | 7d | 1.5 million | 41 | Myocarditis and pericarditis<br><br>All ages RR 6.94 (3.57–14.13) |
| Karlstad et al. (2022) | 12+ | Europe (4 countries) | Unvaccinated control | Adjustment | ICD codes | 28d | 15.1 million | 220 | Myocarditis only<br><br>Higher risk for males, second dose, and 16–24 age group<br><br>mRNA-1273 risk greater than BNT162b2 |
| Le Vu et al. (2022) | 12–50 | France | Case-control | Adjustment | ICD codes | 21d | 21.2 million | 405 | Myocarditis only RR 8.1 (6.7–9.9)<br><br>Higher risk for males, second dose, and 18–24 age group<br><br>mRNA-1273 risk greater than BNT162b2 |

**TABLE 7-2** Continued

| Author | Age | Setting | Design | Confounding | Outcome | Interval | N | Vaccinated Cases | Results (95% CI) |
|---|---|---|---|---|---|---|---|---|---|
| Massari et al. (2022) | 12–39 | Italy | Self-controlled | Self-controlled | ICD codes | 21d | 2.4 million | 74 | Myocarditis or pericarditis RR 3.39 (2.02–5.68)<br><br>Higher risk for males, second dose, and 12–17 and 18–29 age groups<br><br>mRNA-1273 risk greater than BNT162b2 |
| Patone et al. (2022a) | 13+ | England | Self-controlled | Self-controlled | ICD codes | 28d | 21.0 million | 243 | Myocarditis only RR 1.57 (1.28–1.92)<br><br>Higher risk for males, second dose, and <40 age group<br><br>mRNA-1273 risk greater than BNT162b2 |

NOTES: BNT162b2 refers to the COVID-19 vaccine manufactured by Pfizer-BioNTech under the name Comirnaty®. mRNA-1273 refers to the COVID-19 vaccine manufactured by Moderna under the name Spikevax®. CI: confidence interval; d: days; ICD: International Classification of Diseases; RR: relative risk; VSD: Vaccine Safety Datalink.
SOURCES: Bots et al., 2022; Goddard et al., 2022a,b; Karlstad et al., 2022; Le Vu et al., 2022; Massari et al., 2022; Patone et al., 2022a.

reporting rates were orders of magnitude greater than the estimated background rate. Specifically, the rate of validated cases was much higher in male than in female vaccinees, higher after the second dose, and highest in the 12–15, 16–17, and 18–24 age groups.

**TABLE 7-3** Selected Epidemiological Studies of Risk of Pericarditis Associated with BNT162b2

| Author | Age | Setting | Design | Confounding | Outcome | Interval | N | Vaccinated Cases | Results (95% CI) |
|---|---|---|---|---|---|---|---|---|---|
| Bots et al. (2022) | 5+ | Europe (4 countries) | Self-controlled | Self-controlled | ICD codes | 28d | 12.4 million | 244 | RR 0.90 (0.67–1.21) No increased risk |
| Corrao et al. (2022) | 12+ | Italy | Cohort vs. unvaccinated | Adjustment | ICD codes | 28d | 8.9 million | 146 | No increased risk |
| Karlstad et al. (2022) | 12+ | Europe (4 countries) | Unvaccinated control | Adjustment | ICD codes | 28d | 15.1 million | 267 | Increased risk in males RR 1.38 (1.1–1.74) and females RR 1.47 (1.05–2.05)<br><br>Higher RR under age 40 compared to 40 and over<br><br>mRNA-1273 risk greater than BNT162b2 |
| Le Vu et al. (2022) | 12–50 | France | Case-control | Adjustment | ICD codes | 21d | 21.2 million | 288 | RR 2.9 (2.3–3.8).<br><br>Increased risk under age 40 in males, under age 30 if females |
| Patone et al. (2022b) | 13+ | England | Self-controlled | Self-controlled | ICD codes | 28d | 17.0 million | 134 | No increased risk |

NOTES: BNT162b2 refers to the COVID-19 vaccine manufactured by Pfizer-BioNTech under the name Comirnaty®. mRNA-1273 refers to the COVID-19 vaccine manufactured by Moderna under the name Spikevax®. d: days; ICD: International Classification of Diseases; RR: relative risk.
SOURCES: Bots et al., 2022; Corrao et al., 2022; Karlstad et al., 2022; Le Vu et al., 2022; Patone et al., 2022b.

## mRNA-1273

*RCTs, mRNA-1273*

The committee reviewed myocarditis/pericarditis events from published and unpublished reports of individual RCTs of mRNA-1273. The primary unpublished sources include the FDA advisory committee, EUA, and biologic license application materials, which reported individual counts of myocarditis/pericarditis events in each arm of each trial and details about these cases. These counts sometimes changed with additional follow-up and clinical review, so counts from the most recent FDA review documents were used when possible.

In the Phase 2/3 RCT P301, among individuals ages 18+ ($n = 15,206$), no myocarditis was observed, and two pericarditis events were observed that were considered at least possibly related (FDA, 2020c, 2022c). In the Phase 2/3 RCT P203, among individuals aged 12–17 ($n = 2,486$), no myocarditis or pericarditis events were observed that were judged to be at least possibly related (FDA, 2022b).

In the Phase 2/3 RCT P204, among children ages 6–11 ($n = 3,007$), no myocarditis or pericarditis events were observed that were judged to be at least possibly related (FDA, 2023a). In the Phase 2/3 RCT P204, among children

**TABLE 7-4** Reports to the Vaccine Adverse Event Reporting System After mRNA-Based COVID-19 Vaccination That Met the Centers for Disease Control and Prevention's Case Definition for Myocarditis Within a 7-Day Risk Interval per Million Doses of Vaccine Administered

| Reported Cases of Myocarditis Within a 7-Day Risk Interval per Million Doses of Vaccine Administered (95% CI) | | | | | Expected Cases of Myocarditis in a 7-Day Risk Interval per Million Doses |
|---|---|---|---|---|---|
| Age Group (years) | Vaccination with BNT162b2 | | Vaccination with mRNA-1273 | | |
| | First Dose | Second Dose | First Dose | Second Dose | |
| Males | | | | | |
| 12–15 | 7.06 (4.88–10.23) | 70.73 (61.68–81.11) | — | — | 0.53 (0.40–0.70) |
| 16–17 | 7.26 (4.45–11.86) | 105.86 (91.65–122.27) | — | — | 1.34 (1.05–1.72) |
| 18–24 | 3.82 (2.40–6.06) | 52.43 (45.56–60.33) | 10.73 (7.50–15.34) | 56.31 (47.08–67.34) | 1.76 (1.58–1.98) |
| 25–29 | 1.74 (0.78–3.87) | 17.28 (13.02–22.93) | 4.88 (2.70–8.80) | 24.18 (17.93–32.61) | 1.45 (1.21–1.74) |
| 30–39 | 0.54 (0.20–1.44) | 7.10 (5.26–9.57) | 3.00 (1.81–4.97) | 7.93 (5.61–11.21) | 0.63 (0.54–0.73) |
| 40–49 | 0.55 (0.21–1.48) | 3.50 (2.28–5.36) | 0.59 (0.19–1.82) | 4.27 (2.69–6.78) | 0.78 (0.67–0.90) |
| 50–64 | 0.42 (0.17–1.01) | 0.68 (0.33–1.43) | 0.62 (0.28–1.39) | 0.85 (0.41–1.79) | 0.77 (0.68–0.86) |
| ≥65 | 0.19 (0.05–0.76) | 0.32 (0.10–1.00) | 0.18 (0.05–0.72) | 0.51 (0.21–1.23) | — |
| Females | | | | | |
| 12–15 | 0.49 (0.12–1.98) | 6.35 (4.05–9.96) | — | — | 0.17 (0.11–0.29) |
| 16–17 | 0.84 (0.21–3.37) | 10.98 (7.16–16.84) | — | — | 0.42 (0.27–0.66) |
| 18–24 | 0.18 (0.03–1.31) | 4.12 (2.60–6.54) | 0.96 (0.31–2.96) | 6.87 (4.24–11.05) | 0.38 (0.30–0.49) |
| 25–29 | 0.26 (0.04–1.84) | 2.23 (1.07–4.69) | 0.41 (0.06–2.94) | 8.22 (5.03–13.41) | 0.48 (0.35–0.65) |
| 30–39 | 0.72 (0.32–1.60) | 1.02 (0.49–2.14) | 0.74 (0.28–1.98) | 0.68 (0.22–2.10) | 0.47 (0.39–0.57) |
| 40–49 | 0.24 (0.06–0.97) | 1.73 (0.98–3.05) | 0.18 (0.02–1.25) | 1.89 (0.98–3.63) | 0.89 (0.77–1.04) |
| 50–64 | 0.37 (0.15–0.88) | 0.51 (0.23–1.14) | 0.65 (0.31–1.36) | 0.43 (0.16–1.15) | 01.00 (0.89–1.13) |
| ≥65 | 0.08 (0.01–0.54) | 0.35 (0.13–0.92) | — | 0.26 (0.08–0.81) | — |

NOTES: BNT162b2 refers to the COVID-19 vaccine manufactured by Pfizer-BioNTech under the name Comirnaty®. mRNA-1273 refers to the COVID-19 vaccine manufactured by Moderna under the name Spikevax®. CI: confidence interval.
SOURCE: Table adapted from Oster et al., 2022.

ages 6 months to 5 years ($n$ = 4,792), no myocarditis or pericarditis events were observed that were judged to be at least possibly related (FDA, 2023a).

The count of myocarditis and pericarditis events in these trials was so low (two pericarditis events across all trial populations) that no statistical inference could be made. The lack of a clear signal for myocarditis or pericarditis in these trials effectively excludes a large average increase in risk in broad populations studied but not the possibility of a causal effect that results in one case per tens of thousands of vaccine exposures. Based on the RCT evidence alone, no conclusion was made about a potential causal effect of mRNA-1273 on these outcomes.

*Observational Studies, mRNA-1273*

As described, the Living Evidence Synthesis provided strong evidence that mRNA vaccines likely increase the risk of myocarditis, and the same age, sex, and dose trends were observed for BNT162b2 and mRNA-1273. Moreover, the evidence reflected moderate to higher certainty that the risk is greater with mRNA-1273 in the older age groups.

Results from the SPOR review (Gaudet et al., 2023) were consistent with results from the most informative individual epidemiological studies (Table 7-5). Collectively, these studies strongly suggested an increased risk of myocarditis with mRNA-1273, which is likely to be larger compared to BNT162b2.

**TABLE 7-5** Selected Epidemiological Studies of Risk of Myocarditis Associated with mRNA-1273

| Author | Age | Setting | Design | Confounding | Outcome | Interval | N | Vaccinated Cases | Results (95% CI) |
|---|---|---|---|---|---|---|---|---|---|
| Bots et al. (2022) | 5+ | Europe (4 countries) | Self-controlled | Self-controlled | ICD codes | 28d | 1.5 million | 20 | Myocarditis only<br><br>All ages: RR 5.28 (1.68–16.6)<br><br>Men: RR 5.80 (1.62–20.7)<br><br>Men aged 12–29: RR 6.05 (1.09–33.5) |
| Goddard et al. (2022a) | 5–39 | VSD | Vaccinated only | None | Record review | 7d | 949,272 | 36 | Myocarditis/ pericarditis<br><br>Higher risk for males, second dose, and 18–29 age group |
| Goddard et al. (2022b) | 18–39 | VSD | Self-controlled | Self-controlled | Record review | 7d | 923,711 | 38 | Myocarditis and pericarditis<br><br>All ages: RR 18.75 (6.73–64.94)<br><br>mRNA-1273 vs. BNT162b2 RR 1.61 (1.02–2.54) |
| Karlstad et al. (2022) | 12+ | Europe (4 countries) | Unvaccinated control | Adjustment | ICD codes | 28d | 2.4 million | 78 | Myocarditis only<br><br>Higher risk for males, second dose, and aged 16–24<br><br>mRNA-1273 risk greater than BNT162b2 |

**TABLE 7-5** Continued

| Author | Age | Setting | Design | Confounding | Outcome | Interval | N | Vaccinated Cases | Results (95% CI) |
|---|---|---|---|---|---|---|---|---|---|
| Le Vu et al. (2022) | 12–50 | France | Case-control | Adjustment | ICD codes | 21d | 2.9 million | 129 | Myocarditis only<br><br>RR 30 (21–43) Higher risk for males, second dose, and 18–24 age group<br><br>mRNA-1273 risk greater than BNT162b2 |
| Massari et al. (2022) | 12–39 | Italy | Self-controlled | Self-controlled | ICD codes | 21d | 456,050 | 40 | Myocarditis or pericarditis<br><br>RR 7.59 (3.26–17.65) Higher risk for males, second dose, and 18–29 age groups<br><br>mRNA-1273 risk greater than BNT162b2 |
| Patone et al. (2022a) | 13+ | England | Self-controlled | Self-controlled | ICD codes | 28d | 1.2 million | 51 | Myocarditis only<br><br>RR 11.76 (7.25–19.08)<br><br>Higher risk for males, second dose, and <40 age group<br><br>mRNA-1273 risk greater than BNT162b2 |

NOTES: BNT162b2 refers to the COVID-19 vaccine manufactured by Pfizer-BioNTech under the name Comirnaty®. mRNA-1273 refers to the COVID-19 vaccine manufactured by Moderna under the name Spikevax®. CI: confidence interval; d: days; ICD: International Classification of Diseases; RR: relative risk; VSD: Vaccine Safety Datalink.
SOURCES: Bots et al., 2022; Goddard et al., 2022a,b; Karlstad et al., 2022; Le Vu et al., 2022; Massari et al., 2022; Patone et al., 2022a.

Few high-quality epidemiological studies of myocarditis without pericarditis were identified; two found no increased risk, and three found an increased risk for mRNA-1273 (Table 7-6). The relative risk estimates for pericarditis in the positive studies were larger than the risk estimates for BNT162b2 but much lower than the corresponding ones for myocarditis. The analysis of cases of myocarditis related to VAERS also corroborated these findings (Oster et al., 2022).

**TABLE 7-6** Selected Epidemiological Studies of Risk of Pericarditis Associated with mRNA-1273

| Author | Age | Setting | Design | Confounding | Outcome | Interval | N | Vaccinated Cases | Results (95% CI) |
|--------|-----|---------|--------|-------------|---------|----------|---|-----------------|------------------|
| Bots et al. (2022) | 5+ | Europe (4 countries) | Self-controlled | Self-controlled | ICD codes | 28d | 1.5 million | 46 | No increased risk |
| Corrao et al. (2022) | 12+ | Italy | Cohort vs. unvaccinated | Adjustment | ICD codes | 28d | 1.6 million | 52 | RR 1.9 (1.5–2.5) |
| Karlstad et al. (2022) | 12+ | Europe (4 countries) | Unvaccinated control | Adjustment | ICD codes | 28d | 2.4 million | 62 | Increased risk in males RR 2.99 (2.02–4.44) Females RR 3.41 (1.98–5.87) Higher RR under age 40 compared to 40 and over mRNA-1273 risk greater than BNT162b2 |
| Le Vu et al. (2022) | 12–50 | France | Case-control | Adjustment | ICD codes | 21d | 2.9 million | 54 | RR 5.5 (3.3–9.0) |
| Patone et al. (2022b) | 13+ | England | Self-controlled | Self-controlled | ICD codes | 28d | 1.0 million | 0 | No increased risk |

NOTES: BNT162b2 refers to the COVID-19 vaccine manufactured by Pfizer-BioNTech under the name Comirnaty®. mRNA-1273 refers to the COVID-19 vaccine manufactured by Moderna under the name Spikevax®. CI: confidence interval; d: days; ICD: International Classification of Diseases; RR: relative risk.
SOURCES: Bots et al., 2022; Corrao et al., 2022; Karlstad et al., 2022; Le Vu et al., 2022; Patone et al., 2022b.

## Ad26.COV2.S

*RCTs, Ad26.COV2.S*

The committee reviewed myocarditis/pericarditis events from published and unpublished reports of individual RCTs of Ad26.COV2.S.[3] The primary unpublished data sources include the FDA advisory committee and EUA. In the Phase 3 RCT 3001, among individuals aged 18+ ($n = 21,895$), no myocarditis events were observed, and one pericarditis event was observed that was judged to be at least possibly related (FDA, 2021d,e).

The count of myocarditis and pericarditis events was so low (one pericarditis event) that no statistical inference could be made. The lack of a clear signal for myocarditis or pericarditis in these trials effectively excludes a large average increase in risk in broad populations studied but not the possibility of a causal effect that results in one case per tens of thousands of vaccine exposures. Based on the RCT evidence alone, no conclusion was made about a potential causal effect of Ad26.COV2.S on these outcomes.

---

[3] Ad26.COV2.S refers to the COVID-19 vaccine manufactured by Janssen.

*Observational Studies, Ad26.COV2.S*

Few epidemiological studies have attempted to evaluate whether Ad26.COV2.S is associated with myocarditis or pericarditis. The committee identified no studies that included a large number of vaccine-related myocarditis or pericarditis cases, used an appropriate control group, and attempted to address confounding by factors that may be associated with Ad26.COV2.S. For example, in Bots et al. (2022), cited in the BNT162b2 vaccine evidence review, fewer than five cases of myocarditis were reported after Ad26.COV2.S, resulting in a risk estimate that was uninformative (incidence rate ratio 1.6, 95% CI: 0.1–21.6).

In the pharmacovigilance literature, the committee identified only two studies that evaluated the potential myocarditis risks associated with Ad26.COV2.S. One used a global database of spontaneous adverse event reports to evaluate a disproportionality ratio for various COVID-19 vaccines, comparing vaccine exposure in myocarditis cases to other adverse event reports (Macías Saint-Gerons et al., 2023). This study design is highly susceptible to bias and provides no information about the absolute magnitude of risk; the reporting odds ratio for Ad26. COV2.S was 1.9 (95% CI: 1.7–2.1) compared to 17 (95% CI: 16–17) for BNT162b2 and 7.6 (95% CI: 7.4–7.8) for mRNA-1273.

In the second pharmacovigilance study conducted using VAERS data through February 2022, 189 cases of myopericarditis were identified, but only 52 met the CDC case definition for a validated event (Woo et al., 2023). The observed incidence was compared to background rates of myocarditis estimated in two different studies: the relative risk estimates for myopericarditis with Ad26.COV2.S were 3.2 (95% CI: 2.0–4.8) and 1.1 (95% CI: 0.7–1.7), depending on which of the two data sources was used to estimate the background rate.

## NVX-CoV2373

*RCTs, NVX-CoV2373*

The committee reviewed myocarditis/pericarditis events from published and unpublished reports of individual RCTs of NVX-CoV2373.[4] The primary unpublished data source was the EUA memoranda, which included a detailed accounting of the events observed.

In RCT 301, among individuals aged 18+ ($n = 19,735$), one myocarditis and one pericarditis event were judged to be at least possibly related (FDA, 2023b; Marks, 2023). In RCT 302, among individuals age 18+ ($n = 7,750$), one myocarditis and one pericarditis event were judged to be at least possibly related (FDA, 2023b). In RCT 301, among individuals aged 12–17 ($n = 1,487$), one myocarditis event and no pericarditis events were judged to be at least possibly related (FDA, 2023b).

Across all of these trial populations, the number of myocarditis and pericarditis events observed (six) out of approximately 42,000 vaccine exposures raises the possibility of a signal for rare events that typically would not be observed in trials of this size. However, the number of events was inadequate for statistical inference. Based on the RCT evidence alone, no conclusion was made about a potential causal effect of NVX-CoV2373 on these outcomes.

*Observational Studies, NVX-CoV2373*

In the United States, only 89,000 doses of NVX-CoV2373 were administered as of May 11, 2023 (CDC, 2023), approximately double the population that received the vaccine in the Phase 3 trials. The committee did not identify any epidemiological studies of the risk of myocarditis associated with this vaccine. The global pharmacovigilance study cited earlier identified 61 cases of myopericarditis, 50 of which were from Australia (Macías Saint-Gerons et al., 2023). The reported odds ratio for NVX-CoV2373 was 15 (95% CI: 11–19), compared to 17 (95% CI: 17–17) for BNT162b2 and 6.9 (95% CI: 6.8–7.1) for mRNA-1273.

---

[4] Refers to the COVID-19 vaccine manufactured by Novavax.

## From Evidence to Conclusions

The committee identified consistent findings of a large relative risk of myocarditis after either mRNA vaccine in numerous high-quality observational studies, an absolute risk that is orders of magnitude greater than the background rate in certain age and sex subgroups, and a plausible biological mechanism for mRNA vaccines. The strong and substantial body of evidence indicates that the risk of harm varies by age and sex, but it does not exclude the presence of a causal effect in any particular group defined by age or sex.

**Conclusion 7-1: The evidence establishes a causal relationship between the BNT162b2 vaccine and myocarditis.**

**Conclusion 7-2: The evidence establishes a causal relationship between the mRNA-1273 vaccine and myocarditis.**

Evidence of a clear association from any well-designed and adequately powered observational studies and compelling mechanistic evidence was lacking for both Ad26.COV2.S and NVX-CoV2373 and myocarditis.

**Conclusion 7-3: The evidence is inadequate to accept or reject a causal relationship between the Ad26.COV2.S vaccine and myocarditis.**

**Conclusion 7-4: The evidence is inadequate to accept or reject a causal relationship between the NVX-CoV2373 vaccine and myocarditis.**

In contrast to the abundance of evidence regarding the risk of myocarditis and mRNA COVID-19 vaccines, few high-quality epidemiological studies have investigated the risk of pericarditis without myocarditis. Several studies did not find an increased risk, and those that did estimated much lower relative risk of pericarditis than what was observed for myocarditis. Additionally, very few events were observed in RCTs, with uncertainty as to whether all events were related to COVID-19 vaccines.

**Conclusion 7-5: The evidence is inadequate to accept or reject a causal relationship between the BNT162b2 vaccine and pericarditis without myocarditis.**

**Conclusion 7-6: The evidence is inadequate to accept or reject a causal relationship between the mRNA-1273 vaccine and pericarditis without myocarditis.**

**Conclusion 7-7: The evidence is inadequate to accept or reject a causal relationship between the Ad26.COV2.S vaccine and pericarditis without myocarditis.**

**Conclusion 7-8: The evidence is inadequate to accept or reject a causal relationship between the NVX-CoV2373 vaccine and pericarditis without myocarditis.**

## REFERENCES

Abston, E. D., J. G. Barin, D. Cihákova, A. Bucek, M. J. Coronado, J. E. Brandt, D. Bedja, J. B. Kim, D. Georgakopoulos, K. L. Gabrielson, W. Mitzner, and D. Fairweather. 2012a. IL-33 independently induces eosinophilic pericarditis and cardiac dilation: ST2 improves cardiac function. *Circulation: Heart Failure* 5(3):366–375. https://doi.org/10.1161/circheartfailure.111.963769.

Abston, E. D., M. J. Coronado, A. Bucek, D. Bedja, J. Shin, J. B. Kim, E. Kim, K. L. Gabrielson, D. Georgakopoulos, W. Mitzner, and D. Fairweather. 2012b. TH2 regulation of viral myocarditis in mice: Different roles for TLR3 versus TRIF in progression to chronic disease. *Clinical & Developmental Immunology* 2012:129486. https://doi.org/10.1155/2012/129486.

Abston, E. D., M. J. Coronado, A. Bucek, J. A. Onyimba, J. E. Brandt, J. A. Frisancho, E. Kim, D. Bedja, Y. K. Sung, A. J. Radtke, K. L. Gabrielson, W. Mitzner, and D. Fairweather. 2013. TLR3 deficiency induces chronic inflammatory cardiomyopathy in resistant mice following coxsackievirus B3 infection: Role for IL-4. *American Journal of Physiology: Regulatory, Integrative and Comparative Physiology* 304(4):R267–R277. https://doi.org/10.1152/ajpregu.00516.2011.

Adler, Y., P. Charron, M. Imazio, L. Badano, G. Barón-Esquivias, J. Bogaert, A. Brucato, P. Gueret, K. Klingel, C. Lionis, B. Maisch, B. Mayosi, A. Pavie, A. D. Ristic, M. Sabaté Tenas, P. Seferovic, K. Swedberg, and W. Tomkowski. 2015. 2015 ESC guidelines for the diagnosis and management of pericardial diseases: The task force for the diagnosis and management of pericardial diseases of the European Society of Cardiology (ESC) endorsed by: The European Association for Cardio-Thoracic Surgery (EACTS). *European Heart Journal* 36(42):2921–2964. https://doi.org/10.1093/eurheartj/ehv318.

Afanasyeva, M., Y. Wang, Z. Kaya, S. Park, M. J. Zilliox, B. H. Schofield, S. L. Hill, and N. R. Rose. 2001. Experimental autoimmune myocarditis in A/J mice is an interleukin-4-dependent disease with a TH2 phenotype. *American Journal of Pathology* 159(1):193–203. https://doi.org/10.1016/s0002-9440(10)61685-9.

Aljohani, O. A., D. Mackie, A. Bratincsak, J. S. Bradley, and J. C. Perry. 2022. Spectrum of viral pathogens identified in children with clinical myocarditis (pre-coronavirus disease-2019, 2000–2018): Etiologic agent versus innocent bystander. *Journal of Pediatrics* 242:18–24. https://doi.org/10.1016/j.jpeds.2021.11.011.

Amin, S., S. Aktar, M. M. Rahman, and M. M. H. Chowdhury. 2022. NLRP3 inflammasome activation in COVID-19: An interlink between risk factors and disease severity. *Microbes and Infection* 24(1):104913. https://doi.org/10.1016/j.micinf.2021.104913.

Ammirati, E., G. Veronese, M. Brambatti, M. Merlo, M. Cipriani, L. Potena, P. Sormani, T. Aoki, K. Sugimura, A. Sawamura, T. Okumura, S. Pinney, K. Hong, P. Shah, Ö. Braun, C. M. Van de Heyning, S. Montero, D. Petrella, F. Huang, M. Schmidt, C. Raineri, A. Lala, M. Varrenti, A. Foà, O. Leone, P. Gentile, J. Artico, V. Agostini, R. Patel, A. Garascia, E. M. Van Craenenbroeck, K. Hirose, A. Isotani, T. Murohara, Y. Arita, A. Sionis, E. Fabris, S. Hashem, V. Garcia-Hernando, F. Oliva, B. Greenberg, H. Shimokawa, G. Sinagra, E. D. Adler, M. Frigerio, and P. G. Camici. 2019. Fulminant versus acute nonfulminant myocarditis in patients with left ventricular systolic dysfunction. *Journal of the American College of Cardiology* 74(3):299–311. https://doi.org/10.1016/j.jacc.2019.04.063.

Ammirati, E., L. Lupi, M. Palazzini, N. S. Hendren, J. L. Grodin, C. V. Cannistraci, M. Schmidt, G. Hekimian, G. Peretto, T. Bochaton, A. Hayek, N. Piriou, S. Leonardi, S. Guida, A. Turco, S. Sala, A. Uribarri, C. M. Van de Heyning, M. Mapelli, J. Campodonico, P. Pedrotti, M. I. Barrionuevo Sánchez, A. Ariza Sole, M. Marini, M. V. Matassini, M. Vourc'h, A. Cannatà, D. I. Bromage, D. Briguglia, J. Salamanca, P. Diez-Villanueva, J. Lehtonen, F. Huang, S. Russel, F. Soriano, F. Turrini, M. Cipriani, M. Bramerio, M. Di Pasquale, A. Grosu, M. Senni, D. Farina, P. Agostoni, S. Rizzo, M. De Gaspari, F. Marzo, J. M. Durán, E. D. Adler, C. Giannattasio, C. Basso, T. McDonagh, M. Kerneis, A. Combes, P. G. Camici, J. A. de Lemos, and M. Metra. 2022. Prevalence, characteristics, and outcomes of COVID-19-associated acute myocarditis. *Circulation* 145(15):1123–1139. https://doi.org/10.1161/circulationaha.121.056817.

Arunachalam, P. S., M. K. D. Scott, T. Hagan, C. Li, Y. Feng, F. Wimmers, L. Grigoryan, M. Trisal, V. V. Edara, L. Lai, S. E. Chang, A. Feng, S. Dhingra, M. Shah, A. S. Lee, S. Chinthrajah, S. B. Sindher, V. Mallajosyula, F. Gao, N. Sigal, S. Kowli, S. Gupta, K. Pellegrini, G. Tharp, S. Maysel-Auslender, S. Hamilton, H. Aoued, K. Hrusovsky, M. Roskey, S. E. Bosinger, H. T. Maecker, S. D. Boyd, M. M. Davis, P. J. Utz, M. S. Suthar, P. Khatri, K. C. Nadeau, and B. Pulendran. 2021. Systems vaccinology of the BNT162b2 mRNA vaccine in humans. *Nature* 596(7872):410–416. https://doi.org/10.1038/s41586-021-03791-x.

Baldeviano, G. C., J. G. Barin, M. V. Talor, S. Srinivasan, D. Bedja, D. Zheng, K. Gabrielson, Y. Iwakura, N. R. Rose, and D. Cihákova. 2010. Interleukin-17a is dispensable for myocarditis but essential for the progression to dilated cardiomyopathy. *Circulation Research* 106(10):1646–1655. https://doi.org/10.1161/circresaha.109.213157.

Ball, S., R. K. Ghosh, S. Wongsaengsak, D. Bandyopadhyay, G. C. Ghosh, W. S. Aronow, G. C. Fonarow, D. J. Lenihan, and D. L. Bhatt. 2019. Cardiovascular toxicities of immune checkpoint inhibitors: JACC review topic of the week. *Journal of the American College of Cardiology* 74(13):1714–1727. https://doi.org/10.1016/j.jacc.2019.07.079.

Bansal, S., S. Perincheri, T. Fleming, C. Poulson, B. Tiffany, R. M. Bremner, and T. Mohanakumar. 2021. Cutting edge: Circulating exosomes with COVID spike protein are induced by BNT162b2 (Pfizer-BioNTech) vaccination prior to development of antibodies: A novel mechanism for immune activation by mRNA vaccines. *Journal of Immunology* 207(10):2405–2410. https://doi.org/10.4049/jimmunol.2100637.

Basso, C., O. Leone, S. Rizzo, M. De Gaspari, A. C. van der Wal, M. C. Aubry, M. C. Bois, P. T. Lin, J. J. Maleszewski, and J. R. Stone. 2020. Pathological features of COVID-19-associated myocardial injury: A multicentre cardiovascular pathology study. *European Heart Journal* 41(39):3827–3835. https://doi.org/10.1093/eurheartj/ehaa664.

Baumeier, C., G. Aleshcheva, D. Harms, U. Gross, C. Hamm, B. Assmus, R. Westenfeld, M. Kelm, S. Rammos, P. Wenzel, T. Münzel, A. Elsässer, M. Gailani, C. Perings, A. Bourakkadi, M. Flesch, T. Kempf, J. Bauersachs, F. Escher, and H. P. Schultheiss. 2022. Intramyocardial inflammation after COVID-19 vaccination: An endomyocardial biopsy-proven case series. *International Journal of Molecular Sciences* 23(13). https://doi.org/10.3390/ijms23136940.

Beetler, D. J., K. A. Bruno, M. M. Watkins, V. Xu, I. Chekuri, P. Giresi, D. N. Di Florio, E. R. Whelan, B. H. Edenfield, S. A. Walker, A. C. Morales-Lara, A. R. Hill, A. Jain, M. E. Auda, L. P. Macomb, K. A. Shapiro, K. C. Keegan, J. Wolfram, A. Behfar, P. G. Stalboerger, A. Terzic, H. Farres, L. T. Cooper, and D. Fairweather. 2023. Reconstituted extracellular vesicles from human platelets decrease viral myocarditis in mice. *Small* e2303317. https://doi.org/10.1002/smll.202303317.

Boehmer, T. K., L. Kompaniyets, A. M. Lavery, J. Hsu, J. Y. Ko, H. Yusuf, S. D. Romano, A. V. Gundlapalli, M. E. Oster, and A. M. Harris. 2021. Association between COVID-19 and myocarditis using hospital-based administrative data—United States, March 2020–January 2021. *MMWR: Morbidity and Mortality Weekly Report* 70(35):1228–1232. https://doi.org/10.15585/mmwr.mm7035e5.

Bots, S. H., J. Riera-Arnau, S. V. Belitser, D. Messina, M. Aragón, E. Alsina, I. J. Douglas, C. E. Durán, P. García-Poza, R. Gini, R. M. C. Herings, C. Huerta, M. M. Sisay, M. Martín-Pérez, I. Martin, J. A. Overbeek, O. Paoletti, M. Pallejà-Millán, A. Schultze, P. Souverein, K. M. A. Swart, F. Villalobos, O. H. Klungel, and M. Sturkenboom. 2022. Myocarditis and pericarditis associated with SARS-CoV-2 vaccines: A population-based descriptive cohort and a nested self-controlled risk interval study using electronic health care data from four European countries. *Frontiers in Pharmacology* 13:1038043. https://doi.org/10.3389/fphar.2022.1038043.

Bruno, K. A., J. E. Mathews, A. L. Yang, J. A. Frisancho, A. J. Scott, H. D. Greyner, F. A. Molina, M. S. Greenaway, G. M. Cooper, A. Bucek, A. C. Morales-Lara, A. R. Hill, A. A. Mease, D. N. Di Florio, J. M. Sousou, A. C. Coronado, A. R. Stafford, and D. Fairweather. 2019. BPA alters estrogen receptor expression in the heart after viral infection activating cardiac mast cells and T cells leading to perimyocarditis and fibrosis. *Frontiers in Endocrinology* 10:598. https://doi.org/10.3389/fendo.2019.00598.

Bruno, K. A., L. P. Macomb, A. C. Morales-Lara, J. E. Mathews, J. A. Frisancho, A. L. Yang, D. N. Di Florio, B. H. Edenfield, E. R. Whelan, G. R. Salomon, A. R. Hill, C. C. Hewa-Rahinduwage, A. J. Scott, H. D. Greyner, F. A. Molina, M. S. Greenaway, G. M. Cooper, and D. Fairweather. 2021. Sex-specific effects of plastic caging in murine viral myocarditis. *International Journal of Molecular Sciences* 22(16). https://doi.org/10.3390/ijms22168834.

Caforio, A. L., S. Pankuweit, E. Arbustini, C. Basso, J. Gimeno-Blanes, S. B. Felix, M. Fu, T. Heliö, S. Heymans, R. Jahns, K. Klingel, A. Linhart, B. Maisch, W. McKenna, J. Mogensen, Y. M. Pinto, A. Ristic, H. P. Schultheiss, H. Seggewiss, L. Tavazzi, G. Thiene, A. Yılmaz, P. Charron, and P. M. Elliott. 2013. Current state of knowledge on aetiology, diagnosis, management, and therapy of myocarditis: A position statement of the European Society of Cardiology Working Group on myocardial and pericardial diseases. *European Heart Journal* 34(33):2636–2648, 2648a–2648d. https://doi.org/10.1093/eurheartj/eht210.

Cai, G., R. Kastelein, and C. A. Hunter. 2000. Interleukin-18 (IL-18) enhances innate IL-12-mediated resistance to toxoplasma gondii. *Infection and Immunity* 68(12):6932–6938. https://doi.org/10.1128/iai.68.12.6932-6938.2000.

Carvelli, J., O. Demaria, F. Vély, L. Batista, N. Chouaki Benmansour, J. Fares, S. Carpentier, M. L. Thibult, A. Morel, R. Remark, P. André, A. Represa, C. Piperoglou, P. Y. Cordier, E. Le Dault, C. Guervilly, P. Simeone, M. Gainnier, Y. Morel, M. Ebbo, N. Schleinitz, and E. Vivier. 2020. Association of COVID-19 inflammation with activation of the C5A-C5AR1 axis. *Nature* 588(7836):146–150. https://doi.org/10.1038/s41586-020-2600-6.

CDC (Centers for Disease Control and Prevention). 2023. Covid data tracker. https://covid.cdc.gov/covid-data-tracker/#vaccinations_vacc-people-booster-percent-pop5 (accessed December 20, 2023).

Chaudhary, J. K., R. Yadav, P. K. Chaudhary, A. Maurya, N. Kant, O. A. Rugaie, H. R. Haokip, D. Yadav, R. Roshan, R. Prasad, A. Chatrath, D. Singh, N. Jain, and P. Dhamija. 2021. Insights into COVID-19 vaccine development based on immunogenic structural proteins of SARS-CoV-2, host immune responses, and herd immunity. *Cells* 10(11). https://doi.org/10.3390/cells10112949.

Chen, L., X. Li, M. Chen, Y. Feng, and C. Xiong. 2020. The ACE2 expression in human heart indicates new potential mechanism of heart injury among patients infected with SARS-CoV-2. *Cardiovascular Research* 116(6):1097–1100. https://doi.org/10.1093/cvr/cvaa078.

Chiabrando, J. G., A. Bonaventura, A. Vecchié, G. F. Wohlford, A. G. Mauro, J. H. Jordan, J. D. Grizzard, F. Montecucco, D. H. Berrocal, A. Brucato, M. Imazio, and A. Abbate. 2020. Management of acute and recurrent pericarditis: JACC state-of-the-art review. *Journal of the American College of Cardiology* 75(1):76–92. https://doi.org/10.1016/j.jacc.2019.11.021.

Ciháková, D., R. B. Sharma, D. Fairweather, M. Afanasyeva, and N. R. Rose. 2004. Animal models for autoimmune myocarditis and autoimmune thyroiditis. *Methods in Molecular Medicine* 102:175–193. https://doi.org/10.1385/1-59259-805-6:175.

Cihákova, D., J. G. Barin, M. Afanasyeva, M. Kimura, D. Fairweather, M. Berg, M. V. Talor, G. C. Baldeviano, S. Frisancho, K. Gabrielson, D. Bedja, and N. R. Rose. 2008. Interleukin-13 protects against experimental autoimmune myocarditis by regulating macrophage differentiation. *American Journal of Pathology* 172(5):1195–1208. https://doi.org/10.2353/ajpath.2008.070207.

Cooper, L. T., Jr. 2009. Myocarditis. *New England Journal of Medicine* 360(15):1526–1538. https://doi.org/10.1056/NEJMra0800028.

Cooper, L. T., Jr., G. J. Berry, and R. Shabetai for the Multicenter Giant Cell Myocarditis Study Group investigators. 1997. Idiopathic giant-cell myocarditis—natural history and treatment. *New England Journal of Medicine* 336(26):1860–1866. https://doi.org/10.1056/nejm199706263362603.

Cooper, L. T., Jr., O. K. Onuma, S. Sagar, A. L. Oberg, D. W. Mahoney, Y. W. Asmann, and P. Liu. 2010. Genomic and proteomic analysis of myocarditis and dilated cardiomyopathy. *Heart Failure Clinics* 6(1):75–85. https://doi.org/10.1016/j.hfc.2009.08.012.

Coronado, M. J., J. E. Brandt, E. Kim, A. Bucek, D. Bedja, E. D. Abston, J. Shin, K. L. Gabrielson, W. Mitzner, and D. Fairweather. 2012. Testosterone and interleukin-1β increase cardiac remodeling during coxsackievirus B3 myocarditis via serpin A 3n. *American Journal of Physiology: Heart and Circulatory Physiology* 302(8):H1726–H1736. https://doi.org/10.1152/ajpheart.00783.2011.

Coronado, M. J., K. A. Bruno, L. A. Blauwet, C. Tschöpe, M. W. Cunningham, S. Pankuweit, S. van Linthout, E. S. Jeon, D. M. McNamara, J. Krejčí, J. Bienertová-Vašků, E. J. Douglass, E. D. Abston, A. Bucek, J. A. Frisancho, M. S. Greenaway, A. R. Hill, H. P. Schultheiss, L. T. Cooper, Jr., and D. Fairweather. 2019. Elevated sera sST2 is associated with heart failure in men ≤50 years old with myocarditis. *Journal of the American Heart Association* 8(2):e008968. https://doi.org/10.1161/jaha.118.008968.

Corrao, G., M. Franchi, D. Cereda, F. Bortolan, O. Leoni, E. Vignati, G. Pavesi, and A. Gori. 2022. Increased risk of myocarditis and pericarditis and reduced likelihood of severe clinical outcomes associated with COVID-19 vaccination: A cohort study in Lombardy, Italy. *BMC Infectious Diseases* 22(1):844. https://doi.org/10.1186/s12879-022-07823-3.

Diaz, G. A., G. T. Parsons, S. K. Gering, A. R. Meier, I. V. Hutchinson, and A. Robicsek. 2021. Myocarditis and pericarditis after vaccination for COVID-19. *JAMA* 326(12):1210–1212. https://doi.org/10.1001/jama.2021.13443.

Fairweather, D., Z. Kaya, G. R. Shellam, C. M. Lawson, and N. R. Rose. 2001. From infection to autoimmunity. *Journal of Autoimmunity* 16(3):175–186. https://doi.org/10.1006/jaut.2000.0492.

Fairweather, D., S. Yusung, S. Frisancho, M. Barrett, S. Gatewood, R. Steele, and N. R. Rose. 2003. IL-12 receptor beta 1 and Toll-like receptor 4 increase IL-1 beta- and IL-18-associated myocarditis and coxsackievirus replication. *Journal of Immunology* 170(9):4731–4737. https://doi.org/10.4049/jimmunol.170.9.4731.

Fairweather, D., S. Frisancho-Kiss, S. Gatewood, D. Njoku, R. Steele, M. Barrett, and N. R. Rose. 2004a. Mast cells and innate cytokines are associated with susceptibility to autoimmune heart disease following coxsackievirus B3 infection. *Autoimmunity* 37(2):131–145. https://doi.org/10.1080/0891693042000196200.

Fairweather, D., S. Frisancho-Kiss, S. A. Yusung, M. A. Barrett, S. E. Davis, S. J. Gatewood, D. B. Njoku, and N. R. Rose. 2004b. Interferon-gamma protects against chronic viral myocarditis by reducing mast cell degranulation, fibrosis, and the profibrotic cytokines transforming growth factor-beta 1, interleukin-1 beta, and interleukin-4 in the heart. *American Journal of Pathology* 165(6):1883–1894. https://doi.org/10.1016/s0002-9440(10)63241-5.

Fairweather, D., S. Frisancho-Kiss, D. B. Njoku, J. F. Nyland, Z. Kaya, S. A. Yusung, S. E. Davis, J. A. Frisancho, M. A. Barrett, and N. R. Rose. 2006. Complement receptor 1 and 2 deficiency increases coxsackievirus B3-induced myocarditis, dilated cardiomyopathy, and heart failure by increasing macrophages, IL-1beta, and immune complex deposition in the heart. *Journal of Immunology* 176(6):3516–3524. https://doi.org/10.4049/jimmunol.176.6.3516.

Fairweather, D., K. A. Stafford, and Y. K. Sung. 2012. Update on coxsackievirus B3 myocarditis. *Current Opinion in Rheumatology* 24(4):401–407. https://doi.org/10.1097/BOR.0b013e328353372d.

Fairweather, D., L. T. Cooper, Jr., and L. A. Blauwet. 2013. Sex and gender differences in myocarditis and dilated cardiomyopathy. *Current Problems in Cardiology* 38(1):7–46. https://doi.org/10.1016/j.cpcardiol.2012.07.003.

Fairweather, D., M. J. Coronado, A. E. Garton, J. L. Dziedzic, A. Bucek, L. T. Cooper, Jr., J. E. Brandt, F. S. Alikhan, H. Wang, C. J. Endres, J. Choi, M. G. Pomper, and T. R. Guilarte. 2014. Sex differences in translocator protein 18 kDa (TSPO) in the heart: Implications for imaging myocardial inflammation. *Journal of Cardiovascular Translational Research* 7(2):192–202. https://doi.org/10.1007/s12265-013-9538-0.

Fairweather, D., D. J. Beetler, N. Musigk, B. Heidecker, M. A. Lyle, L. T. Cooper, Jr., and K. A. Bruno. 2023a. Sex and gender differences in myocarditis and dilated cardiomyopathy: An update. *Frontiers in Cardiovascular Medicine* 10:1129348. https://doi.org/10.3389/fcvm.2023.1129348.

Fairweather, D., D. J. Beetler, D. N. Di Florio, N. Musigk, B. Heidecker, and L. T. Cooper, Jr. 2023b. COVID-19, myocarditis and pericarditis. *Circulation Research* 132(10):1302–1319. https://doi.org/10.1161/circresaha.123.321878.

FDA (Food and Drug Administration). 2020a. *Emergency use authorization (EUA) for an unapproved product review memorandum—Pfizer-BioNTech COVID-19 vaccine emergency use authorization review memorandum.* Food and Drug Administration. https://www.fda.gov/media/144416/download (accessed December 5, 2023).

FDA. 2020b. *Vaccines and Related Biological Products Advisory Committee meeting December 10, 2020—Pfizer-BioNTech COVID-19 vaccine.* Food and Drug Administration. https://www.fda.gov/media/144245/download (accessed December 5, 2023).

FDA. 2020c. *Vaccines and Related Biological Products Advisory Committee meeting December 17, 2020—Moderna COVID-19 vaccine.* Food and Drug Administration. https://www.fda.gov/media/144434/download (accessed December 5, 2023).

FDA. 2021a. *Summary basis for regulatory action - Pfizer BioNTech.* https://www.fda.gov/media/151733/download (accessed December 5, 2023).

FDA. 2021b. *Emergency use authorization (EUA) amendment for an unapproved product review memorandum—Pfizer-BioNTech COVID-19 vaccine/BNT162b2.* Food and Drug Administration. https://www.fda.gov/media/148542/download (accessed December 5, 2023).

FDA. 2021c. *Emergency use authorization (EUA) for an unapproved product review memorandum—Pfizer-BioNTech.* Food and Drug Administration. https://www.fda.gov/media/153947/download (accessed December 5, 2023).

FDA. 2021d. *Emergency use authorization (EUA) for an unapproved product review memorandum—Janssen Biotech.* Food and Drug Administration. https://www.fda.gov/media/146338/download (accessed May 3, 2023).

FDA. 2021e. *Vaccines and Related Biological Products Advisory Committee meeting—February 26, 2021—Janssen Ad26. COV2.S vaccine for the prevention of COVID-19.* Food and Drug Administration. https://www.fda.gov/media/146217/download (accessed December 13, 2023).

FDA. 2022a. *Vaccines and Related Biological Products Advisory Committee meeting June 15, 2022—EUA amendment request for Pfizer-BioNTech COVID-19 vaccine for use in children 6 months through 4 years of age.* Food and Drug Administration. https://www.fda.gov/media/159195/download (accessed December 13, 2023).

FDA. 2022b. *Vaccines and Related Biological Products Advisory Committee meeting - June 14–15, 2022: EUA amendment request for the use of Moderna COVID-19 vaccine in children 6 months through 17 years of age.* Food and Drug Administration. https://www.fda.gov/media/159189/download (accessed December 19, 2023).

FDA. 2022c. *Emergency use authorization (EUA) for an unapproved product review memorandum amendment 645—Pfizer-BioNTech.* Food and Drug Administration. https://www.fda.gov/media/162410/download (accessed December 13, 2023).

FDA. 2023a. *Emergency use authorization (EUA) for an unapproved product review memorandum—ModernaTX COVID-19 vaccine.* Food and Drug Administration. https://www.fda.gov/media/167306/download?attachment (accessed December 5, 2023).

FDA. 2023b. *Emergency use authorization (EUA) for an unapproved product review memorandum.* Food and Drug Administration. https://www.fda.gov/media/168233/download?attachment (accessed December 5, 2023).

Ferreira, V. M., J. Schulz-Menger, G. Holmvang, C. M. Kramer, I. Carbone, U. Sechtem, I. Kindermann, M. Gutberlet, L. T. Cooper, P. Liu, and M. G. Friedrich. 2018. Cardiovascular magnetic resonance in nonischemic myocardial inflammation: Expert recommendations. *Journal of the American College of Cardiology* 72(24):3158–3176. https://doi.org/10.1016/j.jacc.2018.09.072.

Fraiman, J., J. Erviti, M. Jones, S. Greenland, P. Whelan, R. M. Kaplan, and P. Doshi. 2022. Serious adverse events of special interest following mRNA COVID-19 vaccination in randomized trials in adults. *Vaccine* 40(40):5798–5805. https://doi.org/10.1016/j.vaccine.2022.08.036.

Frisancho-Kiss, S., J. F. Nyland, S. E. Davis, M. A. Barrett, S. J. Gatewood, D. B. Njoku, D. Ciháková, E. K. Silbergeld, N. R. Rose, and D. Fairweather. 2006a. Cutting edge: T cell IG mucin-3 reduces inflammatory heart disease by increasing CTLA-4 during innate immunity. *Journal of Immunology* 176(11):6411–6415. https://doi.org/10.4049/jimmunol.176.11.6411.

Frisancho-Kiss, S., J. F. Nyland, S. E. Davis, J. A. Frisancho, M. A. Barrett, N. R. Rose, and D. Fairweather. 2006b. Sex differences in coxsackievirus B3–induced myocarditis: IL-12rbeta1 signaling and IFN-gamma increase inflammation in males independent from STAT4. *Brain Research* 1126(1):139–147. https://doi.org/10.1016/j.brainres.2006.08.003.

Frisancho-Kiss, S., S. E. Davis, J. F. Nyland, J. A. Frisancho, D. Ciháková, M. A. Barrett, N. R. Rose, and D. Fairweather. 2007. Cutting edge: Cross-regulation by TLR4 and T cell IG mucin-3 determines sex differences in inflammatory heart disease. *Journal of Immunology* 178(11):6710–6714. https://doi.org/10.4049/jimmunol.178.11.6710.

Frisancho-Kiss, S., M. J. Coronado, J. A. Frisancho, V. M. Lau, N. R. Rose, S. L. Klein, and D. Fairweather. 2009. Gonadectomy of male BALB/c mice increases tim-3(+) alternatively activated M2 macrophages, tim-3(+) T cells, Th2 cells and Treg in the heart during acute coxsackievirus-induced myocarditis. *Brain, Behavior, and Immunity* 23(5):649–657. https://doi.org/10.1016/j.bbi.2008.12.002.

Frustaci, A., R. Verardo, N. Galea, C. Lavalle, G. Bagnato, R. Scialla, and C. Chimenti. 2022. Hypersensitivity myocarditis after COVID-19 mRNA vaccination. *Journal of Clinical Medicine* 11(6). https://doi.org/10.3390/jcm11061660.

Gaudet, L., S. Saba, L. Bialy, A. Mackie, I. Paterson, B. Skidmore, and L. Harting. 2023. *Incidence, natural history, specific populations and hypothesized mechanisms of myocarditis and pericarditis following mRNA COVID-19 vaccination: Living evidence synthesis*. Strategy for Patient-Oriented Research.

Goddard, K., K. E. Hanson, N. Lewis, E. Weintraub, B. Fireman, and N. P. Klein. 2022a. Incidence of myocarditis/pericarditis following mRNA COVID-19 vaccination among children and younger adults in the United States. *Annals of Internal Medicine* 175(12):1769–1771. https://doi.org/10.7326/M22-2274.

Goddard, K., N. Lewis, B. Fireman, E. Weintraub, T. Shimabukuro, O. Zerbo, T. G. Boyce, M. E. Oster, K. E. Hanson, J. G. Donahue, P. Ross, A. Naleway, J. C. Nelson, B. Lewin, J. M. Glanz, J. T. B. Williams, E. O. Kharbanda, W. Katherine Yih, and N. P. Klein. 2022b. Risk of myocarditis and pericarditis following BNT162b2 and mRNA-1273 COVID-19 vaccination. *Vaccine* 40(35):5153–5159. https://doi.org/10.1016/j.vaccine.2022.07.007.

Graña, C., L. Ghosn, T. Evrenoglou, A. Jarde, S. Minozzi, H. Bergman, B. S. Buckley, K. Probyn, G. Villanueva, N. Henschke, H. Bonnet, R. Assi, S. Menon, M. Marti, D. Devane, P. Mallon, J. D. Lelievre, L. M. Askie, T. Kredo, G. Ferrand, M. Davidson, C. Riveros, D. Tovey, J. J. Meerpohl, G. Grasselli, G. Rada, A. Hróbjartsson, P. Ravaud, A. Chaimani, and I. Boutron. 2022. Efficacy and safety of COVID-19 vaccines. *Cochrane Database of Systematic Reviews* 12(12):Cd015477. https://doi.org/10.1002/14651858.Cd015477.

Halamoda-Kenzaoui, B., and S. Bremer-Hoffmann. 2018. Main trends of immune effects triggered by nanomedicines in pre-clinical studies. *International Journal of Nanomedicine* 13:5419–5431. https://doi.org/10.2147/ijn.S168808.

Halsell, J. S., J. R. Riddle, J. E. Atwood, P. Gardner, R. Shope, G. A. Poland, G. C. Gray, S. Ostroff, R. E. Eckart, D. R. Hospenthal, R. L. Gibson, J. D. Grabenstein, M. K. Arness, and D. N. Tornberg. 2003. Myopericarditis following small-pox vaccination among vaccinia-naive U.S. military personnel. *JAMA* 289(24):3283–3289. https://doi.org/10.1001/jama.289.24.3283.

Heidecker, B., N. Dagan, R. Balicer, U. Eriksson, G. Rosano, A. Coats, C. Tschöpe, S. Kelle, G. A. Poland, A. Frustaci, K. Klingel, P. Martin, J. M. Hare, L. T. Cooper, A. Pantazis, M. Imazio, S. Prasad, and T. F. Lüscher. 2022. Myocarditis following COVID-19 vaccine: Incidence, presentation, diagnosis, pathophysiology, therapy, and outcomes put into perspective. A clinical consensus document supported by the Heart Failure Association of the European Society of Cardiology (ESC) and the ESC Working Group on Myocardial and Pericardial Diseases. *European Journal of Heart Failure* 24(11):2000–2018. https://doi.org/10.1002/ejhf.2669.

Hikmet, F., L. Méar, Å. Edvinsson, P. Micke, M. Uhlén, and C. Lindskog. 2020. The protein expression profile of ACE2 in human tissues. *Molecular Systems Biology* 16(7):e9610. https://doi.org/10.15252/msb.20209610.

Hoffmann, M., H. Kleine-Weber, S. Schroeder, N. Krüger, T. Herrler, S. Erichsen, T. S. Schiergens, G. Herrler, N. H. Wu, A. Nitsche, M. A. Müller, C. Drosten, and S. Pöhlmann. 2020. SARS-CoV-2 cell entry depends on ACE2 and TMPRSS2 and is blocked by a clinically proven protease inhibitor. *Cell* 181(2):271–280. https://doi.org/10.1016/j.cell.2020.02.052.

Hou, X., T. Zaks, R. Langer, and Y. Dong. 2021. Lipid nanoparticles for mRNA delivery. *Nature Reviews Materials* 6(12):1078–1094. https://doi.org/10.1038/s41578-021-00358-0.

Huber, S., M. Massri, M. Grasse, V. Fleischer, S. Kellnerová, V. Harpf, L. Knabl, L. Knabl, Sr., T. Heiner, M. Kummann, M. Neurauter, G. Rambach, C. Speth, and R. Würzner. 2021. Systemic inflammation and complement activation parameters predict clinical outcome of severe SARS-CoV-2 infections. *Viruses* 13(12). https://doi.org/10.3390/v13122376.

Huber, S. A., and L. P. Job. 1983. Cellular immune mechanisms in coxsackievirus group b, type 3 induced myocarditis in BALB/c mice. *Advances in Experimental Medicine and Biology* 161:491–508. https://doi.org/10.1007/978-1-4684-4472-8_29.

Hugues, B., H. Ben Amer, F. Bril, M. Groh, and F. Huang. 2022. Interleukin-1/6 blockade for the treatment of severe steroid-refractory BNT162b2 vaccine-induced adult-onset Still's disease. *European Journal of Case Reports in Internal Medicine* 9(8):003469. https://doi.org/10.12890/2022_003469.

Husby, A., J. V. Hansen, E. Fosbøl, E. M. Thiesson, M. Madsen, R. W. Thomsen, H. T. Sørensen, M. Andersen, J. Wohlfahrt, G. Gislason, C. Torp-Pedersen, L. Køber, and A. Hviid. 2021. SARS-CoV-2 vaccination and myocarditis or myopericarditis: Population based cohort study. *British Journal of Medicine* 375:e068665. https://doi.org/10.1136/bmj-2021-068665.

Imazio, M., M. Bobbio, E. Cecchi, D. Demarie, B. Demichelis, F. Pomari, M. Moratti, G. Gaschino, M. Giammaria, A. Ghisio, R. Belli, and R. Trinchero. 2005a. Colchicine in addition to conventional therapy for acute pericarditis: Results of the Colchicine for Acute Pericarditis (COPE) trial. *Circulation* 112(13):2012–2016. https://doi.org/10.1161/circulationaha.105.542738.

Imazio, M., M. Bobbio, E. Cecchi, D. Demarie, F. Pomari, M. Moratti, A. Ghisio, R. Belli, and R. Trinchero. 2005b. Colchicine as first-choice therapy for recurrent pericarditis: Results of the CORE (colchicine for recurrent pericarditis) trial. *Archives of Internal Medicine* 165(17):1987–1991. https://doi.org/10.1001/archinte.165.17.1987.

Imazio, M., A. Brucato, R. Cemin, S. Ferrua, R. Belli, S. Maestroni, R. Trinchero, D. H. Spodick, and Y. Adler. 2011. Colchicine for Recurrent Pericarditis (CORP): A randomized trial. *Annals of Internal Medicine* 155(7):409–414. https://doi.org/10.7326/0003-4819-155-7-201110040-00359.

Imazio, M., A. Brucato, R. Cemin, S. Ferrua, S. Maggiolini, F. Beqaraj, D. Demarie, D. Forno, S. Ferro, S. Maestroni, R. Belli, R. Trinchero, D. H. Spodick, and Y. Adler. 2013. A randomized trial of colchicine for acute pericarditis. *New England Journal of Medicine* 369(16):1522–1528. https://doi.org/10.1056/NEJMoa1208536.

Imazio, M., R. Belli, A. Brucato, R. Cemin, S. Ferrua, F. Beqaraj, D. Demarie, S. Ferro, D. Forno, S. Maestroni, D. Cumetti, F. Varbella, R. Trinchero, D. H. Spodick, and Y. Adler. 2014. Efficacy and safety of colchicine for treatment of multiple recurrences of pericarditis (CORP-2): A multicentre, double-blind, placebo-controlled, randomised trial. *Lancet* 383(9936):2232–2237. https://doi.org/10.1016/s0140-6736(13)62709-9.

Imazio, M., F. Gaita, and M. LeWinter. 2015. Evaluation and treatment of pericarditis: A systematic review. *JAMA* 314(14):1498–1506. https://doi.org/10.1001/jama.2015.12763.

Jain, A., K. A. Bruno, A. Matsumori, L. T. Cooper, M. Yamani, and D. Fairweather. 2022. 4.18—myocarditis and pericarditis. In *Comprehensive pharmacology*, edited by T. Kenakin. Oxford: Elsevier. Pp. 413–431.

Karlstad, Ø., P. Hovi, A. Husby, T. Härkänen, R. M. Selmer, N. Pihlström, J. V. Hansen, H. Nohynek, N. Gunnes, A. Sundström, J. Wohlfahrt, T. A. Nieminen, M. Grünewald, H. L. Gulseth, A. Hviid, and R. Ljung. 2022. SARS-CoV-2 vaccination and myocarditis in a Nordic cohort study of 23 million residents. *JAMA Cardiology* 7(6):600–612. https://doi.org/10.1001/jamacardio.2022.0583.

Kauffman, K. J., F. F. Mir, S. Jhunjhunwala, J. C. Kaczmarek, J. E. Hurtado, J. H. Yang, M. J. Webber, P. S. Kowalski, M. W. Heartlein, F. DeRosa, and D. G. Anderson. 2016. Efficacy and immunogenicity of unmodified and pseudouridine-modified mRNA delivered systemically with lipid nanoparticles in vivo. *Biomaterials* 109:78–87. https://doi.org/10.1016/j.biomaterials.2016.09.006.

Kracalik, I., M. E. Oster, K. R. Broder, M. M. Cortese, M. Glover, K. Shields, C. B. Creech, B. Romanson, S. Novosad, J. Soslow, E. B. Walter, P. Marquez, J. M. Dendy, J. Woo, A. L. Valderrama, A. Ramirez-Cardenas, A. Assefa, M. J. Campbell, J. R. Su, S. S. Magill, D. K. Shay, T. T. Shimabukuro, S. V. Basavaraju, P. Campbell, C. Anugwom, C. Arvelo Jefferson, K. Badger, N. Bafford, C. Barnes, S. Boles, E. Collins, M. Desai, T. Dulski, B. Dyleski, K. Edwards, M. Feyereisen, S. Gonsahn, T. Gregory, J. Gunta, K. Jacobs Slifka, C. Kabore, B. K. Kapella, S. Karol, K. Kennebrew, N. Kluisza, S. Lang, L. Lanier Gholston, M. Law, J. Lehman, J. M. Mazurek, H. McGruder, K. McNamara, M.-L. Moore, P. Moro, J. F. Moroney, O. Museru, C. Nale, A. Neiman, K. Newsome, E. Odom, B. Pantazides, S. Patel, A. Rao, L. Reynolds, S. Robinson, F. L. Ruberg, T. Schaeffer, D. Solanky, L. Sperling, T. Stanley, R. Sullivan, A. Taylor, K. Thomas, S. Thompson, J. Tola, C. H. Tran, S. Wiersma, and K. Works. 2022. Outcomes at least 90 days since onset of myocarditis after mRNA COVID-19 vaccination in adolescents and young adults in the USA: A follow-up surveillance study. *The Lancet Child & Adolescent Health* 6(11):788–798. https://doi.org/https://doi.org/10.1016/S2352-4642(22)00244-9.

Kytö, V., J. Sipilä, and P. Rautava. 2014. Clinical profile and influences on outcomes in patients hospitalized for acute pericarditis. *Circulation* 130(18):1601–1606. https://doi.org/10.1161/circulationaha.114.010376.

Lai, F. T. T., E. W. W. Chan, L. Huang, C. L. Cheung, C. S. L. Chui, X. Li, E. Y. F. Wan, C. K. H. Wong, E. W. Y. Chan, K. H. Yiu, and I. C. K. Wong. 2022. Prognosis of myocarditis developing after mRNA COVID-19 vaccination compared with viral myocarditis. *Journal of the American College of Cardiology* 80(24):2255–2265. https://doi.org/https://doi.org/10.1016/j.jacc.2022.09.049.

Lamerton, R. E., E. Marcial-Juarez, S. E. Faustini, M. Perez-Toledo, M. Goodall, S. E. Jossi, M. L. Newby, I. Chapple, T. Dietrich, T. Veenith, A. M. Shields, L. Harper, I. R. Henderson, J. Rayes, D. C. Wraith, S. P. Watson, M. Crispin, M. T. Drayson, A. G. Richter, and A. F. Cunningham. 2022. SARS-CoV-2 spike- and nucleoprotein-specific antibodies induced after vaccination or infection promote classical complement activation. *Frontiers in Immunology* 13:838780. https://doi.org/10.3389/fimmu.2022.838780.

Lan, J., J. Ge, J. Yu, S. Shan, H. Zhou, S. Fan, Q. Zhang, X. Shi, Q. Wang, L. Zhang, and X. Wang. 2020. Structure of the SARS-CoV-2 spike receptor-binding domain bound to the ACE2 receptor. *Nature* 581(7807):215–220. https://doi.org/10.1038/s41586-020-2180-5.

Lau, E. S., J. N. McNeill, S. M. Paniagua, E. E. Liu, J. K. Wang, I. V. Bassett, C. A. Selvaggi, S. A. Lubitz, A. S. Foulkes, and J. E. Ho. 2021. Sex differences in inflammatory markers in patients hospitalized with COVID-19 infection: Insights from the MGH COVID-19 patient registry. *PLoS One* 16(4):e0250774. https://doi.org/10.1371/journal.pone.0250774.

Law, Y. M., A. K. Lal, S. Chen, D. Čihaková, L. T. Cooper, Jr., S. Deshpande, J. Godown, L. Grosse-Wortmann, J. D. Robinson, and J. A. Towbin. 2021. Diagnosis and management of myocarditis in children: A scientific statement from the American Heart Association. *Circulation* 144(6):e123–e135. https://doi.org/10.1161/cir.0000000000001001.

Le Vu, S., M. Bertrand, M. J. Jabagi, J. Botton, J. Drouin, B. Baricault, A. Weill, R. Dray-Spira, and M. Zureik. 2022. Age and sex-specific risks of myocarditis and pericarditis following COVID-19 messenger RNA vaccines. *Nature Communications* 13(1):3633. https://doi.org/10.1038/s41467-022-31401-5.

Li, C., Y. Chen, Y. Zhao, D. C. Lung, Z. Ye, W. Song, F. F. Liu, J. P. Cai, W. M. Wong, C. C. Yip, J. F. Chan, K. K. To, S. Sridhar, I. F. Hung, H. Chu, K. H. Kok, D. Y. Jin, A. J. Zhang, and K. Y. Yuen. 2022. Intravenous injection of coronavirus disease 2019 (COVID-19) mRNA vaccine can induce acute myopericarditis in mouse model. *Clinical Infectious Diseases* 74(11):1933–1950. https://doi.org/10.1093/cid/ciab707.

Liu, W., M. Moussawi, B. Roberts, J. E. Boyson, and S. A. Huber. 2013. Cross-regulation of T regulatory-cell response after coxsackievirus B3 infection by NKT and γδ T cells in the mouse. *American Journal of Pathology* 183(2):441–449. https://doi.org/10.1016/j.ajpath.2013.04.015.

Lovell, J. P., D. Čihaková, and N. A. Gilotra. 2022. COVID-19 and myocarditis: Review of clinical presentations, pathogenesis and management. *Heart International* 16(1):20–27. https://doi.org/10.17925/hi.2022.16.1.20.

Lüscher, T. F., and M. M. Akhtar. 2022. Looking deeper into Takotsubo's heart. *Cardiovascular Research* 118(8):1851–1853. https://doi.org/10.1093/cvr/cvac069.

Macías Saint-Gerons, D., M. T. Ibarz, J. L. Castro, J. Forés-Martos, and R. Tabarés-Seisdedos. 2023. Myopericarditis associated with the Novavax COVID-19 vaccine (NVX-CoV2373): A retrospective analysis of individual case safety reports from VigiBase. *Drugs—Real World Outcomes* 10(2):263–270. https://doi.org/10.1007/s40801-023-00355-5.

Maleszewski, J. J., V. M. Orellana, D. O. Hodge, U. Kuhl, H. P. Schultheiss, and L. T. Cooper. 2015. Long-term risk of recurrence, morbidity and mortality in giant cell myocarditis. *American Journal of Cardiology* 115(12):1733–1738. https://doi.org/10.1016/j.amjcard.2015.03.023.

Marks, P. 2023. Notice of emergency use authorization (EUA) for an unapproved product—Novavax COVID-19 vaccine, adjuvanted, October 3, 2023. https://www.fda.gov/media/159902/download (accessed December 20, 2023).

Martinon, F., V. Pétrilli, A. Mayor, A. Tardivel, and J. Tschopp. 2006. Gout-associated uric acid crystals activate the NALP3 inflammasome. *Nature* 440(7081):237–241. https://doi.org/10.1038/nature04516.

Massari, M., S. Spila Alegiani, C. Morciano, M. Spuri, P. Marchione, P. Felicetti, V. Belleudi, F. R. Poggi, M. Lazzeretti, M. Ercolanoni, E. Clagnan, E. Bovo, G. Trifirò, U. Moretti, G. Monaco, O. Leoni, R. Da Cas, F. Petronzelli, L. Tartaglia, N. Mores, G. Zanoni, P. Rossi, S. Samez, C. Zappetti, A. R. Marra, and F. Menniti Ippolito. 2022. Postmarketing active surveillance of myocarditis and pericarditis following vaccination with COVID-19 mRNA vaccines in persons aged 12 to 39 years in Italy: A multi-database, self-controlled case series study. *PLoS Medicine* 19(7):e1004056. https://doi.org/10.1371/journal.pmed.1004056.

Matsumori, A. 2003. *Cardiomyopathies and heart failure: Biomolecular, infectious, and immune mechanisms.* Boston: Kluwer Academic Publishers.

McNamara, D. M., R. C. Starling, L. T. Cooper, J. P. Boehmer, P. J. Mather, K. M. Janosko, J. Gorcsan, III, K. E. Kip, and G. W. Dec. 2011. Clinical and demographic predictors of outcomes in recent onset dilated cardiomyopathy: Results of the IMAC (Intervention in Myocarditis and Acute Cardiomyopathy)-2 study. *Journal of the American College of Cardiology* 58(11):1112–1118. https://doi.org/10.1016/j.jacc.2011.05.033.

Miteva, K., K. Pappritz, M. Sosnowski, M. El-Shafeey, I. Müller, F. Dong, K. Savvatis, J. Ringe, C. Tschöpe, and S. Van Linthout. 2018. Mesenchymal stromal cells inhibit NLRP3 inflammasome activation in a model of coxsackievirus B3–induced inflammatory cardiomyopathy. *Scientific Reports* 8(1):2820. https://doi.org/10.1038/s41598-018-20686-6.

Moorlag, S., R. J. Röring, L. A. B. Joosten, and M. G. Netea. 2018. The role of the interleukin-1 family in trained immunity. *Immunological Reviews* 281(1):28–39. https://doi.org/10.1111/imr.12617.

Myers, J. M., L. T. Cooper, D. C. Kem, S. Stavrakis, S. D. Kosanke, E. M. Shevach, D. Fairweather, J. A. Stoner, C. J. Cox, and M. W. Cunningham. 2016. Cardiac myosin-TH17 responses promote heart failure in human myocarditis. *JCI Insight* 1(9). https://doi.org/10.1172/jci.insight.85851.

Ndeupen, S., Z. Qin, S. Jacobsen, A. Bouteau, H. Estanbouli, and B. Z. Igyarto. 2021. The mRNA-LNP platform's lipid nanoparticle component used in preclinical vaccine studies is highly inflammatory. *iScience* 24(12):103479. https://doi.org/10.1016/j.isci.2021.103479.

Neu, N., N. R. Rose, K. W. Beisel, A. Herskowitz, G. Gurri-Glass, and S. W. Craig. 1987. Cardiac myosin induces myocarditis in genetically predisposed mice. *Journal of Immunology* 139(11):3630–3636.

Oster, M. E., D. K. Shay, J. R. Su, J. Gee, C. B. Creech, K. R. Broder, K. Edwards, J. H. Soslow, J. M. Dendy, E. Schlaudecker, S. M. Lang, E. D. Barnett, F. L. Ruberg, M. J. Smith, M. J. Campbell, R. D. Lopes, L. S. Sperling, J. A. Baumblatt, D. L. Thompson, P. L. Marquez, P. Strid, J. Woo, R. Pugsley, S. Reagan-Steiner, F. DeStefano, and T. T. Shimabukuro. 2022. Myocarditis cases reported after mRNA-based COVID-19 vaccination in the U.S. from December 2020 to August 2021. *JAMA* 327(4):331–340. https://doi.org/10.1001/jama.2021.24110.

Pappritz, K., J. Lin, M. El-Shafeey, H. Fechner, U. Kühl, A. Alogna, F. Spillmann, A. Elsanhoury, R. Schulz, C. Tschöpe, and S. Van Linthout. 2022. Colchicine prevents disease progression in viral myocarditis via modulating the NLRP3 inflammasome in the cardiosplenic axis. *ESC Heart Failure* 9(2):925–941. https://doi.org/10.1002/ehf2.13845.

Patone, M., X. W. Mei, L. Handunnetthi, S. Dixon, F. Zaccardi, M. Shankar-Hari, P. Watkinson, K. Khunti, A. Harnden, C. A. C. Coupland, K. M. Channon, N. L. Mills, A. Sheikh, and J. Hippisley-Cox. 2022a. Risk of myocarditis after sequential doses of COVID-19 vaccine and SARS-CoV-2 infection by age and sex. *Circulation* 146(10):743–754. https://doi.org/10.1161/circulationaha.122.059970.

Patone, M., X. W. Mei, L. Handunnetthi, S. Dixon, F. Zaccardi, M. Shankar-Hari, P. Watkinson, K. Khunti, A. Harnden, C. A. C. Coupland, K. M. Channon, N. L. Mills, A. Sheikh, and J. Hippisley-Cox. 2022b. Risks of myocarditis, pericarditis, and cardiac arrhythmias associated with COVID-19 vaccination or SARS-CoV-2 infection. *Nature Medicine* 28(2):410–422. https://doi.org/10.1038/s41591-021-01630-0.

Pillay, J., L. Gaudet, A. Wingert, L. Bialy, A. S. Mackie, D. I. Paterson, and L. Hartling. 2022. Incidence, risk factors, natural history, and hypothesised mechanisms of myocarditis and pericarditis following COVID-19 vaccination: Living evidence syntheses and review. *British Journal of Medicine* 378:e069445. https://doi.org/10.1136/bmj-2021-069445.

Poli, V., K. A. Bruno, and D. Fairweather. 2020. Autoimmune myocarditis: Animal models. In *Myocarditis: Pathogenesis, diagnosis and treatment*, edited by A. L. P. Caforio. Cham: Springer International Publishing. Pp. 111–127.

Potere, N., A. Abbate, Y. Kanthi, M. Carrier, S. Toldo, E. Porreca, and M. Di Nisio. 2023. Inflammasome signaling, thromboinflammation, and venous thromboembolism. *JACC Basic Translational Science* 8(9):1245–1261. https://doi.org/10.1016/j.jacbts.2023.03.017.

Power, J. R., L. K. Keyt, and E. D. Adler. 2022. Myocarditis following COVID-19 vaccination: Incidence, mechanisms, and clinical considerations. *Expert Review of Cardiovascular Therapy* 20(4):241–251. https://doi.org/10.1080/14779072.2022.2066522.

Roberts, B. J., M. Moussawi, and S. A. Huber. 2013. Sex differences in TLR2 and TLR4 expression and their effect on coxsackievirus-induced autoimmune myocarditis. *Experimental and Molecular Pathology* 94(1):58–64. https://doi.org/10.1016/j.yexmp.2012.06.005.

Root-Bernstein, R., and D. Fairweather. 2014. Complexities in the relationship between infection and autoimmunity. *Current Allergy and Asthma Reports* 14(1):407. https://doi.org/10.1007/s11882-013-0407-3.

Root-Bernstein, R., J. Huber, A. Ziehl, and M. Pietrowicz. 2023. SARS-CoV-2 and its bacterial co- or super-infections synergize to trigger COVID-19 autoimmune cardiopathies. *International Journal of Molecular Sciences* 24(15). https://doi.org/10.3390/ijms241512177.

Roth, G. A., G. A. Mensah, C. O. Johnson, G. Addolorato, E. Ammirati, L. M. Baddour, N. C. Barengo, A. Z. Beaton, E. J. Benjamin, C. P. Benziger, A. Bonny, M. Brauer, M. Brodmann, T. J. Cahill, J. Carapetis, A. L. Catapano, S. S. Chugh, L. T. Cooper, J. Coresh, M. Criqui, N. DeCleene, K. A. Eagle, S. Emmons-Bell, V. L. Feigin, J. Fernández-Solà, G. Fowkes, E. Gakidou, S. M. Grundy, F. J. He, G. Howard, F. Hu, L. Inker, G. Karthikeyan, N. Kassebaum, W. Koroshetz, C. Lavie, D. Lloyd-Jones, H. S. Lu, A. Mirijello, A. M. Temesgen, A. Mokdad, A. E. Moran, P. Muntner, J. Narula, B. Neal, M. Ntsekhe, G. Moraes de Oliveira, C. Otto, M. Owolabi, M. Pratt, S. Rajagopalan, M. Reitsma, A. L. P. Ribeiro, N. Rigotti, A. Rodgers, C. Sable, S. Shakil, K. Sliwa-Hahnle, B. Stark, J. Sundström, P. Timpel, I. M. Tleyjeh, M. Valgimigli, T. Vos, P. K. Whelton, M. Yacoub, L. Zuhlke, C. Murray, and V. Fuster. 2020. Global burden of cardiovascular diseases and risk factors, 1990–2019: Update from the GBD 2019 study. *Journal of the American College of Cardiology* 76(25):2982–3021. https://doi.org/10.1016/j.jacc.2020.11.010.

Samaridou, E., J. Heyes, and P. Lutwyche. 2020. Lipid nanoparticles for nucleic acid delivery: Current perspectives. *Advanced Drug Delivery Reviews* 154–155:37–63. https://doi.org/10.1016/j.addr.2020.06.002.

Schultheiss, H. P., D. Fairweather, A. L. P. Caforio, F. Escher, R. E. Hershberger, S. E. Lipshultz, P. P. Liu, A. Matsumori, A. Mazzanti, J. McMurray, and S. G. Priori. 2019. Dilated cardiomyopathy. *Nature Reviews Disease Primers* 5(1):32. https://doi.org/10.1038/s41572-019-0084-1.

Seneff, S., G. Nigh, A. M. Kyriakopoulos, and P. A. McCullough. 2022. Innate immune suppression by SARS-CoV-2 mRNA vaccinations: The role of G-quadruplexes, exosomes, and micrornas. *Food and Chemical Toxicology* 164:113008. https://doi.org/10.1016/j.fct.2022.113008.

Shahbazi, F., M. Karami, M. Mirzaei, and Y. Mohammadi. 2021. Survival rates and prognostic factors in patients with coronavirus disease 2019: A registry-based retrospective cohort study. *Journal of Research in Health Sciences* 21(2):e00515. https://doi.org/10.34172/jrhs.2021.47.

Siemieniuk, R., and G. Guyatt. 2024. *What is GRADE?* https://bestpractice.bmj.com/info/us/toolkit/learn-ebm/what-is-grade (accessed March 7, 2024).

Straus, W., V. Urdaneta, D. B. Esposito, J. A. Mansi, C. Sanz Rodriguez, P. Burton, and J. M. Vega. 2023. Analysis of myocarditis among 252 million mRNA-1273 recipients worldwide. *Clinical Infectious Diseases* 76(3):e544–e552. https://doi.org/10.1093/cid/ciac446.

Takahashi, T., M. K. Ellingson, P. Wong, B. Israelow, C. Lucas, J. Klein, J. Silva, T. Mao, J. E. Oh, M. Tokuyama, P. Lu, A. Venkataraman, A. Park, F. Liu, A. Meir, J. Sun, E. Y. Wang, A. Casanovas-Massana, A. L. Wyllie, C. B. F. Vogels, R. Earnest, S. Lapidus, I. M. Ott, A. J. Moore, A. Shaw, J. B. Fournier, C. D. Odio, S. Farhadian, C. Dela Cruz, N. D. Grubaugh, W. L. Schulz, A. M. Ring, A. I. Ko, S. B. Omer, and A. Iwasaki. 2020. Sex differences in immune responses that underlie COVID-19 disease outcomes. *Nature* 588(7837):315–320. https://doi.org/10.1038/s41586-020-2700-3.

Theoharides, T. C. 2021. Potential association of mast cells with coronavirus disease 2019. *Annals of Allergy, Asthma, and Immunology* 126(3):217–218. https://doi.org/10.1016/j.anai.2020.11.003.

Thurner, L., C. Kessel, N. Fadle, E. Regitz, F. Seidel, I. Kindermann, S. Lohse, I. Kos, C. Tschöpe, P. Kheiroddin, D. Kiblboeck, M. C. Hoffmann, B. Bette, G. Carbon, O. Cetin, K. D. Preuss, K. Christofyllakis, J. T. Bittenbring, T. Pickardt, Y. Fischer, H. Thiele, S. Baldus, K. Stangl, S. Steiner, F. Gietzen, S. Kerber, T. Deneke, S. Jellinghaus, A. Linke, K. Ibrahim, U. Grabmaier, S. Massberg, C. Thilo, S. Greulich, M. Gawaz, E. Mayatepek, L. Meyer-Dobkowitz, M. Kindermann, E. Birk, M. Birk, M. Lainscak, D. Foell, P. M. Lepper, R. Bals, M. Krawczyk, D. Mevorach, T. Hasin, A. Keren, M. Kabesch, H. Abdul-Khaliq, S. Smola, M. Bewarder, B. Thurner, M. Böhm, J. Pfeifer, and K. Klingel. 2022. IL-1RA antibodies in myocarditis after SARS-CoV-2 vaccination. *New England Journal of Medicine* 387(16):1524–1527. https://doi.org/10.1056/NEJMc2205667.

Toldo, S., R. Bussani, V. Nuzzi, A. Bonaventura, A. G. Mauro, A. Cannatà, R. Pillappa, G. Sinagra, P. Nana-Sinkam, P. Sime, and A. Abbate. 2021. Inflammasome formation in the lungs of patients with fatal COVID-19. *Inflammation Research* 70(1):7–10. https://doi.org/10.1007/s00011-020-01413-2.

Toldo, S., and A. Abbate. 2023. The role of the NLRP3 inflammasome and pyroptosis in cardiovascular diseases. *Nature Reviews: Cardiology* 21:219–237. https://doi.org/10.1038/s41569-023-00946-3.

Tschöpe, C., I. Müller, Y. Xia, K. Savvatis, K. Pappritz, S. Pinkert, D. Lassner, M. M. Heimesaat, F. Spillmann, K. Miteva, S. Bereswill, H. P. Schultheiss, H. Fechner, B. Pieske, U. Kühl, and S. Van Linthout. 2017. NOD2 (nucleotide-binding oligomerization domain 2) is a major pathogenic mediator of coxsackievirus B3–induced myocarditis. *Circulation: Heart Failure* 10(9). https://doi.org/10.1161/circheartfailure.117.003870.

Tschöpe, C., E. Ammirati, B. Bozkurt, A. L. P. Caforio, L. T. Cooper, S. B. Felix, J. M. Hare, B. Heidecker, S. Heymans, N. Hübner, S. Kelle, K. Klingel, H. Maatz, A. S. Parwani, F. Spillmann, R. C. Starling, H. Tsutsui, P. Seferovic, and S. Van Linthout. 2021. Myocarditis and inflammatory cardiomyopathy: Current evidence and future directions. *Nature Reviews: Cardiology* 18(3):169–193. https://doi.org/10.1038/s41569-020-00435-x.

Tsilingiris, D., N. G. Vallianou, I. Karampela, J. Liu, and M. Dalamaga. 2022. Potential implications of lipid nanoparticles in the pathogenesis of myocarditis associated with the use of mRNA vaccines against SARS-CoV-2. *Metabolism Open* 13:100159. https://doi.org/10.1016/j.metop.2021.100159.

Van Linthout, S., and C. Tschöpe. 2018. Viral myocarditis: A prime example for endomyocardial biopsy-guided diagnosis and therapy. *Current Opinion in Cardiology* 33(3):325–333. https://doi.org/10.1097/hco.0000000000000515.

Won, T., N. A. Gilotra, M. K. Wood, D. M. Hughes, M. V. Talor, J. Lovell, A. M. Milstone, C. Steenbergen, and D. Cihákova. 2022. Increased interleukin 18-dependent immune responses are associated with myopericarditis after COVID-19 mRNA vaccination. *Frontiers in Immunology* 13:851620. https://doi.org/10.3389/fimmu.2022.851620.

Woo, E. J., J. Gee, P. Marquez, J. Baggs, W. E. Abara, M. M. McNeil, R. B. Dimova, and J. R. Su. 2023. Post-authorization safety surveillance of Ad.26.COV2.S vaccine: Reports to the Vaccine Adverse Event Reporting System and V-Safe, February 2021–February 2022. *Vaccine* 41(30):4422–4430. https://doi.org/10.1016/j.vaccine.2023.06.023.

Wu, L. Y., S. C. Shao, and S. C. Liao. 2023. Positive predictive value of ICD-10-CM codes for myocarditis in claims data: A multi-institutional study in Taiwan. *Clinical Epidemiology* 15:459–468. https://doi.org/10.2147/clep.S405660.

Yonker, L. M., Z. Swank, Y. C. Bartsch, M. D. Burns, A. Kane, B. P. Boribong, J. P. Davis, M. Loiselle, T. Novak, Y. Senussi, C. A. Cheng, E. Burgess, A. G. Edlow, J. Chou, A. Dionne, D. Balaguru, M. Lahoud-Rahme, M. Arditi, B. Julg, A. G. Randolph, G. Alter, A. Fasano, and D. R. Walt. 2023. Circulating spike protein detected in post-COVID-19 mRNA vaccine myocarditis. *Circulation* 147(11):867–876. https://doi.org/10.1161/CIRCULATIONAHA.122.061025.

# 8

# Sudden Death and COVID-19 Vaccines

This chapter describes the potential relationship between COVID-19 vaccines and sudden death (see Box 8-1 for conclusions).

---

**BOX 8-1**
**Conclusions for Sudden Death**

**Conclusion 8-1: The evidence is inadequate to accept or reject a causal relationship between the BNT162b2 vaccine and sudden death.**

**Conclusion 8-2: The evidence is inadequate to accept or reject a causal relationship between the mRNA-1273 vaccine and sudden death.**

**Conclusion 8-3: The evidence is inadequate to accept or reject a causal relationship between the Ad26.COV2.S vaccine and sudden death.**

**Conclusion 8-4: The evidence is inadequate to accept or reject a causal relationship between the NVX-CoV2373 vaccine and sudden death.**

---

## BACKGROUND

The conceptualization, definition, and clinical assignment of a "sudden death" or a "sudden unexpected death" (SUD) is complex and challenging despite useful attempts to define "sudden death" in the general case, and several public health applications have been advanced. This whole area will not be reviewed in detail, but some relevant dimensions will be addressed.

Sudden death is subject to considerable definitional variation; most epidemiological studies have been limited to individual countries or subregions. One example of SUD is offered by the World Health Organization (WHO): "sudden, unexpected, natural deaths either witnessed, and within one hour of symptom onset or, if unwitnessed, within 24 hours of having been last seen alive and symptom-free" (Sefton et al., 2023). This definition highlights

*159*

some of the definitional challenges. Whether a death is "witnessed" depends in part on social, geographic, and residential characteristics (Taylor et al., 2023). It also depends on the underlying medical conditions of the decedent and access to health care. In forensic and pathological studies and series, underlying causes of death can often be identified, but these studies (autopsies of certain types) are only variably performed, in part due to their substantial costs and whether certain legal, regulatory, clinical, or public health issues are in play, such as possible homicide, suicide, environmental exposures, vehicular crashes, poisonings, or other "suspicious" circumstances.

The rates of designating SUDs in a given community will likely also depend on its health, social, and economic status, likely to vary among geographic areas. A central determinant of the accuracy of discovering SUD causes is the level of professional forensic skills and resources a community devotes to these services, including access to toxicologic, microbiologic, and other laboratory and technical services. Only about half of the U.S. population lives in a jurisdiction where coroner and medical examiner services are accredited by the National Association of Medical Examiners. Some U.S. communities, and others globally, have geographic sudden death registries. However, differences in definitions may occur when conducting SUD surveillance, such as time since apparent death or special topical areas of emphasis, including sudden cardiac death, acute drug poisonings, or a focus on adolescents and young adults. These registries may have other public health value, such as in assessing the efficacy of community-based cardiopulmonary resuscitation programs.

However, estimates of community SUD incidence rates have been made. For example, in 2019, an estimate was published of 49 and 21.7 per 100,000 men and women aged 20–64, respectively (Mirzaei et al., 2019). In this same study, the years of life lost in this age group was estimated to be higher than all but combined cancer, heart disease, and unintentional injury deaths. This estimate may also reflect the lesser interest or greater complexity of assessing SUDs among older persons.

In the past several years, there has been more emphasis on "sudden cardiac death," due perhaps to increased attention to SUDs among younger people and to technical and scientific advances in understanding the mechanisms and treatments of SUDs. However, with the advent of COVID-19 vaccines, their distribution in public health programs often favored targeting older people, because of their greater mortality risks, and underlying causes of SUDs are at least somewhat different in this age group.

With regard to COVID-19 distribution and overall population mortality trends, there was no difference in non-COVID-19 mortality between those who were or were not vaccinated as the pandemic worsened in 2020 and 2021 in the United States. For example, a report from the U.S. Vaccine Safety Datalink (Xu et al., 2021) found that vaccine recipients have lower mortality than those unvaccinated. Similarly, a report using data from the Vaccine Adverse Event Reporting System found that in those receiving vaccines, death events within 7 and 42 days following vaccination occurred at lower rates than all-cause expected rates (Day et al., 2023). Despite limitations, this finding suggested lower mortality event rates among vaccinees.

## MECHANISMS AND CAUSES OF SUDS

The WHO definition does not imply a particular cause or mechanism of death per se, and in many instances, evidence must often be gathered in multiple ways, including investigation of the death scene and the general environment, autopsies and related laboratory investigations, interviews with witnesses and other informants, and medical histories from informants and medical records. It has been estimated that about two-thirds of persons with SUDs have medical records from a visit to a health care provider in the 2 years prior to their unexpected death (Husain et al., 2021). However, identifying useful informants and accessing relevant medical records can be challenging, and cultural and legal impediments and other logistical or technical challenges may occur. For example, underreporting in patients with epilepsy has been suggested. Acute myocardial infarction, pulmonary embolism, stroke, and myocarditis can all cause SUD, as discussed in Chapters 6 and 7.

The role of various COVID-19 vaccines in causing SUD is complex as well. The extent to which vaccines may cause particular medical conditions that may lead to an SUD is discussed in other chapters in this report. For example, it would seem that acute allergic vaccine reactions, such as anaphylaxis, would be immediate and likely detected at the time of vaccination, although some delays are possible. Such delays could conceivably relate to unattended deaths.

SUDs may also occur in the context of COVID-19 vaccines in other ways. First and probably most important is that vaccinees may have various underlying conditions that could coincidentally lead to an SUD. Under most circumstances, it would seem possible to identify such situations using informants, autopsy, and other forensic procedures and medical records; most persons with SUDs are likely to have a notable medical history.

Another circumstance that is likely to lead to SUDs is infection with various strains of severe acute respiratory syndrome coronavirus-2 (SARS-CoV-2) itself. This virus, and possibly other viruses circulating in the community, may cause cardiomyopathies of various types, which are known to cause SUDs (Kyuno et al., 2023). The possibility of SUDs in association with post-COVID-19 syndrome has also been raised (Spartalis et al., 2024). In this situation, many cases may be suspected or identified using conventional virus detection techniques, and incumbent pathological findings may be seen at autopsy. However, if viral testing was not performed in the community, and the infected cases had asymptomatic or presymptomatic infections, the infection may never have been identified.

## Epidemiological Evidence

Clinical trial results submitted to the Food and Drug Administration for Emergency Use Authorization and/or full approval do not indicate a signal regarding sudden death and any of the vaccines under study (FDA, 2021, 2023a,b,c). Table 8-1 presents one study that contributed to the causality assessment.

The committee explored Paratz et al. (2023), who used an Australian population study of one type of SUD, out-of-hospital cardiac arrest (OHCA), obtained from a registry of about 4.49 million persons, 4.2 million of whom were 5–50 years old and eligible for vaccination. The authors report unexplained deaths by month, April 2019–March 2022. Deaths when vaccines (BNT162b2, mRNA-1273, and ChAdOx1-S[1]) were available were compared to immediate earlier time periods. The vaccines available and used during the period of analysis varied, and the data do not identify which vaccines were given to any specific individual.

During the study period, 2,242 people experienced OHCA; the authors noted no variation in median monthly rates during the three time periods. Within 30 days of their COVID-19 vaccination (type not documented), 38 people died and were referred for forensic assessment: "No differences were seen in underlying causes of death compared with previously published age-matched data" (Paratz et al., 2023).

The authors only assessed sudden cardiac arrest, unascertained sudden cardiac arrest, and myocarditis, and it was not clear how many deaths resulted from each type of OHCA. They used a clear definition of OHCA, and in one analysis, they linked the history of COVID-19 vaccination within 30 days. The number of deaths was modest, and it was not clear which vaccines were associated with those deaths. The report showed no evidence of an association between the SUD syndrome and vaccination. Paratz et al. (2023) also included an analysis of sudden death within 30 days of vaccination in "young people" without specifying the age. They reported that causes of death in that population "were consistent with pre-pandemic causative profiles," but specific data were not included in the paper.

---

[1] The COVID-19 vaccine manufactured by Oxford-AstraZeneca.

**TABLE 8-1** Epidemiological Study in the Sudden Death Evidence Review

| Author | Study Design and Comparison Group | Location | Data Source | Vaccine(s) | Age Range | N | Number of Events | Results |
|---|---|---|---|---|---|---|---|---|
| Paratz et al. (2023) | Ecological, previously published age-matched data | Australia | Out-of-hospital cardiac arrest registry | BNT162b2, mRNA-1273 | 5–50 | 4.2 million eligible for vaccination  8.8 million doses | 38 | "No difference was seen in underlying causes of sudden death compared with previously published age-matched data ($p = 0.235$)" |

SOURCE: Paratz et al., 2023.

## FROM EVIDENCE TO CONCLUSIONS

The informative literature that critically assessed the association of SUD with COVID-19 immunizations was sparse, with many methodological limitations. Only one paper, which included BNT162b2 and mRNA-1273, was relevant. The authors found a modest number of SUDs and noted no difference from the comparators. No studies assessed the relationship between Ad26.COV2.S and NVX-CoV2373 and sudden death.

> **Conclusion 8-1: The evidence is inadequate to accept or reject a causal relationship between the BNT162b2 vaccine and sudden death.**

> **Conclusion 8-2: The evidence is inadequate to accept or reject a causal relationship between the mRNA-1273 vaccine and sudden death.**

> **Conclusion 8-3: The evidence is inadequate to accept or reject a causal relationship between the Ad26.COV2.S vaccine and sudden death.**

> **Conclusion 8-4: The evidence is inadequate to accept or reject a causal relationship between the NVX-CoV2373 vaccine and sudden death.**

## REFERENCES

Day, B., D. Menschik, D. Thompson, C. Jankosky, J. Su, P. Moro, C. Zinderman, K. Welsh, R. B. Dimova, and N. Nair. 2023. Reporting rates for VAERS death reports following COVID-19 vaccination, December 14, 2020–November 17, 2021. *Pharmacoepidemiology and Drug Safety* 32(7):763–772.

FDA (Food and Drug Administration). 2021. *Emergency use authorization (EUA) amendment for an unapproved product review memorandum.* Food and Drug Administration. https://www.fda.gov/media/153439/download (accessed May 3, 2023).

FDA. 2023a. *BLA clinical review memorandum—COMIRNATY.* Food and Drug Administration. https://www.fda.gov/media/172333/download?attachment (accessed December 5, 2023).

FDA. 2023b. *BLA clinical review memorandum—SPIKEVAX.* Food and Drug Administration. https://www.fda.gov/media/172357/download?attachment (accessed December 5, 2023).

FDA. 2023c. *Emergency use authorization (EUA) for an unapproved product review memorandum.* Food and Drug Administration. https://www.fda.gov/media/168233/download?attachment (accessed December 5, 2023).

Husain, A., E. A. Masoudi, M. Mirzaei, G. Joodi, M. I. Sadaf, F.-C. Lin, and R. J. Simpson, Jr. 2021. Missed opportunities for prevention of sudden death. *North Carolina Medical Journal* 82(2):95–99. https://doi.org/10.18043/ncm.82.2.95.

Kyuno, D., M. Tateno, Y. Ono, K. Magara, K. Takasawa, A. Takasawa, and M. Osanai. 2023. Common pathological findings in the heart in COVID-19-related sudden death cases: An autopsy case series. *Heliyon* 9(10):e20564. https://doi.org/10.1016/j.heliyon.2023.e20564.

Mirzaei, M., G. Joodi, B. Bogle, S. Chen, and R. J. Simpson, Jr. 2019. Years of life and productivity loss due to adult sudden unexpected death in the United States. *Medical Care* 57(7):498–502. https://doi.org/10.1097/mlr.0000000000001129.

Paratz, E. D., Z. Nehme, D. Stub, and A. La Gerche. 2023. No association between out-of-hospital cardiac arrest and COVID-19 vaccination. *Circulation* 147(17):1309–1311. https://doi.org/10.1161/circulationaha.122.063753.

Sefton, C., S. Keen, C. Tybout, F. C. Lin, H. Jiang, G. Joodi, J. G. Williams, and R. J. Simpson, Jr. 2023. Characteristics of sudden death by clinical criteria. *Medicine (Baltimore)* 102(16):e33029. https://doi.org/10.1097/md.0000000000033029.

Spartalis, M., D. Zweiker, E. Spartalis, D. C. Iliopoulos, and G. Siasos. 2024. Long COVID-19 syndrome and sudden cardiac death: The phantom menace. *Current Medicinal Chemistry* 31(1):2–6. https://doi.org/10.2174/0929867330666230515145041.

Taylor, C. T., L. Campbell-Sills, R. C. Kessler, X. Sun, M. K. Nock, R. J. Ursano, S. Jain, and M. B. Stein. 2023. Social network size and personality traits independently and prospectively predict distress disorders and suicidal behavior in U.S. Army soldiers. *Psychological Medicine* 53(11):5081–5090. https://doi.org/10.1017/s0033291722002082.

Xu, S., R. Huang, L. S. Sy, S. C. Glenn, D. S. Ryan, K. Morrissette, D. K. Shay, G. Vazquez-Benitez, J. M. Glanz, N. P. Klein, D. McClure, E. G. Liles, E. S. Weintraub, H. F. Tseng, and L. Qian. 2021. COVID-19 vaccination and non-COVID-19 mortality risk—seven integrated health care organizations, United States, December 14, 2020–July 31, 2021. *Morbidity and Mortality Weekly Report* 70(43):1520–1524. https://doi.org/10.15585/mmwr.mm7043e2.

# 9

# Female Infertility and COVID-19 Vaccines

This chapter describes the potential relationship between COVID-19 vaccines and female infertility (see Box 9-1 for conclusions).

---

**BOX 9-1**
**Conclusions for Female Infertility**

**Conclusion 9-1: The evidence favors rejection of a causal relationship between the BNT162b2 vaccine and female infertility.**

**Conclusion 9-2: The evidence favors rejection of a causal relationship between the mRNA-1273 vaccine and female infertility.**

**Conclusion 9-3: The evidence is inadequate to accept or reject a causal relationship between the Ad26.COV2.S vaccine and female infertility.**

**Conclusion 9-4: The evidence is inadequate to accept or reject a causal relationship between the NVX-CoV2373 vaccine and female infertility.**

---

## BACKGROUND

Infertility is defined as not being able to conceive after 1 year of unprotected sex in couples with opposite-sex gametes or donor insemination in those under the age of 35 years or within 6 months in those over 35 years (ACOG, 2019). In the United States, among married females aged 15 to 49 years with no prior births, about 1 in 5 (19 percent) are unable to get pregnant after 1 year of trying (CDC, 2023).

Unassisted conception is complex. At minimum, it requires ovulation, sperm that is capable of fertilizing an oocyte, functional female pelvic anatomy including patent fallopian tubes, and uterine endometrium that can support embryo implantation.

Fertility may be impacted by a number of different biologic factors, in either the male or female reproductive systems. For females, there is an age-related decline in ovarian reserve (decrease in oocyte number) (Sharma et al., 2013). There is also an age-related decline in oocyte quality with an associated increase in aneuploidy. This decline can be exacerbated by exposure to things like cytotoxic chemotherapy, or alcohol or tobacco use. Metabolic (e.g., obesity) or lifestyle (e.g., alcohol or tobacco use) factors can also contribute to infertility (Sharma et al., 2013). In addition to issues related to the oocyte and ovulation, the fallopian tubes, uterus, and endometrium also need to be considered.

The study of biologic factors impacting natural reproduction is challenging given the complexity of the process. Investigating the cause of infertility is challenging given the latency to diagnose and its heterogeneous nature. Therefore, this review incorporates studies with measurable outcomes for specific elements of the reproductive process including ovarian reserve (expected female response to exogenous gonadotropins as measured by anti-Müllerian hormone [AMH] levels, and/or antral follicle count [AFC], fertilization, and embryo implantation).

## MECHANISMS

Syncytin-1, a crucial membrane glycoprotein, facilitates the fusion of trophoblasts into syncytiotrophoblasts, which are essential for the early development of the placenta during pregnancy (Gallagher, 2020; Lavillette et al., 2002). Initial theories posited that COVID-19 vaccines might trigger autoantibodies against Syncytin-1, potentially leading to female infertility due to its structural resemblance to the severe acute respiratory syndrome coronavirus-2 (SARS-CoV-2) spike protein (Prasad et al., 2021). However, these concerns were primarily rooted in the interaction of the virus with the angiotensin-converting enzyme 2 (ACE2) receptor, which is expressed in reproductive tissues such as the testes, ovaries, and placenta.

The paper by Segars et al. (2020) underscores the biological plausibility of SARS-CoV-2 affecting reproductive health, given its mode of cell entry through the S1 domain of the spike protein to receptors present in reproductive tissues, including ACE2, CD26, Ezrin, and cyclophilins. This connection is particularly concerning, as previous instances of coronaviruses, like SARS-CoV-1, have been associated with severe orchitis and the loss of germ cells in males, potentially affecting sperm quality for up to 90 days post-infection. Although ACE2 expression in human ovaries is dependent on gonadotropins, the exact impact of SARS-CoV-2 on female gametogenesis remains to be clarified.

Contradicting the initial speculations about Syncytin-1 autoantibodies, subsequent investigations into the potential cross-reactivity between antibodies generated against the SARS-CoV-2 spike protein and Syncytin-1 revealed no detection of such autoantibodies in human plasma (Prasad et al., 2021). Moreover, studies by Lu-Culligan et al. (2022) in both animal models and humans confirmed that vaccination does not induce anti-Syncytin-1 antibodies, dispelling concerns over vaccine-related female infertility through this mechanism.

Another hypothesized mechanism of female infertility is the effect of messenger ribonucleic acid (mRNA) vaccines on AMH, a critical biomarker for assessing ovarian reserve, providing measurable insight into remaining egg count and, by extension, fertility potential. This hormone plays a vital role in evaluating ovarian health and predicting responses to fertility treatments like assisted reproductive technologies. The potential impact of mRNA vaccines on reproductive health, specifically whether the immune response they provoke could inadvertently affect ovarian tissues or hormonal balance, thus influencing AMH levels and fertility, was a concern.

In a longitudinal cohort study, AMH in participants pre- and post-administration of mRNA-based COVID-19 vaccines was quantified to assess its impact on ovarian reserve and fertility potential. The study accounted for established confounding variables that are known to affect AMH concentrations, including age, body mass index, and the phase of the menstrual cycle. There were no significant alterations in AMH levels post-vaccination, thus providing evidence against the hypothesis that mRNA COVID-19 vaccines compromise ovarian reserve (Chen et al., 2021).

## CLINICAL AND EPIDEMIOLOGICAL EVIDENCE

In evaluating the literature on whether COVID-19 vaccines impact female fertility, the committee considered three types of studies that included important biologic measures known to be associated with reproduction:

- Epidemiologic studies of populations that may or may have not included females with infertility,
- Studies among oocyte donors, and
- Studies among females going through in vitro fertilization.

The last type of study does not provide direct evidence but is used to support clinical and epidemiological evidence. These studies evaluate treatment outcomes, not the development of female infertility. Female infertility was not an outcome studied in the clinical trials submitted for authorization or approval (FDA, 2021, 2023a,b,c). Table 9-1 presents eight studies that contributed to the causality assessment.

Although all oocyte donors do not have proven fertility, they are screened for a number of infertility factors. Because oocyte donors are young, they do not have age-related infertility. Donor oocyte studies provide the strongest available evidence about the absence of a relationship between COVID-19 vaccines and female infertility. Oocyte donors are healthy females, usually 18–33 years old, who have undergone intensive medical, psychological, and genetic testing. Potential oocyte donors are screened for expected ovarian response to stimulation to exogeneous gonadotropin via AMH and/or AFC. They undergo ovarian stimulation therapy, to develop multiple oocytes, followed by oocyte retrieval. The oocytes are fertilized by sperm in the laboratory, and, after several days, the best resulting embryo(s) is (are) placed in the uterus of the recipient, whose uterine lining has been appropriately prepared. Studies of in vitro fertilization provide an opportunity to study measurable outcomes in specific steps of the reproductive process including markers of ovarian reserve (AMH, AFC, oocyte count), fertilization, embryo development, and embryo implantation.

Bosch et al. (2023) conducted a self-controlled study on a number of factors related to fertility pre- and post-vaccination with an mRNA vaccine (BNT162b2,[1] mRNA-1273[2]), among 115 oocyte donors serving as their own controls. More oocytes were retrieved post-vaccination (16.62 ± 7.1, 95% confidence interval [CI]: 15–18) versus prevaccination (15.38 ± 7.0, 95% CI: 14–17), with no difference in the mean fertilization rate comparing pre- to post-vaccination (82.69 percent vs. 78.84 percent, respectively), or high-quality embryos (2.29 vs. 2.32, respectively) (Bosch et al., 2023). Although the sample was small, the findings support the absence of a causal relationship between mRNA vaccines and female infertility.

In a study of women undergoing elective oocyte cryopreservation, Karavani et al. (2022) compared 224 women aged 30–39 or older from before (January 2019 to February 2020) or during (December 2020 to January 2022) the pandemic who were unvaccinated with those vaccinated with BNT162b2. They found that the vaccinated group had comparable mean numbers of retrieved and mature oocytes compared with the two unvaccinated groups (12.6 ± 8.0 versus 13.0 ± 8.2 and 12.5 ± 7.4 retrieved, and 10.1 ± 6.9 versus 9.5 ± 6.4 and 10.1 ± 6.3 mature oocytes, respectively; not significant for both) (Karavani et al., 2022). They included women who had been screened to identify and exclude pre-existing infertility factors.

To assess whether COVID-19 vaccine had an effect on the levels of AMH, Mohr-Sasson et al. (2022) conducted a self-controlled study among 129 reproductive-age women (18–42) who were evaluated for infertility before vaccination with BNT162b2. They found no difference between mean AMH levels (µg/L) pre- and post-vaccination (5.3 ± 4.2 versus 5.2 ± 4.5, respectively).

Yildiz et al. (2023) conducted a prospective case-control study of 104 women (74 vaccinated with an mRNA vaccine, and 30 unvaccinated) without known infertility who presented for routine follow-up. Their mean AMH levels (µg/L) were assessed as an indirect measure of ovarian reserve before two doses of mRNA vaccines, with no difference pre- and post-vaccination (vaccinated group baseline versus 6 months post-vaccination: 3.37 ± 2.23 versus 3.40 ± 2.26; unvaccinated group baseline versus 6 months post vaccination: 3.17 ± 2.17 versus 3.32 ± 2.13).

---

[1] Refers to the COVID-19 vaccine manufactured by Pfizer-BioNTech under the name Comirnaty®.
[2] The COVID-19 vaccine manufactured by Moderna under the name Spikevax®.

**TABLE 9-1** Clinical and Epidemiological Studies in the Female Infertility Evidence Review

| Author | N | Vaccine Type | Study Type | Comparison Group/ Control | Outcome Variable(s) | Results |
|---|---|---|---|---|---|---|
| Bosch et al. (2023) | 115 oocyte donors | mRNA (BNT162b2, mRNA-1273) | Cohort with pre- and postexposure | Self-controlled | Mean number of oocytes retrieved | Prevaccination: 15.38 ± 7.0 (95% CI: 14–17) Post-vaccination: 16.62 ± 7.1 (95% CI: 15–18) Mean difference: −1.24 ± 6.0 (95% CI 2.34–0.14) |
| | | | | | Mean fertilization rate | Prevaccination: 82.69% (95% CI: 79.23–86.15) Post-vaccination: 78.84% (95% CI: 75.21–82.47) |
| | | | | | Mean number of high-quality embryos (Grade A) | Prevaccination: 2.29 (95% CI: 1.85–2.73) Post-vaccination: 2.32 (95% CI: 1.96–2.68) |
| Karavani et al. (2022) | 224 women Pre-pandemic: 103 Intra-pandemic unvaccinated: 52 Vaccinated: 69 | BNT162b2 | Retrospective cohort | Unvaccinated (pre- and intrapandemic) | Mean number of oocytes retrieved | Pre-pandemic: 13.0 ± 8.2 Intra-pandemic unvaccinated: 12.5 ± 7.4 Vaccinated: 12.6 ± 8.0 $p = 0.892$ |
| | | | | | Number of mature oocytes | Pre-pandemic: 9.5 ± 6.4 Intra-pandemic unvaccinated: 10.1 ± 6.3 Vaccinated: 10.1 ± 6.9 $p = 0.744$ |
| Kolatorova et al. (2022) | 25 healthy fertile women before and after third vaccination | BNT162b2, mRNA-1273 | Cohort | Self-controlled | LH, FSH, SHBG, AMH, AFC | LH: Before dose 3: 6.36 IU/L After dose 3: 6.11 IU/L $p = 0.424$ FSH: Before dose 3: 6.2 IU/L After dose 3: 6.49 IU/L $p = 0.424$ SHBG: Before dose 3: 67.4 nmol/L After dose 3: 70.17 nmol/L $p = 0.75$ AMH: Before dose 3: 3.25 ng/mL After dose 3: 3.03 ng/mL $p = 0.689$ AFC: Before dose 3: 23 After dose 3: 24 $p = 0.19$ |
| Mohr-Sasson et al. (2022) | 129 without known infertility | BNT162b2 | Self-controlled | Self-controlled | Mean AMH levels | Prevaccination: 5.3 ± 4.2 µg/L Post-vaccination: 5.2 ± 4.5 µg/L $p = 0.11$ |

**TABLE 9-1** Continued

| Author | N | Vaccine Type | Study Type | Comparison Group/ Control | Outcome Variable(s) | Results |
|---|---|---|---|---|---|---|
| Soysal and Yilmaz (2022) | 30 vaccinated and 30 unvaccinated with no history of infertility | BNT162b2 | Prospective cross sectional | Unvaccinated women and pre- and post-vaccination among the same vaccinated people (self-controlled) | AMH | Control group: 4.14 ± 2.79 Pre-vaccine group: 4.17 ± 1.87 Post-vaccine study group: 4.13 ± 1.94 $p > 0.05$, between control group and post-vaccine group, and pre- and post-vaccine group |
| Wesselink et al. (2022) | 2,126 women aged 21–45 vaccinated: 1,229 unvaccinated: 897 | BNT162b2, mRNA-1273, Ad26.COV2.S | Cohort | Unvaccinated | Per cycle fecundity rate | First dose for any vaccine, compared with unvaccinated: FR 1.09 (95% CI: 0.92–1.30)<br><br>BNT162b2: FR 1.06 (95% CI: 0.92–1.22)<br><br>mRNA-1273: FR 1.11 (95% CI: 0.95–1.29)<br><br>Ad26.COV2.S: FR 1.06 (95% CI: 0.78–1.43) |
| Yang et al. (2023) | 836 patients prevaccination, 138 patients post-vaccination | BNT162b2, mRNA-1273, Ad26.COV2.S | Retrospective cohort | Self-controlled pre-vaccination | Mean AMH, median AFC | Mean AMH Prevaccination: 3.83 ± 4.56 ng/mL Post-vaccination: 3.86 ± 4.31 ng/mL (95% CI: 0.491–0.566)<br><br>Median AFC Prevaccination: 18 (IQR, 11–28) Post-vaccination: 20 (IQR, 12–29) |
| Yildiz et al. (2023) | 104 women: 74 vaccinated and 30 unvaccinated | mRNA (BNT162b2, mRNA-1273) | Prospective case control | Unvaccinated | Mean AMH levels | Vaccinated group: Baseline: 3.37 ± 2.23 µg/L After 6 months: 3.40 ± 2.26 µg/L $p = 0.127$<br><br>Unvaccinated group: Baseline: 3.17 ± 2.17 µg/L After 6 months: 3.32 ± 2.13 µg/L $p = 0.166$ |

NOTES: BNT162b2 refers to the COVID-19 vaccine manufactured by Pfizer-BioNTech under the name Comirnaty®. mRNA-1273 refers to the COVID-19 vaccine manufactured by Moderna under the name Spikevax®. Ad26.COV2.S refers to the COVID-19 vaccine manufactured by Janssen. AFC: antral follicle count; AMH: anti-Müllerian hormone; CI: confidence interval; FR: fecundability rate; FSH: follicle-stimulating hormone; IQR: interquartile range; IU/L: international units per liter; LH: luteinizing hormone; mRNA: messenger ribonucleic acid; ng/mL: nanograms per mililiter; nmol/L = nanomoles per liter; SHBG: sex hormone binding globulin; µg/L: microgram per liter.
SOURCES: Bosch et al., 2023; Karavani et al., 2022; Kolatorova et al., 2022; Mohr-Sasson et al., 2022; Soysal and Yılmaz, 2022; Wesselink et al., 2022; Yang et al., 2023; Yildiz et al., 2023.

One retrospective cohort study evaluated the impact of mRNA vaccines (BNT162]b2 and mRNA-1273) and Ad26.COV2.S[3] on ovarian function, measured by mean AMH (ng/mL) and median AFC (Yang et al., 2023). Results were aggregated. Baseline AMH levels were 3.83 ± 4.56 prevaccination compared to 3.86 ± 4.31 post-vaccination (95% CI: 0.491–0.566), and median AFC were 18 (interquartile range [IQR], 11–28) prevaccination compared to 20 (IQR, 12–29) post-vaccination. The investigators found no difference in ovarian function pre- and post-vaccination; however, this study was carried out among women who may have had pre-existing infertility (Yang et al., 2023).

In a self-controlled study of women without known infertility, no difference appeared in ovarian function as measured by luteinizing hormone, follicle-stimulating hormone, sex hormone binding globulin, AMH, and AFC before and after the third mRNA vaccine (Kolatorova et al., 2022).

Soysal and Yılmaz (2022) also evaluated the effect of the BNT162b2 vaccine on ovarian reserve by comparing AMH levels pre- and post-COVID-19 vaccination in 30 young women 60–90 days after vaccination and comparing levels between vaccinated and unvaccinated women. The study excluded women with a history of infertility. The 30 women showed no difference in the mean AMH before and after vaccination (4.17 vs. 4.13; $p = 0.785$). The authors also found no difference in the mean AMH comparing vaccinated with unvaccinated women (4.13 vs. 4.14; $p = 1.0$) (Soysal and Yılmaz, 2022).

A cohort study of 2,126 women found no decreased fecundability in either partner after BNT162b2 (fecundity rate [FR] 1.06, 95% CI: 0.92–1.22), mRNA-1273 (FR 1.11, 95% CI: 0.95–1.29), or Ad26.COV2.S (FR 1.06, 95% CI: 0.78–1.43) (Wesselink et al., 2022); it was one of very few studies to include Ad26.COV2.S. The study was limited by self-report of both exposure and outcomes. The authors also noted that approximately 11 percent of the participants had a prior history of female infertility (Wesselink et al., 2022). None of the studies reported an adverse effect on fertility after vaccination.

Most studies that examined whether COVID-19 vaccines affect the treatment outcomes of female infertility found no association. These studies have been summarized in few systematic reviews. Although they were not the focus of this review, they provided reassurance and context that COVID-19 vaccines do not affect fertility.

All systematic reviews focused on whether COVID-19 vaccines affected female infertility (Chamani et al., 2022; Huang et al., 2023; Zaçe et al., 2022; Zhang et al., 2023). None of these studies reported that COVID-19 vaccines negatively affected in vitro fertilization treatment outcomes.

## FROM EVIDENCE TO CONCLUSIONS

The studies reviewed reported no effect of COVID-19 vaccines on fertility. The donor oocyte studies provide the strongest clinical evidence, although the sample sizes were small (Bosch et al., 2023; Karavani et al., 2022). The lack of an adverse impact on ovarian function further suggests no effect on fertility. This conclusion was further supported by animal and human data that disprove a hypothesized mechanism (Lu-Culligan et al., 2022; Prasad et al., 2021).

**Conclusion 9-1: The evidence favors rejection of a causal relationship between the BNT162b2 vaccine and female infertility.**

**Conclusion 9-2: The evidence favors rejection of a causal relationship between the mRNA-1273 vaccine and female infertility.**

Very few studies examined Ad26.COV2.S and female infertility; the only epidemiological study that did so did not find an association. The study was limited by the inclusion of people with known infertility and because measures of infertility and exposure to vaccines were both self-reported (Wesselink et al., 2022). No studies examined NVX-CoV2373[4] and female infertility.

---

[3] Refers to the COVID-19 vaccine manufactured by Janssen.
[4] The COVID-19 vaccine manufactured by Novavax.

**Conclusion 9-3: The evidence is inadequate to accept or reject a causal relationship between the Ad26.COV2.S vaccine and female infertility.**

**Conclusion 9-4: The evidence is inadequate to accept or reject a causal relationship between the NVX-CoV2373 vaccine and female infertility.**

# REFERENCES

ACOG (American College of Obstetricians and Gynecologists). 2019. Committee opinion: Infertility workup for the women's health specialist. Paper read at Committee on Gynecologic Practice, American Society for Reproductive Medicine, May 23, 2019. https://www.acog.org/clinical/clinical-guidance/committee-opinion/articles/2019/06/infertility-workup-for-the-womens-health-specialist.

Bosch, A., S. Albero, J. C. Castillo, J. Ten, J. Guerrero, J. A. Ortiz, A. Bernabeu, and R. Bernabeu. 2023. Does mRNA COVID-19 vaccination in oocyte donors impact ovarian stimulation parameters or IVF outcomes for recipients? *Reproductive Biomedicine Online* 46(4):697–704. https://doi.org/10.1016/j.rbmo.2023.01.002.

CDC (Centers for Disease Control and Prevention). 2023. *Infertility.* https://www.cdc.gov/reproductivehealth/infertility/index.htm (accessed December 18, 2023).

Chamani, I. J., L. McKenzie, F. Licciardi, and D. H. McCulloh. 2022. COVID-19 vaccination and assisted reproduction outcomes: A literature review and meta-analysis. *Fertility and Sterility* 118(4):e82. https://doi.org/10.1016/j.fertnstert.2022.08.249.

Chen, F., S. Zhu, Z. Dai, L. Hao, C. Luan, Q. Guo, C. Meng, and Y. Zhang. 2021. Effects of COVID-19 and mRNA vaccines on human fertility. *Human Reproduction* 37(1):5–13. https://doi.org/10.1093/humrep/deab238.

FDA (Food and Drug Administration). 2021. *Emergency use authorization (EUA) amendment for an unapproved product review memorandum.* Food and Drug Administration. https://www.fda.gov/media/153439/download (accessed May 3, 2023).

FDA. 2023a. *BLA clinical review memorandum—COMIRNATY.* Food and Drug Administration. https://www.fda.gov/media/172333/download?attachment (accessed December 5, 2023).

FDA. 2023b. *BLA clinical review memorandum—SPIKEVAX.* Food and Drug Administration. https://www.fda.gov/media/172357/download?attachment (accessed December 5, 2023).

FDA. 2023c. *Emergency use authorization (EUA) for an unapproved product review memorandum.* Food and Drug Administration. https://www.fda.gov/media/168233/download?attachment (accessed December 5, 2023).

Gallagher, B. 2020. Response to nCoV-2019 against backdrop of endogenous retroviruses. https://virological.org/t/response-to-ncov2019-against-backdrop-of-endogenous-retroviruses/396 (accessed December 12, 2023).

Huang, J., Z. Fang, Y. Liu, C. Xing, L. Huang, J. Mao, H. Chen, Z. Huang, L. Xia, L. Tang, Z. Zhang, B. Liu, H. Huang, L. Tian, X. Ai, and Q. Wu. 2023. Effect of female coronavirus disease 2019 vaccination on assisted reproductive outcomes: A systematic review and meta-analysis. *Fertility and Sterility* 119(5):772–783. https://doi.org/10.1016/j.fertnstert.2023.01.024.

Karavani, G., H. H. Chill, A. Dick, C. Meirman, E. Gutman-Ido, S. Herzberg, A. Ben-Meir, and T. Imbar. 2022. Pfizer SARS-CoV-2 BNT162b2 mRNA vaccination (BNT162b2) has no adverse effect on elective oocyte cryopreservation outcomes. *Reproductive Biomedicine Online* 45(5):987–994. https://doi.org/10.1016/j.rbmo.2022.06.001.

Kolatorova, L., K. Adamcova, J. Vitku, L. Horackova, M. Simkova, M. Hornova, M. Vosatkova, V. Vaisova, A. Parizek, and M. Duskova. 2022. COVID-19, vaccination, and female fertility in the Czech Republic. *International Journal of Molecular Sciences* 23(18). https://doi.org/10.3390/ijms231810909.

Lavillette, D., M. Marin, A. Ruggieri, F. Mallet, F. L. Cosset, and D. Kabat. 2002. The envelope glycoprotein of human endogenous retrovirus type W uses a divergent family of amino acid transporters/cell surface receptors. *Journal of Virology* 76(13):6442–6452. https://doi.org/10.1128/jvi.76.13.6442-6452.2002.

Lu-Culligan, A., A. Tabachnikova, E. Pérez-Then, M. Tokuyama, H. J. Lee, C. Lucas, V. Silva Monteiro, M. Miric, V. Brache, L. Cochon, M. C. Muenker, S. Mohanty, J. Huang, I. Kang, C. Dela Cruz, S. Farhadian, M. Campbell, I. Yildirim, A. C. Shaw, S. Ma, S. H. Vermund, A. I. Ko, S. B. Omer, and A. Iwasaki. 2022. No evidence of fetal defects or anti-syncytin-1 antibody induction following COVID-19 mRNA vaccination. *PLoS Biology* 20(5):e3001506. https://doi.org/10.1371/journal.pbio.3001506.

Mohr-Sasson, A., J. Haas, S. Abuhasira, M. Sivan, H. Doitch Amdurski, T. Dadon, S. Blumenfeld, E. Derazne, R. Hemi, R. Orvieto, A. Afek, and J. Rabinovici. 2022. The effect of COVID-19 mRNA vaccine on serum anti-Müllerian hormone levels. *Human Reproduction* 37(3):534–541. https://doi.org/10.1093/humrep/deab282.

Prasad, M., J. L. Lin, Y. Gu, R. Gupta, P. Macary, and H. Schwarz. 2021. No crossreactivity of anti-SARS-CoV-2 spike protein antibodies with syncytin-1. *Cellular & Molecular Immunology* 18(11):2566–2568. https://doi.org/10.1038/s41423-021-00773-x.

Segars, J., Q. Katler, D. B. McQueen, A. Kotlyar, T. Glenn, Z. Knight, E. C. Feinberg, H. S. Taylor, J. P. Toner, and J. F. Kawwass. 2020. Prior and novel coronaviruses, coronavirus disease 2019 (COVID-19), and human reproduction: What is known? *Fertility and Sterility* 113(6):1140-1149. https://doi.org/10.1016/j.fertnstert.2020.04.025.

Sharma, R., K. R. Biedenharn, J. M. Fedor, and A. Agarwal. 2013. Lifestyle factors and reproductive health: Taking control of your fertility. *Reproductive Biology and Endocrinology* 11:66. https://doi.org/10.1186/1477-7827-11-66.

Soysal, Ç., and E. Yılmaz. 2022. The effect of COVID-19 vaccine on ovarian reserve. *Saudi Medical Journal* 43(5):486–490. https://doi.org/10.15537/smj.2022.43.5.20220007.

Wesselink, A. K., E. E. Hatch, K. J. Rothman, T. R. Wang, M. D. Willis, J. Yland, H. M. Crowe, R. J. Geller, S. K. Willis, R. B. Perkins, A. K. Regan, J. Levinson, E. M. Mikkelsen, and L. A. Wise. 2022. A prospective cohort study of COVID-19 vaccination, SARS-CoV-2 infection, and fertility. *American Journal of Epidemiology* 191(8):1383–1395. https://doi.org/10.1093/aje/kwac011.

Yang, L., S. Neal, T. Lee, A. Chou, A. K. Schutt, and W. Gibbons. 2023. Comparison of female ovarian reserve before vs. after COVID-19 vaccination. *JAMA Network Open* 6(6):e2318804. https://doi.org/10.1001/jamanetworkopen.2023.18804.

Yildiz, E., B. Timur, G. Guney, and H. Timur. 2023. Does the SARS-CoV-2 mRNA vaccine damage the ovarian reserve? *Medicine* 102(20):e33824. https://doi.org/10.1097/md.0000000000033824.

Zaçe, D., E. La Gatta, L. Petrella, and M. L. Di Pietro. 2022. The impact of COVID-19 vaccines on fertility—a systematic review and meta-analysis. *Vaccine* 40(42):6023–6034. https://doi.org/10.1016/j.vaccine.2022.09.019.

Zang, L., X. Sun, R. Wang, and F. Ma. 2023. Effect of COVID-19 vaccination on the outcome of in vitro fertilization: A systematic review and meta-analysis. *Frontiers in Public Health* 11. https://doi.org/10.3389/fpubh.2023.1151999.

# 10

# Shoulder Injuries and Vaccines

## INTRODUCTION

The deltoid muscle is the preferred location for vaccination because of an apparent lower risk of subcutaneous injection, and the immunogenicity is higher compared to gluteal injections (Shaw et al., 1989). The committee was tasked with reviewing the evidence regarding vaccination and specific injuries to the shoulder (see Chapter 1). Before doing so, for completeness, the committee provides background information on nonspecific shoulder injuries associated with vaccination but does not make conclusions. Unlike the previous chapters in this report, this chapter is not restricted to COVID-19 vaccines. Therefore, the literature search spans from 2011 to 2023, ensuring inclusion of material released subsequent to the last report by the Institute of Medicine (IOM) in 2012 (IOM, 2012).

The first report of a relationship between vaccination and shoulder injury profiled two patients who developed shoulder pain and dysfunction after injection into the deltoid (Bodor and Montalvo, 2007). Atanasoff et al. (2010) offered a case series of 13 patients who developed prolonged shoulder pain after vaccination and offered the term "SIRVA," for "shoulder injury related to vaccine administration," characterized by shoulder pain with limited motion that develops within a few minutes to <24 hours of vaccine administration and lasts more than 6 months, which distinguishes it from the typical transient soreness after vaccination administration (Atanasoff et al., 2010; Cagle, 2021).

SIRVA represents a clinical syndrome, is not a specific diagnosis, and may have a number of causes. There are no specific objective tests to diagnose the condition and no specific International Classification of Diseases (ICD)-10 codes exist for "SIRVA" (Zheng et al., 2022). In fact, "SIRVA represents a constellation of different pain-causing diagnoses" (Atanasoff et al., 2010; Cagle, 2021; MacMahon et al., 2022; Slette et al., 2022; Wood and Ilyas, 2022; Wright et al., 2023). As a result, "SIRVA" is considered confusing (Petrakis et al., 2023), is controversial (MacMahon et al., 2022), leads to conflicting reports in the literature (Leopold, 2022), and may be best described as a medico-legal term instead of a diagnosis (Mackenzie et al., 2022). The American Academy of Orthopaedic Surgeons offered a position statement (AAOS, 2017) that does not use the term "SIRVA" and states, "The members of the American Academy of Orthopaedic Surgeons (AAOS) take the position that vaccination administered to the shoulder cannot cause or contribute to common shoulder pathologies such as rotator cuff tendinopathy, glenohumeral arthritis, and adhesive capsulitis."

In the absence of epidemiological studies, the committee chose to focus on case reports as the primary source of analysis, especially in this chapter. Despite being regarded as the lowest level of evidence, well-defined case reports can provide compelling evidence, which is what the committee aims to present in this context.

The committee has reviewed evidence on the etiology of shoulder injuries following vaccination, considering three possible mechanisms of injury. The first encompasses direct trauma from improper placement within the arm, potentially due to deviations from the optimal injection technique. The second mechanism involves injury following the needle or fluid injection, even when the vaccination is correctly placed, suggesting a reaction independent of the technique. The third potential mechanism is the constituents of the vaccine, such as antigens or adjuvants, which might induce harms without any error in the administration process. The committee will discern the most likely causative factors for shoulder injuries or related structural damage when possible.

The committee avoids "SIRVA" and, in response to the Statement of Task, instead focuses on the specific shoulder-related diagnoses that have been associated with vaccine administration. See Box 10-1 for all conclusions in this chapter.

---

### BOX 10-1
### Conclusions for Shoulder Injuries

**Conclusion 10-1:** The evidence establishes a causal relationship between vaccine administration and subacromial/subdeltoid bursitis caused by direct injection into the bursa.

**Conclusion 10-2:** The evidence establishes a causal relationship between vaccine administration and acute rotator cuff or acute biceps tendinopathy caused by direct injection into or adjacent to the tendon.

**Conclusion 10-3:** The evidence favors rejection of a causal relationship between vaccine administration and chronic rotator cuff disease.

**Conclusion 10-4:** The evidence is inadequate to accept or reject a causal relationship between vaccine administration and adhesive capsulitis.

**Conclusion 10-5:** The evidence is inadequate to accept or reject a causal relationship between vaccine administration and septic arthritis.

**Conclusion 10-6:** The evidence establishes a causal relationship between vaccine administration and bone injury caused by direct injection into or adjacent to the bone.

**Conclusion 10-7:** The evidence establishes a causal relationship between vaccine administration and axillary or radial nerve injury caused by direct injection into or adjacent to the nerve.

**Conclusion 10-8:** The evidence is inadequate to accept or reject a causal relationship between vaccine administration and Parsonage-Turner syndrome.

**Conclusion 10-9:** The evidence is inadequate to accept or reject a causal relationship between vaccine administration and complex regional pain syndrome.

---

### SUBACROMIAL/SUBDELTOID BURSITIS

Subacromial/subdeltoid bursitis is characterized by inflammation of the subacromial and subdeltoid bursae located in the shoulder. Bursae are small, fluid-filled sacs that serve as cushions and lubricating structures between bones (see Figure 10-1), tendons, and muscles to reduce friction and enable smooth movement. Bursitis typically results from factors such as overuse, trauma, or underlying issues, such as rotator cuff injuries, tendonitis, or arthritis.

Common symptoms of subacromial/subdeltoid bursitis include shoulder pain, especially when performing overhead movements or lifting the arm, along with swelling, tenderness, reduced range of motion, radiating pain into the upper arm, and weakness (due to pain or disuse) in the affected shoulder. Diagnosis involves a physical examination by a health care provider and may include imaging studies, such as X-rays, ultrasonography, or magnetic resonance imaging (MRI) scans, to confirm the presence of bursitis and rule out other shoulder conditions.

The prevalence of subacromial/subdeltoid bursitis varies by age group. Although it can affect individuals of all ages, it is more commonly observed in adults, particularly those over the age of 30. This is largely due to age-related changes in the shoulder, such as degeneration of tendons and bursa, which can increase the risk of developing bursitis. The prevalence is not strongly biased toward one gender. Some studies have suggested that it may be slightly more common in men, but the gender difference is not significant.

The underlying causes often involve factors such as repetitive overhead activities, trauma, and pre-existing shoulder problems, including rotator cuff injuries and tendonitis. Individuals engaged in activities that place increased stress on the shoulder, such as athletes or manual laborers, may be at higher risk.

## Evidence from Epidemiological Studies and Case Reports

In recent years, multiple case reports have documented patients developing acute subacromial bursitis shortly after receiving vaccines. Additionally, Hesse et al. (2020) used the Vaccine Safety Datalink to assess the risk of subdeltoid bursitis after influenza vaccination. They found that an attributable risk of 7.78 (95% confidence interval [CI]: 2.19–13.38) additional cases of bursitis occur per 1 million persons vaccinated. Post-vaccine subdeltoid bursitis has been observed in adults spanning an age range of 23–82 years. A common issue identified was the incorrect injection technique, particularly the placement of injections too high on the arm (see Figure 10-1), underscoring the importance of adherence to proper vaccination procedures to minimize risk of harm.

The evidence most significant to the committee consisted of numerous well-documented case reports in adults (see Table 10-1). No cases of imaging-documented bursitis after vaccine administration were found for the pediatric population.

The prognosis is generally positive, with most experiencing a complete resolution of symptoms. However, the recovery time can vary considerably, from as little as 1 week to as long as over 6 months, underscoring the importance of individualized care and management.

Patients with postvaccine subdeltoid bursitis have commonly reported that the vaccine was administered at a higher site than anticipated, as documented in studies by Atanasoff et al. (2010), Bodor and Montalvo (2007), and Hesse et al. (2020). This inadvertent high placement of the vaccine injection may be a contributing factor due to the proximity of the subacromial and subdeltoid bursae to the injection site.

To mitigate the risk of improper vaccine placement and reduce the likelihood of bursitis, numerous techniques and guidelines have been proposed and discussed in the medical literature. Researchers and health care providers have recognized the importance of ensuring correct vaccine administration to minimize the risk of complications. The literature is replete with reports and recommendations, including studies authored by Bancsi et al. (2018), Cook (2011), Cross et al. (2016), Doppen et al. (2023), Kowatari et al. (2023), Mardourian et al. (2023), Marshall et al. (2022), Nakajima et al. (2017), and Pettyjohn et al. (2022).

These reports and studies highlight the significance of proper injection and emphasize the need to avoid vaccine placement in the proximity of the subacromial and subdeltoid bursae.[1] Inadvertently injecting the vaccine into or too close to these structures can lead to irritation, inflammation, and ultimately bursitis, resulting in pain and difficulty in shoulder motion technique (see Figure 10-1).

---

[1] An IOM committee concluded that "the evidence convincingly supports a causal relationship between the injection of a vaccine and deltoid bursitis" (IOM, 2012).

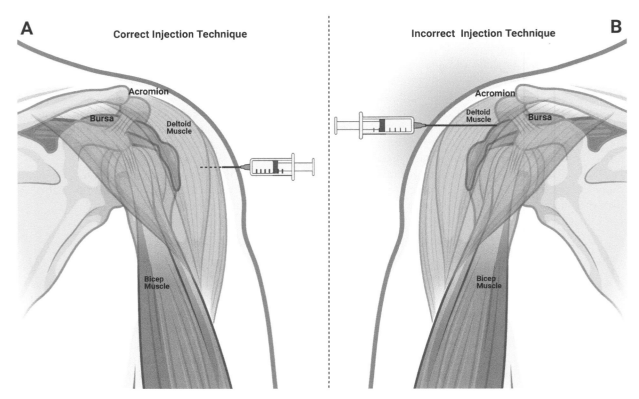

**FIGURE 10-1** Illustration of intramuscular injection techniques.
NOTES: A. Correct injection technique: Demonstrates proper administration of an intramuscular vaccine into the deltoid muscle, utilizing an appropriate anatomical approach for effective delivery. Dotted line indicates needle inside the deltoid muscle. B. Incorrect injection technique: Depicts an erroneous injection leading to inadvertent administration into the subdeltoid bursa, potentially inducing deltoid or subdeltoid bursitis. Solid needle line indicated breach into the bursa. Created with BioRender.com.

### From Evidence to Conclusion

The committee conclusion is derived from a body of evidence, as demonstrated in the 15 case reports described in Table 10-1, that consistently features ultrasound or MRI imaging and symptom onset in the ipsilateral shoulder occurring within a biologically significant time window (typically 0–48 hours after vaccination). Studies that lacked pertinent imaging data or extend beyond this critical time frame present a less compelling connection to vaccination. Many patients report that the injection was "too high" or "too deep," which would put the vaccine material in the subdeltoid bursa. The mechanism behind subacromial/subdeltoid bursitis following vaccine administration is closely tied to the incorrect placement of the needle, particularly when it is higher than expected.

**Conclusion 10-1: The evidence establishes a causal relationship between vaccine administration and subacromial/subdeltoid bursitis caused by direct injection into the bursa.**

**TABLE 10-1** Case Reports Regarding Subacromial/Subdeltoid Bursitis After Vaccination

| Author | Age | Sex | Vaccine(s) | Onset of Symptoms | Symptom Duration Before Evaluation | Imaging |
|---|---|---|---|---|---|---|
| Cantarelli Rodrigues et al. (2021) | 61 | F | ChAdOx1-S | 30 min | 8 weeks | MRI |
| Chow et al. (2022) | 62 | F | ChAdOx1-S | Immediate | 2 weeks | Ultrasound and MRI |
| Chuaychoosakoon et al. (2021) | 52 | M | Sinovac (COVID-19) | 3 days | NR | Ultrasound |
| Chuaychoosakoon and Boonsri (2023) | 52 | F | mRNA COVID-19 | 2 weeks | 17 days | MRI |
| Cook (2014) | 76 | M | Influenza | Immediate | 3 days | Ultrasound |
| Cross et al. (2016) | 82 | F | Pneumococcal (PPSV23) | 2 hours | NR | Ultrasound |
| Cross et al. (2016) | 23 | F | DTaP | 24 hours | 2–3 days | Ultrasound |
| Honarmand et al. (2021) | 42 | M | mRNA-1273 | 2 days | NR | MRI |
| Honarmand et al. (2021) | 38 | M | BNT162b2 | 2 weeks | NR | Ultrasound |
| Jenkins et al. (2020) | 61 | F | Influenza | NR | 3 months | MRI |
| Maliwankul et al. (2022) | 52 | M | Sinovac (COVID-19) | 2 days | 6 days | MRI |
| Maliwankul et al. (2022) | 51 | F | ChAdOx1-S | 3 hours | 4 days | MRI |
| Maliwankul et al. (2022) | 71 | M | ChAdOx1-S | 1 day | 6 weeks | MRI |
| Maliwankul et al. (2022) | 68 | M | ChAdOx1-S | 1 day | 2 weeks | Ultrasound |
| Moya et al. (2022) | 69 | F | Sputnik V (COVID-19) | Immediate | 5 days | MRI |
| Okur et al. (2014) | 66 | F | Influenza | Immediate | NR | MRI |
| Okur et al. (2014) | 39 | M | Influenza | NR | 2 months | MRI |
| Okur et al. (2014) | 36 | M | Influenza | NR | NR | MRI |
| Pearson and Bent (2022) | 74 | M | COVID-19 (unspecified) | 3 days | 3–4 weeks | MRI |
| Salmon et al. (2015) | 26 | F | DTaP | NR | 48 hours | MRI |
| Uchida et al. (2012) | 45 | F | HPV (Cervarix) | 3 hours | 3 days | MRI |
| Wharton et al. (2022) | 31 | M | mRNA-1273 | 1 day | 2.5 weeks | MRI |
| Wong et al. (2021) | 51 | F | Influenza | 48 hours | 3 months | MRI |
| Wright et al. (2019) | 72 | F | Influenza | NR | 2 weeks | MRI |
| Yuen et al. (2022) | 84 | F | mRNA COVID-19 | 3 days | 1 week | MRI |

NOTES: BNT162b2 refers to the COVID-19 vaccine manufactured by Pfizer-BioNTech under the name Comirnaty®. mRNA-1273 refers to the COVID-19 vaccine manufactured by Moderna under the name Spikevax®. ChAdOx1-S refers to the COVID-19 vaccine manufactured by Oxford-AstraZeneca. DTaP: diphtheria, tetanus, and acellular pertussis; F: female; HPV: human papillomavirus; M: male; MRI: magnetic resonance imaging; NR: not reported.
SOURCES: Cantarelli Rodrigues et al., 2021; Chow et al., 2022; Chuaychoosakoon and Boonsri, 2023; Chuaychoosakoon et al., 2021; Cook, 2014; Cross et al., 2016; Honarmand et al., 2021; Jenkins et al., 2020; Maliwankul et al., 2022; Moya et al., 2022; Okur et al., 2014; Pearson and Bent, 2022; Salmon et al., 2015; Uchida et al., 2012; Wharton et al., 2022; Wong et al., 2021; Wright et al., 2019; Yuen et al., 2022.

### ACUTE ROTATOR CUFF OR ACUTE BICEPS TENDINOPATHY

Acute rotator cuff or biceps tendinopathy caused by direct injection into the tendon or tendon sheath is characterized by onset of pain within 24 hours and evidence of acute pathology (such as marked edema in the tendon) on imaging. Imaging of a partial- or full-thickness rotator cuff tear or chronic tendinosis alone is insufficient to demonstrate a direct injury to the tendon.

Acute rotator cuff tendinopathy refers to acute inflammation or irritation of the tendons comprising the rotator cuff, a group of four tendons that surround the shoulder joint: the supraspinatus (SSP), infraspinatus, teres minor, and subscapularis tendons. Acute tendinopathy typically arises from trauma, overuse, or sudden strain on these tendons. Common clinical presentations include shoulder pain, limited range of motion, and localized tenderness. Imaging modalities, such as ultrasound or MRI, are often employed to aid in diagnosis, revealing signs of inflammation and tendon damage. Treatment strategies are rest, anti-inflammatory medication, physical therapy, and sometimes corticosteroid injections to alleviate pain and promote healing.

Acute biceps tendinopathy involves inflammation or injury to the long head of the biceps tendon, which runs through the bicipital groove in the upper arm and attaches to the superior labrum of the glenoid in the shoulder joint. This condition can arise from sudden overexertion, repetitive strain, or direct trauma to the biceps tendon. Clinical manifestations include localized anterior shoulder pain, which may be aggravated by certain movements, such as overhead lifting or reaching. Patients may experience weakness and discomfort during activities that involve the affected tendon. Diagnosis often relies on clinical evaluation, imaging studies (such as ultrasound or MRI), and occasionally, arthroscopy to assess the extent of damage. A consistent hallmark is the conspicuous enlargement of the affected tendon or muscle in diagnostic imaging with a significant increase in signal intensity, indicating pronounced edema. These findings are instrumental in identifying and characterizing the condition.

The clinical outcomes of individuals afflicted with this tendinopathy can be quite diverse. Although some improve in a week or two, others may endure discomfort and functional limitations for an extended period, sometimes beyond 6 months.

### Mechanisms of Injury

In assessing the strength of mechanistic evidence related to this condition, it is important to consider the combination of clinical factors, including the specific demographic characteristics, imaging findings, and observed outcomes. These elements collectively contribute to the overall understanding of the cause of rotator cuff or biceps acute tendinopathy caused by vaccine injection, aiding in evaluation and management.

### Evidence from Case Reports

Rotator cuff or acute biceps tendinopathy induced by inadvertent injection into the rotator cuff tendon or muscle has been notably reported in adults spanning a relatively wide age range, 26–83 years (see Table 10-2). Among these 14 cases, the onset of pain is a particularly salient feature, with the majority of individuals experiencing immediate discomfort. No cases of imaging-documented acute rotator cuff injury have been reported in the pediatric population.

**TABLE 10-2** Case Reports of Acute Rotator Cuff or Acute Biceps Tendinopathy After Vaccination

| Author | Age | Sex | Vaccine | Onset of Symptoms | Symptom Duration Before Evaluation | Imaging | Findings |
|---|---|---|---|---|---|---|---|
| Bansal and DiLorenzo (2020) | 59 | F | DTaP | <24 hours | 6 weeks | MRI | High-grade partial teres minor tear |
| Barnes et al. (2017) | 22 | F | Influenza | 2 hours | 2 months | MRI and ultrasound | Partial supraspinatus tear |
| Bathia and Stitik (2009) | 34 | F | Influenza | Immediate | 3 weeks | MRI | Tendinosis of infraspinatus |
| Chuaychoosakoon and Boonsri (2023) | 52 | F | mRNA COVID-19 | NR | 3 days | MRI | Fluid supraspinatus tendinosis |
| Klabklay et al. (2022) | 50 | M | ChAdOx1-S | 3 hours | 3 days | Ultrasound | Swelling of supraspinatus, calcific tendonitis in subscapularis |
| Maliwankul et al. (2022) | 64 | M | ChAdOx1-S | 2 days | 1 month | Ultrasound | Biceps tenosynovitis |
| Nakajima et al. (2023) | 83 | F | BNT162b2 | Immediate | 8 days | X-ray and MRI | Calcium in supraspinatus inflammatory subdeltoid bursitis |
| Natanzi et al. (2020) | 42 | F | Influenza | Immediate | 7 weeks | MRI | Edema at teres minor insertion |
| Natanzi et al. (2020) | 38 | F | Influenza | Immediate | 2 months | MRI | Edema in humerus and teres minor insertion |
| Sahu and Shetty (2022) | 33 | M | Covaxin (COVID-19) | Immediate | 2 days | X-ray | Calcific tendonitis supraspinatus |
| Shabhaz et al. (2019) | 35 | F | Influenza | Immediate | 1 hour | MRI | Biceps tenosynovitis |
| Sukhija et al. (2022) | 26 | F | Covaxin (COVID-19) | 15 days | 15 days | MRI and ultrasound | Edema in myotendinous junction of teres minor* |
| Szari et al. (2019) | 31 | M | Influenza | Immediate | 4 months | MRI | Partial cuff tear diffuse cuff tendinosis |
| Zeldin et al. (2023) | 53 | F | Influenza | Immediate | 2 months | MRI | Fluid collection lateral to biceps groove with hyperechoic focus, possibly a needle tip |

NOTES: *The committee identified edema in the myotendinous junction of Teres Minor on the MRI images, which was not specifically indicated in the case study. BNT162b2 refers to the COVID-19 vaccine manufactured by Pfizer-BioNTech under the name Comirnaty®. ChAdOx1-S refers to the COVID-19 vaccine manufactured by Oxford-AstraZeneca. DTaP: diphtheria, tetanus, and acellular pertussis; F: female; M: male; MRI: magnetic resonance imaging; NR: not reported.

SOURCES: Bansal and DiLorenzo, 2020; Barnes et al., 2017; Bathia and Stitik, 2009; Chuaychoosakoon and Boonsri, 2023; Klabklay et al., 2022; Maliwankul et al., 2022; Nakajima et al., 2023; Natanzi et al., 2020; Sahu and Shetty, 2022; Shahbaz et al., 2019; Sukhija et al., 2022; Szari et al., 2019; Zeldin et al., 2023.

**From Evidence to Conclusion**

The committee's decision is derived from a body of evidence, as demonstrated in the case reports provided (see Table 10-2). Injection of a vaccine into the biceps or rotator cuff tendon can produce an acute tendinosis characterized by edema and increased signal on ultrasound or MRI imaging.

> **Conclusion 10-2: The evidence establishes a causal relationship between vaccine administration and acute rotator cuff or acute biceps tendinopathy caused by direct administration of vaccine into or adjacent to the tendon.**

## CHRONIC ROTATOR CUFF DISEASE

Chronic rotator cuff disease comprises a diverse range of injuries and pathological conditions, with its prevalence escalating in correlation with age. This encompassing term encapsulates chronic tendinosis as well as partial- and full-thickness tears of the rotator cuff, collectively delineating the multifaceted nature of the condition. Approximately 22 percent of individuals over 40 are affected by full-thickness rotator cuff tears (Kuhn, 2023). The prevalence increases with advancing age: approximately 13 percent of people in their fifth decade, 20 percent in their sixth decade, 30 percent in their seventh decade, and a striking 50 percent in their eighth decade of life have full-thickness rotator cuff tears (Kuhn, 2023; Minagawa et al., 2013; Tempelhof et al., 1999; Teunis et al., 2014; Yamamoto et al., 2011). It is essential to note that the overwhelming majority of these cases are asymptomatic, meaning that individuals may not experience noticeable symptoms despite the presence of these tears (Jeong et al., 2017; Kuhn, 2023; Minagawa et al., 2013; Reilly et al., 2006; Tempelhof et al., 1999). As most patients with rotator cuff tears are asymptomatic it is not surprising that surgical intervention is performed in fewer than 5 percent of all individuals with rotator cuff tears (Kuhn, 2023).

In cases where individuals develop shoulder pain, particularly after vaccination, diagnostic imaging is frequently employed to evaluate the shoulder joint. An investigation of patients who applied for compensation through vaccine injury programs revealed that 80.3 percent of these individuals underwent MRI imaging. Interestingly, partial and complete rotator cuff tears were observed in 44.3 percent of these cases (Hesse et al., 2020). The median age was approximately 51, which aligns with the prevalence data in the general population. Given the high prevalence, especially in older individuals, it has been suggested that the observed rotator cuff pathology after vaccination is not directly related to the vaccine itself (AAOS, 2017; Slette et al., 2022).

### Mechanism of Injury

Chronic tendinosis and partial- and full-thickness tears of the rotator cuff collectively represent common degenerative shoulder conditions (Jeong et al., 2017; Minagawa et al., 2013; Reilly et al., 2006; Tempelhof et al., 1999; Teunis et al., 2014). No plausible mechanism exists whereby vaccine administration would be responsible for chronic rotator cuff disease.

### From Evidence to Conclusion

Chronic rotator cuff disease is typically a degenerative age-related condition and ubiquitous in the adult population. An injection into tendon material may produce increased signal on MRI imaging and an acute tendinosis (see section on acute tendinopathy) but not acute rotator cuff tears or corresponding rotator cuff muscle atrophy. Although it is common for patients with shoulder pain to undergo imaging and identify degeneration in the rotator cuff, these findings are more likely pre-existing and not related to a vaccine. The committee found the lack of a mechanistic explanation for chronic rotator cuff disease compelling.

> **Conclusion 10-3: The evidence favors rejection of a causal relationship between vaccine administration and chronic rotator cuff disease.**

## ADHESIVE CAPSULITIS

Frozen shoulder, also known as "adhesive capsulitis," is a debilitating condition that affects 1–5 percent of the population (Kingston et al., 2018). Certain demographic factors may increase the risk, with higher prevalence rates in females between 40 and 60, who have obesity, or who have diabetes (Huang et al., 2013; Kingston et al., 2018). Despite the higher prevalence in those under 50, reports in pediatric patients are rare (Levin et al., 2021). Furthermore, frozen shoulder can sometimes manifest as a complication after surgical procedures or injuries that require immobilization, such as a proximal humerus fracture. The multifaceted demographic associations highlight the need for careful assessment and tailored management.

Diagnosing frozen shoulder can be a complex process. In the early stages, when the condition may be inflammatory, it is often a clinical diagnosis of exclusion, as it shares symptoms with other shoulder conditions. However, in later stages, where it may be fibrotic, a marked loss of motion becomes a defining feature. Diagnostic imaging, such as MRI, may reveal characteristic signs, including rotator interval thickening and axillary capsule thickening (Choi and Kim, 2020). Early diagnosis is critical for a favorable prognosis, but health care providers often face challenges in accurately diagnosing frozen shoulder in its early stages due to its shared symptoms.

Although frozen shoulder was considered a self-limited issue with a typical duration of 1-year, longer-term studies have revealed that some individuals continue to experience unresolved pain and limited motion beyond this time frame (Hand et al., 2008; Kim et al., 2020). These findings emphasize the importance of ongoing monitoring and management to optimize long-term outcomes. The multifaceted nature of this condition, including its demographic associations, diagnostic challenges, and evolving treatment approaches, underscores the complexity of addressing it effectively.

### Evidence from Case Reports

Data reviewed by the committee regarding frozen shoulder after vaccination are limited (see Table 10-3): four case series ranging in sample size from 3 to 16 cases (Chu, 2022; Ghosh et al., 2023; Sahu and Shetty, 2022; Saleh et al., 2015). Three of the four reported on frozen shoulder with symptom onset within days after either BNT162b2[2] or ChAdOx1-S[3] and diagnosis months to years later (Chu, 2022; Ghosh et al., 2023; Sahu and Shetty, 2022). In addition, three case studies reported frozen shoulder in three patients diagnosed months to a year after BNT162b2, mRNA-1273,[4] or ChAdOx1-S. The fourth case series reported on frozen shoulder 1.5 months to 2 years after unidentified flu ($n = 2$) and pneumonia ($n = 1$) vaccination (Saleh et al., 2015). An additional two case studies reported on frozen shoulder after an unidentified flu vaccine (Thompson and Ensrud, 2020) and a human papillomavirus (HPV) vaccine (Smith et al., 2020); the child who had the HPV vaccine had diagnoses of Parsonage-Turner syndrome (PTS) and osteomyelitis.

### From Evidence to Conclusion

The cause of frozen shoulder is still unclear, and diagnosis often comes at later stages, when a fibrotic process greatly limits motion and function. The clinical diagnosis is least clear early on, and a diagnosis months to years later makes establishing a cause and effect unlikely, given the many confounding factors over time. Thus, attribution to vaccination is difficult if not impossible.

**Conclusion 10-4: The evidence is inadequate to accept or reject a causal relationship between vaccine administration and adhesive capsulitis.**

---

[2] The COVID-19 vaccine manufactured by Pfizer-BioNTech under the name Comirnaty®.

[3] The COVID-19 vaccine manufactured by Oxford-AstraZeneca.

[4] The COVID-19 vaccine manufactured by Moderna under the name Spikevax®.

**TABLE 10-3** Case Reports of Adhesive Capsulitis After Vaccination

| Author | Age | Sex | Vaccine(s) | Onset of Symptoms | Symptom Duration Before Evaluation | Imaging | Findings |
|---|---|---|---|---|---|---|---|
| Aldosary (2022) | 52 | F | ChAdOx1-S | 24 hours | 8 months | MRI | Frozen shoulder 8 months after injection |
| Biglia et al. (2023) | 50 | F | BNT162b2 | 48 hours | 1 month | Ultrasound | Frozen shoulder |
| Chu (2022) | 18+ | 4 M 12 F | BNT162b2 (12/16 patients) | 3.5 ± 2.5 days | >3 months | MRI | Frozen shoulder in 10/16 patients |
| Ghosh et al. (2023) | 48.7 ± 12.7 years | 5 M 4 F | ChAdOx1-S | 12.3 ± 3.1 days | 9.4 ± 2.4 weeks | NR | Frozen shoulder |
| Quinodoz et al. (2023) | "In his 40s" | M | mRNA-1273 | 4 months | 1 year | MRI | Frozen shoulder |
| Sahu and Shetty (2022) | 10 cases, mean 53.8 | 9 F 1 M 4 diabetic or prediabetic and 4 hypothyroid | ChAdOx1-S (9 cases) Covaxin (COVID-19) (1 case) | 24–48 hours | 14+ months | X-rays, MRI in 3 | Frozen shoulder |
| Saleh et al. (2015) | 30 67 69 | 2 M F | Influenza (2) Pneumonia (1) | Following day; soon after; same day | 3 months; 2 years; 6 weeks | Lab work, X-ray, MRI | Frozen shoulder |
| Smith et al. (2020) | 15 | F | HPV (Gardisil) | 11 days | NR | X-ray, MRI | Frozen shoulder, Parsonage-Turner, and osteomyelitis |
| Thompson and Ensrud (2020) | 64 | M | Influenza | 3 days | >9 months | MRI | Frozen shoulder 6 months after injection |

NOTES: BNT162b2 refers to the COVID-19 vaccine manufactured by Pfizer-BioNTech under the name Comirnaty®. mRNA-1273 refers to the COVID-19 vaccine manufactured by Moderna under the name Spikevax®.ChAdOx1-S refers to the COVID-19 vaccine manufactured by Oxford-AstraZeneca. F: female; HPV: human papillomavirus; M: male; MRI: magnetic resonance imaging; NR: not reported.
SOURCES: Aldosary, 2022; Biglia et al., 2023; Chu, 2022; Ghosh et al., 2023; Quinodoz et al., 2023; Sahu andShetty, 2022; Saleh et al., 2015; Smith et al., 2020; Thompson and Ensrud, 2020.

## SEPTIC ARTHRITIS

Septic arthritis of the shoulder, also referred to as "infectious arthritis," is a rare but serious condition characterized by the invasion of the shoulder joint by infectious microorganisms, typically bacteria. A cross-sectional study involving 97 patients indicated that the primary source of infection is often hematogenous, meaning that the bacteria spread through the bloodstream and access the joint (Sweet et al., 2019). However, other contiguous infections (e.g., soft tissue abscess, osteomyelitis) can be a cause. Septic arthritis can also arise from direct inoculation of bacteria into the joint via major trauma or, very rarely, by injection of bacterially contaminated material directly into the joint. The most commonly identified infectious organism in these cases is Staphylococcus aureus. Septic arthritis leads to inflammation and damage within the joint, resulting in significant pain, reduced range of motion, and potential joint destruction if not promptly and effectively managed.

**TABLE 10-4** Case Reports of Septic Arthritis After Vaccination

| Author | Age | Sex | Vaccine | Onset of Symptoms | Symptom Duration Before Evaluation | Imaging | Findings |
|---|---|---|---|---|---|---|---|
| Darnley et al. (2019) | 32 | F | Influenza | 2 weeks | NR | Negative X-rays, positive MRI | Septic arthritis |
| Floyd et al. (2012) | 59 | F | Pneumococcal (PPSV23) | 2 hours | 3 days | MRI and surgical cultures negative | Aseptic inflammatory arthritis |

NOTE: F: female; MRI: magnetic resonance imaging; NR: not reported.
SOURCES: Darnley et al., 2019; Floyd et al., 2012.

Epidemiological data on septic arthritis of the shoulder are limited, but estimates suggest an annual U.S. incidence of approximately 3,200 cases (Jiang et al., 2017). Certain risk factors have been associated with an increased likelihood, including older age, pre-existing joint diseases, lower socioeconomic status, diabetes, and underlying skin infections (Brennan and Hsu, 2012; Favero et al., 2008; Kunutsor et al., 2016).

Diagnosis typically involves a combination of clinical evaluation, laboratory testing, and imaging studies. One key criterion is the presence of a positive synovial fluid culture, which confirms the presence of infectious microorganisms within the joint. Laboratory tests, such as complete blood counts and inflammatory markers, can support the diagnosis.

### Evidence from Case Reports

The evidence reviewed by the committee, two case studies, is meager (see Table 10-4). In the first case (Darnley et al., 2019), the diagnosis was made via surgical pathology 3.5 months after influenza vaccination. Given the long interval between vaccination and diagnosis, it is impossible to rule out other sources of the infection. Furthermore, the initial MRI finding of an SSP tear could have explained the shoulder pain. In the second case, the diagnosis was septic arthritis, but a surgical culture was negative (Floyd et al., 2012). Neither case report was of a child.

### From Evidence to Conclusion

Evidence linking septic arthritis of the shoulder with vaccination is limited to two case studies.

**Conclusion 10-5: The evidence is inadequate to accept or reject a causal relationship between vaccine administration and septic arthritis.**

### BONE INJURY

Bone injuries following vaccinations have been highlighted through numerous case reports, indicating a wide array of bone-related issues in adults. There are diverse symptoms that typically manifest within a few days after vaccination. Advanced diagnostic tools such as MRI have been used in uncovering a range of bone pathologies post-vaccination, including marrow edema, cortical bone erosions, avascular necrosis, and cystic lesions particularly noted in the humeral head (see Table 10-5).

### Mechanism of Injury

The mechanism underlying bone injury after vaccination is supported by one small case series where 12 of 16 adults diagnosed with an influenza vaccine–mediated shoulder injury had ultrasound, immunophenotypic analyses, human leukocyte antigen (HLA) typing, and antigen-specific immunoassays. Vaccine-related bone toxicity and T cell/osteoclast interactions were assessed in vitro. Of these 12 adults, imaging demonstrated inflammatory tissue

**TABLE 10-5** Case Reports of Bone Injury After Vaccination

| Author | Age | Sex | Vaccine | Onset of Symptoms | Symptom Duration Before Evaluation | Imaging | Findings |
|---|---|---|---|---|---|---|---|
| Erickson et al. (2019) | 51 | F | Influenza | 1 day | 10 months | MRI at 2 months and 10 months | 10-month MRI showed humeral head osseous erosion |
| Flores et al. (2022) | 49 | M | Influenza | 1 day | 2 months | MRI | Bone marrow edema |
| Kashkosh et al. (2023) | 40 | M | COVID-19 | 2 days | 12 weeks | MRI, normal CT 3 months prior | Focal avascular necrosis |
| Kuether et al. (2011) | 48 | F | Influenza | 2.5 hours | 10 weeks | MRI | Localized avascular necrosis humeral head |
| Littrell et al. (2020) | 51 | M | Influenza | 2 hours | 6 weeks | MRI 6 weeks | 6 weeks: cortical irregularity, bone edema 9 months : progressive erosive changes of humeral head bone marrow edema |
| Messerschmitt et al. (2012) | 46 | M | Influenza | 3 days | 3 weeks | Bone scan, MRI, X-ray | Humeral head lytic lesion chondrolysis from intraosseous injection |
| Okur et al. (2014) | 39 | M | Influenza | NR | 2 months | MRI | Edema in greater tuberosity |
| Okur et al. (2014) | 36 | M | Influenza | NR | NR | MRI | Edema in greater tuberosity |
| Salmon et al. (2015) | 26 | F | Diptheria, tetanus, polio | NR | 48 hours | MRI | Edema in humeral head |
| Shabhaz et al. (2019) | 35 | F | Influenza | Immediate | 1 hour | MRI 1 week, 6 weeks, 8 months | 1 week effusion 4 weeks biceps tendonitis 8 months reactive bone edema |
| Szari et al. (2019) | 31 | M | Influenza | Immediate | 4 months | MRI | Edema in humeral head |
| Taylor and Hinke (2014) | 55 | F | Influenza | <1 day | 3 months | MRI | Humeral head edema, repeat at 3 months, cortical erosion |

NOTES: CT: computed tomography scan; F: female; M: male; MRI: magnetic resonance imaging; NR: not reported.
SOURCES: Erickson et al., 2019; Flores et al., 2022; Kashkosh et al., 2023; Kuether et al., 2011; Littrell et al., 2021; Messerschmitt et al., 2012; Okur et al., 2014; Salmon et al., 2015; Shabhaz et al., 2019; Szari et al., 2019; Taylor and Hinke, 2014.

damage, including bone erosions, in six. Tissue damage was associated with a strong peripheral blood T and B cell activation and extracellular matrix-reactive autoantibodies (autoantigen microarray). Subjects with erosions were HLA-DRB1*04 positive and showed extracellular matrix-reactive HLA-DRB1*04 restricted T cell responses targeting heparan sulfate proteoglycan. Antigen-specific T cells potently activated osteoclasts via receptor activator of nuclear factor kappa-B (RANK) interaction with its ligand (RANK/RANK-L), and the osteoclast activation marker Trap5b was high in sera of patients with an erosive shoulder injury. In vitro, the vaccine adjuvant alphatocopheryl succinate recapitulated bone toxicity (Hirsiger et al., 2021).

### Evidence from Case Reports

Vaccine-related bone injury has appeared in a number of case reports for adults aged 22–55. No pediatric cases of imaging-documented vaccine-related bone injury have been reported (see Table 10-5). Symptoms typically develop within 3 days. MRI demonstrated a variety of bone pathologies, including marrow edema near the site of the injection, cortical bone erosions (Salmon et al., 2015), avascular necrosis (Kashkosh et al., 2023; Kuether et al., 2011), and humeral head cystic lesions (Erickson et al., 2019). Treatment included nonsteroidal anti-inflammatory drugs, corticosteroid injections, physical therapy, and rarely surgery. The course for recovery of bone changes is variable but typically lasts many months.

### From Evidence to Conclusion

The conclusion is derived from a body of evidence, as demonstrated in the case reports (see Table 10-5), which consistently feature imaging and symptom onset within a biologically significant time window (typically 0–72 hours after vaccination). Studies that lack pertinent imaging data or extend beyond this critical time frame are likely to present a less compelling connection to vaccination. Patients who develop shoulder pain after vaccination will rarely demonstrate bone erosions, new-onset avascular necrosis, or bone marrow edema. These changes occur at the site of the injection and appear acute on imaging. Although the mechanistic data are limited, they do suggest that bone erosions in patients with shoulder pain may have T cell activation of osteoclasts, which would produce these erosions.

**Conclusion 10-6: The evidence establishes a causal relationship between vaccine administration and bone injury caused by direct injection into or adjacent to the bone.**

### AXILLARY OR RADIAL NERVE INJURY

The axillary nerve is a branch of the brachial plexus, a network of nerves in the shoulder and upper arm. It controls the deltoid, a major muscle involved in shoulder movement and stability. Axillary nerve injury can occur due to various causes, including trauma, compression, or surgical procedures in the shoulder area. Common symptoms include weakness or paralysis of the deltoid muscle, leading to difficulty in raising the arm and performing overhead movements.

The radial nerve is another major nerve of the arm, originating from the brachial plexus, connecting to the muscles that control wrist and finger extension, and playing a vital role in hand and forearm function. Radial nerve injuries can result from a variety of factors, including trauma, fractures of the arm bones, compression of the nerve, or complications from medical procedures. Symptoms typically include weakness or loss of function in wrist and finger extension, which can lead to difficulties in gripping objects and performing fine motor tasks.

Nerve injuries, including to the axillary and radial nerves, can vary in severity, from mild and temporary to more severe and long lasting, depending on the cause and extent. Treatment may involve physical therapy, medication, and sometimes surgical intervention to repair the damaged nerve or address underlying issues. Nerve injuries can significantly impact motor function, and management is often focused on restoring as much functionality as possible.

Axillary and radial nerve injuries can also be associated with vaccination, particularly when the vaccine is injected directly into or very close to the nerve. This unusual occurrence is characterized by progressive weakness that typically develops within 24 hours. To support the diagnosis of such injuries related to vaccination, medical professionals often rely on diagnostic tests, such as electromyogram and nerve conduction studies (EMG/NCS), and imaging techniques, such as ultrasound or MRI. These tests can help confirm the presence of nerve damage and its specific location, aiding in the identification and evaluation of the injury.

In these cases, the proximity of the vaccine injection site to the nerves in question can potentially lead to localized trauma or inflammation, resulting in nerve injury and its associated symptoms. Vaccine-related nerve injuries are extremely rare and represent only a small fraction of vaccine-related adverse events. Nonetheless, health care professionals carefully monitor and investigate such cases to ensure vaccine safety and provide appropriate care.

## Mechanism of Injury

The mechanism related to vaccination appears to stem from a direct injury to the nerve or inflammation in the vicinity of the nerve. This typically occurs when the needle placement is in close proximity to the nerve, which may inadvertently traumatize or irritate it, leading to damage. The proximity of the injection to the nerve can result in localized trauma or inflammation, which may trigger nerve injury or lead to nerve compression, irritation, or damage, ultimately resulting in weakness and related symptoms. This mechanism highlights the importance of precise and careful injection techniques to minimize the risk.

## Evidence from Case Reports

Direct nerve injuries related to vaccination have been documented in four case reports (Beredjiklian et al., 2012; Blumstein and Kreithen, 1966; Imran and Hayley, 2013; Meirelles and Motta Filho, 2004) (see Table 10-6). A comprehensive review of these data appears in a systematic review (Wright et al., 2023).

These cases reveal certain demographic patterns: direct nerve injuries have been exclusively reported in adults, spanning a wide age range, 23–73 years. The vaccines included two solitary influenza, one combined influenza and tetanus/diphtheria, and one tetanus. Of the documented cases, two involved injuries to the axillary nerve; the other two affected the radial nerve. All four patients consistently reported developing symptoms within 24 hours after vaccination. These symptoms typically manifested as progressive weakness in the affected limbs. No cases of nerve injury related to vaccination have been reported in children.

Physicians employed a variety of diagnostic techniques. EMG and NCS were used to identify the nerve injuries in two patients, and imaging techniques such as ultrasound or MRI were employed for one patient each.

The treatment approach in all four cases was nonsurgical, emphasizing noninvasive methods to manage the nerve injuries. Ultimately, all four patients experienced a degree of recovery, regaining function, although recuperation time varied significantly. The recovery period ranged from as short as 1 month to as long as 31 months. One patient reported some residual weakness even after recovery, underlining the diversity in outcomes among cases of direct nerve injury associated with vaccination.

**TABLE 10-6** Case Reports of Axillary or Radial Nerve Injury After Vaccination

| Author | Cases | Age | Sex | Vaccine | Onset of Symptoms | Symptom Duration Before Evaluation | Imaging |
|---|---|---|---|---|---|---|---|
| Beredjiklian et al. (2012) | 1 | 26 | M | Influenza | 16 hours | 1 day | MRI edema along radial nerve EMG neuropathy |
| Blumstein and Kreithen (1966) | 1 | 23 | M | Tetanus | <1 day | 7 hours | NR |
| Imran and Hayley (2013) | 1 | 73 | M | Influenza | Immediate | 8 weeks | None |
| Meirelles and Motta Filho (2004) | 1 | 67 | M | Influenza, diphtheria, tetanus | <1 day | 6 months | NCS axillary nerve with reinnervation |

NOTES: EMG: electromyogram; M: male; MRI: magnetic resonance imaging; NCS: nerve conduction study; NR: not reported.
SOURCES: Beredjiklian et al., 2012; Blumstein and Kreithen, 1966; Imran and Hayley, 2013; Meirelles and Motta Filho, 2004.

## From Evidence to Conclusion

The committee conclusion is derived from a body of evidence, as demonstrated in the case reports provided (see Table 10-6), which consistently feature imaging or EMG/NCS and symptom onset occurring within a biologically significant time (typically 0–24 hours after vaccination). Studies that lack pertinent imaging data or extend beyond this critical time frame are likely to present a less compelling connection to vaccine administration.

The axillary and radial nerves are potentially at risk for deltoid vaccine injections. A direct injection of vaccine material into or near a nerve could damage it, producing pain and weakness for its sensory and motor portions. Damage can be confirmed by diagnostic studies.

> **Conclusion 10-7: The evidence establishes a causal relationship between vaccine administration and axillary or radial nerve injury caused by direct injection into or adjacent to the nerve.**

## PARSONAGE-TURNER SYNDROME

PTS is a clinical syndrome classically typified by new onset of pain in the upper quarter followed by, within hours to days, paresis. Also known as "neuralgic amyotrophy" or "idiopathic brachial plexus neuropathy," it presents as a distinctive clinical syndrome characterized by abrupt, intense pain, typically within the shoulder and upper arm regions (Van Eijk et al., 2016). This pain is often described as sharp, burning, or neuralgic. Within a relatively short time frame, typically hours to days, individuals can develop muscle weakness or paralysis that is often localized along the innervation pathway of specific nerves within the brachial plexus, resulting in particular functional impairments (Van Eijk et al., 2016).

Commonly affected nerves include the long thoracic, suprascapular, and anterior interosseous nerves (Van Eijk et al., 2016). Damage to the long thoracic nerve can lead to scapular winging, characterized by the abnormal protrusion of the shoulder blade, which can cause both visible and functional changes in the shoulder region. Injury to the suprascapular nerve often makes it challenging to lift the arm and rotate it outward. Damage to the anterior interosseous nerve may lead to decreased grip strength, impacting the ability to hold and grasp objects effectively. In addition to pain and muscle weakness, individuals may experience tingling sensations and sensory disturbances in the upper extremity. This multifaceted clinical presentation underscores the complexity of PTS.

The diagnosis typically involves a thorough clinical assessment and EMG/NCS. Occasionally, an MRI will show inflammation around the brachial plexus. These diagnostic tests help confirm the presence of nerve damage and assess the extent of neural involvement.

The prevalence of PTS is not well defined and has generated variable estimates. The epidemiology remains uncertain, and incidence rates reported in the literature vary significantly, from 1–3 cases per 1,000 to 1–3 cases per 100,000 (van Alfen et al., 2015; Van Eijk et al., 2016). This disparity highlights the challenges in precisely establishing prevalence.

PTS may be more frequent in certain populations. Some studies have suggested that it may be more common in men than women (Ameer et al., 2023; van Alfen and van Engelen, 2006), but the underlying factors contributing to this difference are not fully explained. Children can be diagnosed with PTS, albeit rarely and more often after immunization or viral infection (van Alfen et al., 2000).

## Mechanism of Injury

The pathophysiology also remains unclear. The evidence does not support a genetic susceptibility or autoimmunity as primary causes. Limited low-level evidence has indicated potential associations between PTS and recent infections, but the causative relationship remains uncertain (van Alfen and van Engelen, 2006). Additionally, there have been reports of PTS after vaccination for various diseases, including COVID-19 (Ameer et al., 2023), influenza (Shaikh et al., 2012), and typhoid (Kim et al., 2021). These associations are still a subject of ongoing investigation and require further research to establish the nature of these links definitively.

**TABLE 10-7** Case Reports of Parsonage-Turner Syndrome After Vaccination

| Author | Age | Sex | Vaccine | Onset of Symptoms | Symptom Duration Before Evaluation | Imaging | Findings |
|---|---|---|---|---|---|---|---|
| Bernheimer and Gasbarro (2022) | 42 | F | mRNA-1273 | 3 weeks | 3 weeks + 1 day | MRI unremarkable | Parsonage-Turner syndrome |
| Chua et al. (2022) | 64 | M | mRNA-1273 | 12–24 hours | 3 weeks | EMG, nerve conduction study, MRI | Brachial neuritis |
| Coffman et al. (2021) | 66 | F | BNT162b2 | 1 month | NR | EMG | Parsonage-Turner syndrome |
| Flikkema and Brossy (2021) | 43 | M | mRNA-1273 | 2 days | NR | MRI of brachial plexus | Parsonage-Turner syndrome |
| Fransz et al. (2014) | 25 | M | Hepatitis B | 1 month | NR | EMG | Parsonage-Turner syndrome |
| Holmes et al. (2019) | 12 | M | Influenza | More than a year | NR | None | Brachial neuritis |
| Kang and Cho (2022) | 63 | M | ChAdOx1-S | Within a week | 1 month | EMG | Brachial neuritis |
| Kawegere and Goldberg (2022) | 62 | F | Influenza | Within hours | NR | X-ray, MRI | Brachial neuritis |
| Kim et al. (2021) | 20 | M | Typhoid | 6 days | 3 days | EMG, MRI | Parsonage-Turner syndrome |
| Koh et al. (2021) | Mean 50.66 with range 44–58 | 3 M | 2 BNT162b2 and 1 mRNA-1273 | 25 days, 4 days, 7 days | NR | MRI, EMG | Parsonage-Turner syndrome |
| Lindgren et al. (2019) | 54 | M | Shingles | A few days | 9+ months | EMG, MRI | Parsonage-Turner syndrome |
| Öncel and Coşkun (2022) | 56 | M | BNT162b2 (second dose) | 24 hours | NR | EMG, MRI | Parsonage-Turner syndrome |
| Shields et al. (2022) | 6 patients aged 36–84 | 3 M 3 F | mRNA-1273 and BNT162b2 | Not stated | NR | EMG | Parsonage-Turner syndrome |
| Sinha and Gupta (2017) | 85 | M | Influenza | 1 week | NR | MRI, EMG | Parsonage-Turner syndrome |
| VanLancker and Sheth (2022) | 29 | M | mRNA COVID-19, Influenza | A few hours | NR | EMG | Brachial neuritis |
| Vitturi et al. (2021) | 51 | M | ChAdOx1-S | Onset of symptoms not reported | A few days | EMG | Brachial neuritis |

NOTES: BNT162b2 refers to the COVID-19 vaccine manufactured by Pfizer-BioNTech under the name Comirnaty®. mRNA-1273 refers to the COVID-19 vaccine manufactured by Moderna under the name Spikevax®. ChAdOx1-S refers to the COVID-19 vaccine manufactured by Oxford-AstraZeneca. EMG: electromyogram; F: female; M: male; MRI: magnetic resonance imaging; NR: not reported.
SOURCES: Bernheimer and Gasbarro, 2022; Chua et al., 2022; Coffman et al., 2021; Flikkema and Brossy, 2021; Fransz et al., 2014; Holmes et al., 2019; Kang and Cho, 2022; Kawegere and Goldberg, 2022; Kim et al., 2021; Koh et al., 2021; Lindgren et al., 2019; Öncel and Coşkun, 2022; Shields et al., 2022; Sinha and Gupta, 2017; VanLancker and Sheth, 2022; Vitturi et al., 2021.

## Evidence from Case Reports

A syndrome is defined by a collection of clinical signs and symptoms where the pathophysiology and cause of a disease are poorly understood. PTS is no exception. The evidence reviewed by the committee is confined to two case series, totaling nine patients, and 14 case studies (see Table 10-7). In the case series of six patients, all of them reported symptoms after COVID-19 messenger ribonucleic acid (mRNA) injection (BNT162b2, mRNA-1273), but when symptoms appeared was not reported in individual patients, making the timeline unknown (mean duration of 17 days, with 5 days–8-week range) (Shields et al., 2022). In the case series of three patients, symptoms appeared 4–25 days after mRNA injection (two BNT162b2 and one mRNA-1273) (Koh et al., 2021). In addition, in nine case studies, symptoms appeared days to months after COVID-19 vaccination, the majority after mRNA vaccines. In five case studies, symptoms appeared after vaccinations for influenza ($n = 3$), hepatitis B ($n = 1$), and typhoid ($n = 1$).[5]

## From Evidence to Conclusion

The committee identified descriptions of PTS after vaccination in 23 people. In several cases, the onset of symptoms was either not reported or months after several different kinds of vaccination. In addition, PTS appears to be rare with a poorly understood pathophysiology; because of these issues, the evidence is limited to case studies, and establishing cause and effect is difficult.

**Conclusion 10-8: The evidence is inadequate to accept or reject a causal relationship between vaccine administration and Parsonage-Turner syndrome.**

## COMPLEX REGIONAL PAIN SYNDROME

Complex regional pain syndrome (CRPS), previously known as "reflex sympathetic dystrophy," is a multifaceted and often debilitating chronic condition that typically affects a limb, although it can spread to other parts of the body. CRPS is characterized by persistent, intense pain, and a range of sensory, motor, and autonomic symptoms.

CRPS exhibits a diverse demographic profile. Its incidence varies widely across studies, estimated at 5–26 individuals per 100,000 per year (de Mos et al., 2007; Elsharydah et al., 2017; Ott and Maihofner, 2018; Sandroni et al., 2003). Certain demographic variables have been associated with a higher risk, including being female and of Caucasian ethnicity and having a higher socioeconomic status, a history of depression, headaches, or drug abuse (Elsharydah et al., 2017). Conversely, diabetes, obesity, and hypothyroidism have been linked to lower rates of CRPS Type 1 (Elsharydah et al., 2017; Harden et al., 2010). Evidence is quite limited in children. A scoping review on CRPS in pediatric athletes (Moretti et al., 2021) identified twelve case studies and three case series implying that sport-related injury may be a causal factor.

Diagnosis can be challenging, given no universally accepted standard. To enhance diagnostic accuracy, the Budapest criteria, developed by Harden and colleagues in 2007 (see Table 10-8), have been used (Harden et al., 2007; Kessler et al., 2020). They include a combination of clinical effects, including sensory, vasomotor, sudomotor/edema, and motor/trophic symptoms, and provide a standardized framework to aid health care providers, promoting more consistent and accurate identification. The fourth criterion seems to indicate that CRPS is a diagnosis of exclusion.

## Mechanism of Injury

The pathological etiology remains complex and multifactorial. Although a definitive cause has not been established, inflammation is considered a potential contributor. Research has indicated elevated levels of proinflammatory

---

[5] An IOM committee concluded that "the evidence favors acceptance of a causal relation between tetanus toxoid and brachial neuritis" (IOM, 1994).

**TABLE 10-8** Budapest Criteria to Diagnose Complex Regional Pain Syndrome

| | |
|---|---|
| 1. Continuing pain that is disproportionate to inciting event | |
| 2. At least one sign in three of four categories by history | **Sensory:** Hyperesthesia or allodynia<br>**Vasomotor:** Temperature abnormalities/asymmetry, skin color changes/asymmetry<br>**Sudomotor:** Edema, sweating changes/asymmetry<br>**Motor/trophic:** Decreased range of motion; weakness; dystonia; hair, nail, or skin changes |
| 3. At least one sign in two of four categories by exam | **Sensory:** Evidence of hyperalgesia (to pinprick) and/or allodynia (to light touch and/or temperature sensation and/or deep somatic pressure and/or joint movement)<br>**Vasomotor:** Evidence of temperature asymmetry > 1 degree C, skin color changes/asymmetry<br>**Sudomotor:** Evidence of edema, sweating changes, asymmetry<br>**Motor/trophic:** Evidence of decreased range of motion; weakness; tremor; dystonia; hair, nail, skin changes |
| 4. There is no other diagnosis that better explains the symptoms | |

SOURCES: Harden et al., 2007; Kessler et al., 2020.

cytokines and decreased levels of the anti-inflammatory protein interleukin (IL)-1RA, suggesting an inflammatory component (Lenz et al., 2013). Trauma has also been implicated as a cause (Beerthuizen et al., 2012).

### Evidence from Case Reports

Evidence reviewed by the committee on the association of CRPS with vaccination is confined to one database study of 120 female vaccinees after HPV (Ozawa et al., 2017) and one after anthrax (Phillips et al., 2017) (see Table 10-9). Unfortunately, the database study (Ozawa et al., 2017) had no report of treatment or outcome, and patients reported onset of symptoms an average of 319 days after vaccination. Over such an extended period, many confounding factors are likely. Another study (Naleway et al., 2023) assessed the incidence of CRPS involving the upper extremity in individuals aged 9-30 years in a single integrated health system during three time periods: 2002–2006, before HPV vaccine licensure; 2007–2012, after licensure but before published case reports; and 2013–2017, after published case reports. Cases were identified using ICD-9/ICD-10 codes and text-based diagnoses

**TABLE 10-9** Case Reports of Complex Regional Pain Syndrome After Vaccination

| Author | Age | Sex | Vaccine | Onset of Symptoms | Symptom Duration Before Evaluation | Imaging | Findings |
|---|---|---|---|---|---|---|---|
| Naleway et al. (2023) | 14 | F | HPV | Same day as vaccination | 49 days | NR | CRPS |
| Ozawa et al. (2017) | Mean 13.6 ±1.6 years; range 11–19 | 120 F | HPV | 1 to 1,532 days (average 319.7 ± 349.3 days) | >8 months | NR | CRPS |
| Phillips et al. (2017) | 21 | F | Anthrax | 2 weeks | >7 months | EMG, MRI | CRPS |

NOTES: CRPS: complex regional pain syndrome; EMG: electromyogram; F: female; HPV: human papillomavirus; MRI: magnetic resonance imaging; NR: not reported.
SOURCES: Naleway et al., 2023; Ozawa et al., 2017; Phillips et al., 2017.

in the electronic health record. There was no difference in the incidence between these three time periods, and out of the total of 113 verified cases identified, only one case was attributed by a practitioner to HPV vaccination.[6]

## From Evidence to Conclusion

A syndrome is defined by a collection of clinical signs and symptoms where the pathophysiology and cause of a disease are poorly understood. CRPS is no exception. The case descriptions in Table 10-9 include sufficiently long times between vaccination and onset of symptoms to cloud interpretation of the role vaccination might have played.

**Conclusion 10-9: The evidence is inadequate to accept or reject a causal relationship between vaccine administration and complex regional pain syndrome.**

## REFERENCES

AAOS (American Academy of Orthopaedic Surgeons). 2017. Position statement 1190: Rotator cuff tendinopathy and glenohumeral arthritis are unlikely to be caused by vaccine administration. American Academy of Orthopaedic Surgeons.

Aldosary, A. H. 2022. Prolonged shoulder dysfunction after coronavirus disease vaccination: A case of shoulder injury related to vaccine administration. *SAGE Open Medical Case Reports* 10:2050313X221089494. https://doi.org/10.1177/2050313x221089494.

Ameer, M. Z., A. U. Haiy, M. H. Bajwa, H. Abeer, B. Mustafa, F. Ameer, Z. Amjad, and A. U. Rehman. 2023. Association of Parsonage-Turner syndrome with COVID-19 infection and vaccination: A systematic review. *Journal of International Medical Research* 51(7):3000605231187939. https://doi.org/10.1177/03000605231187939.

Atanasoff, S., T. Ryan, R. Lightfoot, and R. Johann-Liang. 2010. Shoulder injury related to vaccine administration (SIRVA). *Vaccine* 28(51):8049–8052. https://doi.org/10.1016/j.vaccine.2010.10.005.

Bancsi, A., S. K. D. Houle, and K. A. Grindrod. 2018. Getting it in the right spot: Shoulder injury related to vaccine administration (SIRVA) and other injection site events. *Canadian Pharmacists Journal* 151(5):295–299. https://doi.org/10.1177/1715163518790771.

Bansal, D., and D. R. DiLorenzo. 2020. Shoulder injury related to vaccine administration: Isolated teres minor tear. *Applied Radiology* 49(1):50–52.

Barnes, L. A. F., H. M. Kim, J. M. Caldwell, J. Buza, C. S. Ahmad, L. U. Bigliani, and W. N. Levine. 2017. Satisfaction, function and repair integrity after arthroscopic versus mini-open rotator cuff repair. *The Bone & Joint Journal* 99-B(2):245–249. https://doi.org/10.1302/0301-620X.99B2.BJJ-2016-0055.R1.

Bathia, N. A., and T. Stitik. 2009. Poster 35: "Influenza vaccine shoulder"—vaccination-related traumatic injury to the infraspinatus: A case report. *PM&R* 9(1):S118.

Beerthuizen, A., D. L. Stronks, A. Van't Spijker, A. Yaksh, B. M. Hanraets, J. Klein, and F. J. P. M. Huygen. 2012. Demographic and medical parameters in the development of complex regional pain syndrome type 1 (CRPS1): Prospective study on 596 patients with a fracture. *Pain* 153(6):1187–1192. https://doi.org/10.1016/j.pain.2012.01.026.

Beredjiklian, P. K., L. N. Nazarian, M. J Bercik, M. Gorski, and S. Mandel. 2012. Isolated radial nerve palsy secondary to influenza vaccination: A case report with imaging correlation. *Practical Neurology* 14–16.

Bernheimer, J. H., and G. Gasbarro. 2022. Parsonage-Turner syndrome following vaccination with mRNA-1273 SARS-CoV-2 vaccine. *Journal of Clinical Neuromuscular Disease* 23(4):229–230. https://doi.org/10.1097/cnd.0000000000000411.

Biglia, A., V. Morandi, G. Zanframundo, D. Donati, F. Maggiore, F. Vita, L. Sammarchi, C. Pagani, L. Cavagna, S. Galletti, and C. Montecucco. 2023. Adhesive capsulitis after COVID-19 vaccine injection: A peculiar case treated with combined bursa distention and glenohumeral capsular hydrodilatation. *Journal of Ultrasound* 26(4):909–911. https://doi.org/10.1007/s40477-022-00739-3.

Blumstein, G. I., and H. Kreithen. 1966. Peripheral neuropathy following tetanus toxoid administration. *JAMA* 198(9):1030–1031.

Bodor, M., and E. Montalvo. 2007. Vaccination-related shoulder dysfunction. *Vaccine* 25(4):585–587. https://doi.org/10.1016/j.vaccine.2006.08.034.

Brennan, M. B., and J. L. Hsu. 2012. Septic arthritis in the native joint. *Current Infectious Disease Reports* 14(5):558–565. https://doi.org/10.1007/s11908-012-0285-1.

---

[6] An IOM committee concluded that "the evidence is inadequate to accept or reject a causal relationship between the injection of a vaccine and CRPS" (IOM, 2012).

Cagle, P. J., Jr. 2021. Shoulder injury after vaccination: A systematic review. *Brazilian Journal of Orthopedics* 56(3):299–306. https://doi.org/10.1055/s-0040-1719086.

Cantarelli Rodrigues, T., P. F. Hidalgo, A. Y. Skaf, and A. Serfaty. 2021. Subacromial-subdeltoid bursitis following COVID-19 vaccination: A case of shoulder injury related to vaccine administration (SIRVA). *Skeletal Radiology* 50(11):2293–2297. https://doi.org/10.1007/s00256-021-03803-x.

Choi, Y.-H., and D. H. Kim. 2020. Correlations between clinical features and MRI findings in early adhesive capsulitis of the shoulder: A retrospective observational study. *BMC Musculoskeletal Disorders* 21:1–9.

Chow, J.C.K., S. L. Koles, and A. J. Bois. 2022. Shoulder injury related to SARS-CoV-2 vaccine administration. *Canadian Medical Association Journal* 194(2):E46–E49. https://doi.org/10.1503/cmaj.211162.

Chu, E. C.-P. 2022. Shoulder injury related to vaccine administration (SIRVA) in 16 patients following COVID-19 vaccination who presented to chiropractic, orthopedic, and physiotherapy clinics in Hong Kong during 2021. *Medical Science Monitor* 28:e937430. https://doi.org/10.12659/msm.937430.

Chua, M. M. J., M. T. Hayes, and R. Cosgrove. 2022. Parsonage-Turner syndrome following COVID-19 vaccination and review of the literature. *Surgical Neurology International* 13:152. https://doi.org/10.25259/sni_4_2022.

Chuaychoosakoon, C., and P. Boonsri. 2023. Partial infraspinatus tear with bursitis following an mRNA vaccination: A case report. *Annals of Medicine and Surgery* 85(5):2159–2161. https://doi.org/10.1097/ms9.0000000000000655.

Chuaychoosakoon, C., W. Parinyakhup, P. Tanutit, K. Maliwankul, and P. Klabklay. 2021. Shoulder injury related to Sinovac COVID-19 vaccine: A case report. *Annals of Medicine and Surgery* 68:102622. https://doi.org/10.1016/j.amsu.2021.102622.

Coffman, J. R., A. C. Randolph, and J. S. Somerson. 2021. Parsonage-Turner syndrome after SARS-CoV-2 BNT162b2 vaccine: A case report. *JBJS Case Connector* 11(3). https://doi.org/e21.0037010.2106/jbjs.Cc.21.00370.

Cook, I. F. 2011. An evidence based protocol for the prevention of upper arm injury related to vaccine administration (UAIRVA). *Human Vaccines & Immunotherapeutics* 7(8):845–848. https://doi.org/10.4161/hv.7.8.16271.

Cook, I. F. 2014. Subdeltoid/subacromial bursitis associated with influenza vaccination. *Human Vaccines & Immunotherapeutics* 10(3):605–606. https://doi.org/10.4161/hv.27232.

Cross, G. B., J. Moghaddas, J. Buttery, S. Ayoub, and T. M. Korman. 2016. Don't aim too high: Avoiding shoulder injury related to vaccine administration. *Australian Family Physician* 45(5):303–306.

Darnley, J. E., J. A. Rosenbaum, G. L. Jones, and J. Y. Bishop. 2019. Septic arthritis of the glenohumeral joint following influenza vaccination: Case report and review of the literature. *Current Orthopaedic Practice* 30(5):495–497.

de Mos, M., A. G. de Bruijn, F. J. Huygen, J. P. Dieleman, B. H. Stricker, and M. C. Sturkenboom. 2007. The incidence of complex regional pain syndrome: A population-based study. *Pain* 129(1–2):12–20. https://doi.org/10.1016/j.pain.2006.09.008.

Doppen, M., M. Black, I. Braithwaite, J. Bong, A. Eathorne, L. Kirton, S. Kung, M. Walton, T. Hills, M. Weatherall, R. Beasley, and C. Kearns. 2023. Skin-to-deltoid-muscle distance at three recommended sites for intramuscular vaccination in a population with obesity: An observational study. *New Zealand Medical Journal* 136(1573):67–76.

Elsharydah, A., N. H. Loo, A. Minhajuddin, and E. S. Kandil. 2017. Complex regional pain syndrome type 1 predictors—epidemiological perspective from a national database analysis. *Journal of Clinical Anesthesia* 39:34–37. https://doi.org/10.1016/j.jclinane.2017.03.027.

Erickson, B. J., E. F. DiCarlo, B. Brause, L. Callahan, and J. Hannafin. 2019. Lytic lesion in the proximal humerus after a flu shot: A case report. *JBJS Case Connector* 9(3):e0248.

Favero, M., F. Schiavon, L. Riato, V. Carraro, and L. Punzi. 2008. Rheumatoid arthritis is the major risk factor for septic arthritis in rheumatological settings. *Autoimmunity Reviews* 8(1):59–61. https://doi.org/10.1016/j.autrev.2008.07.018.

Flikkema, K., and K. Brossy. 2021. Parsonage-Turner syndrome after COVID-19 vaccination: A case report. *JBJS Case Connector* 11(4). https://doi.org/e21.0057710.2106/jbjs.Cc.21.00577.

Flores, C., W.S. Choate, and R. Tupler. 2022. Shoulder injury related to vaccine administration. *Ochsner Journal* 22(3). https://doi.org/doi.org/10.31486/toj.21.0114.

Floyd, M. W., B. M. Boyce, R. M. Castellan, and E. B. McDonough. 2012. Pseudoseptic arthritis of the shoulder following pneumococcal vaccination. *Orthopedics* 35(1):e101–e103.

Fransz, D. P., C. P. Schönhuth, T. J. Postma, and B. J. van Royen. 2014. Parsonage-Turner syndrome following post-exposure prophylaxis. *BMC Musculoskeletal Disorders* 15(1):265. https://doi.org/10.1186/1471-2474-15-265.

Ghosh, S., S. K. Pandey, A. Biswas, and J. Pandey. 2023. Adhesive capsulitis after COVID-19 vaccination: A case series. *American Journal of Physical Medicine and Rehabilitation* 102(6):e79–e82. https://doi.org/10.1097/phm.0000000000002194.

Hand, C., K. Clipsham, J. L. Rees, and A. J. Carr. 2008. Long-term outcome of frozen shoulder. *Journal of Shoulder and Elbow Surgery* 17(2):231–236. https://doi.org/10.1016/j.jse.2007.05.009.

Harden, N. R., S. Bruehl, R. Perez, F. Birklein, J. Marinus, C. Maihofner, T. Lubenow, A. Buvanendran, S. Mackey, J. Graciosa, M. Mogilevski, C. Ramsden, M. Chont, and J.-J. Vatine. 2010. Validation of proposed diagnostic criteria (the "Budapest criteria") for complex regional pain syndrome. *Pain* 150(2):268–274. https://doi.org/10.1016/j.pain.2010.04.030.

Harden, R. N., S. Bruehl, M. Stanton-Hicks, and P. R. Wilson. 2007. Proposed new diagnostic criteria for complex regional pain syndrome. *Pain Medicine* 8(4):326–331. https://doi.org/10.1111/j.1526-4637.2006.00169.x.

Hesse, E. M., S. Atanasoff, B. F. Hibbs, O. J. Adegoke, C. Ng, P. Marquez, M. Osborn, J. R. Su, P. L. Moro, T. Shimabukuro, and N. Nair. 2020. Shoulder injury related to vaccine administration (SIRVA): Petitioner claims to the National Vaccine Injury Compensation Program, 2010–2016. *Vaccine* 38(5):1076–1083. https://doi.org/10.1016/j.vaccine.2019.11.032.

Hirsiger, J. R., G. Tamborrini, D. Harder, G. R. Bantug, G. Hoenger, M. Recher, C. Marx, Q.-Z. Li, I. Martin, C. Hess, A. Scherberich, T. Daikeler, and C. T. Berger. 2021. Chronic inflammation and extracellular matrix-specific autoimmunity following inadvertent periarticular influenza vaccination. *Journal of Autoimmunity* 124:102714. https://doi.org/10.1016/j.jaut.2021.102714.

Holmes, R., K. Armon, and P. Bale. 2019. P39 physiotherapy management of long thoracic nerve injury (LTNI) post-flu vaccine in an immunocompromised patient with vasculitis: What is the best strategy? *Rheumatology* 58(Suppl 4):kez416.006.

Honarmand, A. R., J. Mackey, and R. Hayeri. 2021. Shoulder injury related to vaccine administration (SIRVA) following mRNA COVID-19 vaccination: Report of 2 cases of subacromial-subdeltoid bursitis. *Radiology Case Reports* 16(12):3631–3634. https://doi.org/https://doi.org/10.1016/j.radcr.2021.08.019.

HRSA (Health Resources and Services Administration). 2023. *Vaccine injury table.* Health Resources and Services Administration.

Huang, Y.-P., C.-Y. Fann, Y.-H. Chiu, M.-F. Yen, L.-S. Chen, H.-H. Chen, and S.-L. Pan. 2013. Association of diabetes mellitus with the risk of developing adhesive capsulitis of the shoulder: A longitudinal population-based followup study. *Arthritis Care & Research* 65(7):1197–1202. https://doi.org/10.1002/acr.21938.

Imran, M., and D. Hayley. 2013. Injection-induced axillary nerve injury after a drive-through flu shot. *Clinical Geriatrics* 21(12).

IOM (Institute of Medicine). 1994. *Adverse events associated with childhood vaccines: Evidence bearing on causality.* Edited by K. R. Stratton, C. J. Howe, and R. B. Johnston, Jr. Washington, DC: National Academy Press.

IOM. 2012. *Adverse effects of vaccines: Evidence and causality.* Edited by K. Stratton, A. Ford, E. Rusch, and E. W. Clayton. Washington, DC: The National Academies Press.

Jenkins, M., D. Rupp, and L. J. Goebel. 2020. Post-influenza vaccine subdeltoid bursitis. *Cureus* 12(10).

Jeong, J., D.-C. Shin, T.-H. Kim, and K. Kim. 2017. Prevalence of asymptomatic rotator cuff tear and their related factors in the Korean population. *Journal of Shoulder and Elbow Surgery* 26(1):30–35. https://doi.org/10.1016/j.jse.2016.05.003.

Jiang, J. J., H. I. Piponov, D. P. Mass, J. G. Angeles, and L. L. Shi. 2017. Septic arthritis of the shoulder: A comparison of treatment methods. *Journal of the American Academy of Orthopaedic Surgeons* 25(8):e175–e184. https://doi.org/10.5435/JAAOS-D-16-00103.

Kang, J., and J.-Y. Cho. 2022. Diaphragmatic dysfunction due to neuralgic amyotrophy after SARS-CoV-2 vaccination: A case report. *Journal of Korean Medical Science* 37(38):e283. https://doi.org/10.3346/jkms.2022.37.e283.

Kashkosh, A., C. M. Peake, A. A. Narvani, and M. Imam. 2023. Spontaneous avascular necrosis of the humeral head following COVID-19 vaccination. *Archives of Bone and Joint Surgery* 11(2):140.

Kawagere, E., and T. Goldberg. 2022. Shoulder injury related to vaccine administration (SIRVA). *Journal of General Internal Medicine* 37. https://doi.org/covidwho-1995707.

Kessler, A., M. Yoo, and R. Calisoff. 2020. Complex regional pain syndrome: An updated comprehensive review. *NeuroRehabilitation* 47(3):253–264.

Kim, D. H., Y. S. Kim, B.-S. Kim, D. H. Sung, K.-S. Song, and C.-H. Cho. 2020. Is frozen shoulder completely resolved at 2 years after the onset of disease? *Journal of Orthopaedic Science* 25(2):224–228.

Kim, J. G., S. Y. Kim, H. S. Oh, and D. H. Jo. 2021. Parsonage-Turner syndrome following typhoid vaccination. *Yonsei Medical Journal* 62(9):868–871. https://doi.org/10.3349/ymj.2021.62.9.868.

Kingston, K., E. J. Curry, J. W. Galvin, and X. Li. 2018. Shoulder adhesive capsulitis: Epidemiology and predictors of surgery. *Journal of Shoulder and Elbow Surgery* 27(8):1437–1443.

Klabklay, P., P. Boonsri, P. Kanyakool, and C. Chuaychoosakoon. 2022. A COVID-19 vaccination precipitating symptomatic calcific tendinitis: A case report. *Annals of Medicine and Surgery* 74:103347. https://doi.org/https://doi.org/10.1016/j.amsu.2022.103347.

Koh, J. S., Y. Goh, B. Y.-Q. Tan, A. C.-F. Hui, R. H. M. Hoe, A. Makmur, P. L. Kei, J. Vijayan, K. W. P. Ng, A. M. L. Quek, and U. Thirugnanm. 2021. Neuralgic amyotrophy following COVID-19 mRNA vaccination. *QJM: An International Journal of Medicine* 114(7):503–505. https://doi.org/10.1093/qjmed/hcab216.

Kowatari, R., H. Sasaki, K. Murata, K. Sato, K. Sagawa, M. Kudo, and M. Minakawa. 2023. Establishment of prediction equations for subcutaneous tissue thickness in two representative intramuscular deltoid injections. *Vaccine X* 14:100316. https://doi.org/10.1016/j.jvacx.2023.100316.

Kuether, G., B. Dietrich, T. Smith, C. Peter, and S. Gruessner. 2011. Atraumatic osteonecrosis of the humeral head after influenza A-(H1N1) V-2009 vaccination. *Vaccine* 29(40):6830–6833.

Kuhn, J. E. 2023. Prevalence, natural history, and nonoperative treatment of rotator cuff disease. *Operative Techniques in Sports Medicine* 31(1). https://doi.org/ARTN15097810.1016/j.otsm.2023.150978.

Kunutsor, S. K., M. R. Whitehouse, A. W. Blom, A. D. Beswick, and INFORM Team. 2016. Patient-related risk factors for periprosthetic joint infection after total joint arthroplasty: A systematic review and meta-analysis. *PLoS One* 11(3):e0150866. https://doi.org/10.1371/journal.pone.0150866.

Lenz, M., N. Üçeyler, J. Frettlöh, O. Höffken, E. K. Krumova, S. Lissek, A. Reinersmann, C. Sommer, P. Stude, A. M. Waaga-Gasser, M. Tegenthoff, and C. Maier. 2013. Local cytokine changes in complex regional pain syndrome type I (CRPS I) resolve after 6 months. *Pain* 154(10):2142–2149. https://doi.org/10.1016/j.pain.2013.06.039.

Leopold, S. S. 2022. Editor's spotlight/take 5: Discussing two systematic reviews with opposing conclusions on shoulder pain after vaccine administration. *Clinical Orthopaedics and Related Research* 480(7):1234–1240. https://doi.org/10.1097/CORR.0000000000002259.

Levin, J., A. R. Siddiqi, and H. Kim. 2021. Capsular distention for adhesive capsulitis in a pediatric patient with acute flaccid myelitis: A case report. *Journal of Pediatric Rehabilitation Medicine* 14(1):37–40. https://doi.org/10.3233/prm-190640.

Lindgren, B., D. Rivers, and J. Clark. 2019. Bilateral Parsonage-Turner syndrome after initial unilateral presentation: A case report. *Cureus* 11(12):e6422. https://doi.org/10.7759/cureus.6422.

Littrell, L. A., D. F. Leslie, D. M. Bierle, and D. E. Wenger. 2020. Progressive monoarticular inflammatory arthritis following influenza vaccination. *Mayo Clinic Proceedings: Innovations, Quality & Outcomes* 5(1):204–209.

Mackenzie, L. J., M. A. Bushell, P. Newman, and J. A. Bousie. 2022. Shoulder injury related to vaccine administration (SIRVA): What do we know about its incidence and impact? *Exploratory Research in Clinical and Social Pharmacy* 8:100183. https://doi.org/10.1016/j.rcsop.2022.100183.

MacMahon, A., S. K. Nayar, and U. Srikumaran. 2022. What do we know about shoulder injury related to vaccine administration? An updated systematic review. *Clinical Orthopaedics and Related Research* 480(7):1241–1250. https://doi.org/10.1097/Corr.0000000000002181.

Maliwankul, K., P. Boonsri, P. Klabklay, and C. Chuaychoosakoon. 2022. Shoulder injury related to COVID-19 vaccine administration: A case series. *Vaccines* 10(4):588.

Mardourian, M., K. A. Hao, W. Wiggins, J. Arias, J. J. King, T. W. Wright, and J. O. Wright. 2023. Optimizing needle length and site choice for adult immunization. *Vaccine* 41(33):4836–4843. https://doi.org/10.1016/j.vaccine.2023.06.031.

Marshall, T., M. Addison, N. W. Crawford, J. P. Buttery, and D. R. Cheng. 2022. Aiming too high: Shoulder injury related to vaccine administration (SIRVA): A case series. *Vaccine* 40(52):7505–7509. https://doi.org/10.1016/j.vaccine.2022.10.086.

Meirelles, H., and G. R. Motta Filho. 2004. Axillary nerve injury caused by intramuscular injection into the deltoid: Case report. *Brazilian Review of Orthopedics* 39(10).

Messerschmitt, P. J., F. W. Abdul-Karim, J. P. Iannotti, and R. G. Gobezie. 2012. Progressive osteolysis and surface chondrolysis of the proximal humerus following influenza vaccination. *Orthopedics* 35(2):e283–e286.

Minagawa, H., N. Yamamoto, H. Abe, M. Fukuda, N. Seki, K. Kikuchi, H. Kijima, and E. Itoi. 2013. Prevalence of symptomatic and asymptomatic rotator cuff tears in the general population: From mass-screening in one village. *Journal of Orthopaedics* 10(1):8–12. https://doi.org/10.1016/j.jor.2013.01.008.

Moretti, A., A. Palomba, M. Paoletta, S. Liguori, G. Toro, and G. Iolascon. 2021. Complex regional pain syndrome in athletes: Scoping review. *Medicina* 57(11). https://doi.org/10.3390/medicina57111262.

Moya, D., D. Gómez, P. Patiño, N. N. Altamirano, M. Balzarini, and K. Freitag. 2022. Shoulder injury related to vaccine administration following misplaced SARS-CoV-2 vaccination: A case report and review of literature. *Journal of Orthopaedic Case Reports* 12(3):100.

Nakajima, K., A. Miyata, K. Kato, Y. Oshima, and S. Tanaka. 2023. Calcific tendinitis of the shoulder induced by an mRNA vaccine for COVID-19: A case report. *Modern Rheumatology Case Reports* 7(1):211–214. https://doi.org/10.1093/mrcr/rxac006.

Nakajima, Y., K. Mukai, K. Takaoka, T. Hirose, K. Morishita, T. Yamamoto, Y. Yoshida, T. Urai, and T. Nakatani. 2017. Establishing a new appropriate intramuscular injection site in the deltoid muscle. *Human Vaccines & Immunotherapeutics* 13(9):2123–2129. https://doi.org/10.1080/21645515.2017.1334747.

Naleway, A. L., M. L. Henninger, S. A. Irving, S. Bianca Salas, T. L. Kauffman, B. Crane, K. F. Mittendorf, S. Harsh, C. Elder, and J. Gee. 2023. Epidemiology of upper limb complex regional pain syndrome in a retrospective cohort of persons aged 9–30 years, 2002–2017. *Permanente Journal* 27(2):75–86. https://doi.org/10.7812/tpp/22.170.

Natanzi, N., F. Hebroni, and M. Bodor. 2020. Teres minor injury related to vaccine administration. *Radiology Case Reports* 15(5):552–555. https://doi.org/10.1016/j.radcr.2020.02.009.

Okur, G., K. A. Chaney, and L. M. Lomasney. 2014. Magnetic resonance imaging of abnormal shoulder pain following influenza vaccination. *Skeletal Radiology* 43:1325–1331.

Öncel, A., and E. Coşkun. 2022. Parsonage-Turner syndrome after SARS-CoV-2 vaccination: A case report. *Turkish Journal of Physical Medicine and Rehabilitation* 68(3):418–421. https://doi.org/10.5606/tftrd.2022.10456.

Ott, S., and C. Maihöfner. 2018. Signs and symptoms in 1,043 patients with complex regional pain syndrome. *Pain* 19(6):599–611.

Ozawa, K., A. Hineno, T. Kinoshita, S. Ishihara, and S.-I. Ikeda. 2017. Suspected adverse effects after human papillomavirus vaccination: A temporal relationship between vaccine administration and the appearance of symptoms in Japan. *Drug Safety* 40:1219–1229.

Pearson, M., and S. Bent. 2022. Postvaccination subacromial bursitis. *Journal of General Internal Medicine* 37(2):467.

Petrakis, N., M. Addison, B. Penak, S. Schrader, J. Mallard, H. J. Clothier, J. P. Buttery, N. W. Crawford, and D. R. Cheng. 2023. Shoulder injury following COVID-19 vaccine administration: A case series and proposed diagnostic algorithm. *Expert Review of Vaccines* 22(1):299–306. https://doi.org/10.1080/14760584.2023.2189463.

Pettyjohn, E. W., J. R. Clugston, and J. L. Zaremski. 2022. Shoulder injury related to vaccine administration and a growing challenge: A focused review. *Current Sports Medicine Reports* 21(3):78–83. https://doi.org/10.1249/jsr.0000000000000939.

Phillips, C., A. Constanzo, and I. Fowler, 2017. Complex regional pain syndrome following anthrax vaccine. *Pain Medicine* 18(3):52. https://doi.org/10.1093.

Quinodoz, A., F. Luthi, S. Revaz, and M. Konzelmann. 2023. Acute myopericarditis and left shoulder capsulitis following second dose of mRNA SARS-CoV-2 Moderna vaccination. *BMJ Case Reports* 16(6):e254110. https://doi.org/10.1136/bcr-2022-254110.

Reilly, P., I. Macleod, R. Macfarlane, J. Windley, and R. J. Emery. 2006. Dead men and radiologists don't lie: A review of cadaveric and radiological studies of rotator cuff tear prevalence. *Annals of the Royal College of Surgeons of England* 88(2):116–121. https://doi.org/10.1308/003588406X94968.

Sahu, D., and G. Shetty. 2022. Frozen shoulder after COVID-19 vaccination. *JSES International* 6(4):682–685. https://doi.org/10.1016/j.jseint.2022.02.013.

Saleh, Z. M., S. Faruqui, and A. Foad. 2015. Onset of frozen shoulder following pneumococcal and influenza vaccinations. *Journal of Chiropractic Medicine* 14(4):285–289. https://doi.org/10.1016/j.jcm.2015.05.005.

Salmon, J., M. Geoffroy, J. Eschard, and X. Ohl. 2015. Bone erosion and subacromial bursitis caused by diphtheria-tetanus-poliomyelitis vaccine. *Vaccine* 33(46):6152–6155.

Sandroni, P., L. M. Benrud-Larson, R. L. McClelland, and P. A. Low. 2003. Complex regional pain syndrome type I: Incidence and prevalence in Olmsted County, a population-based study. *Pain* 103(1–2):199–207. https://doi.org/10.1016/s0304-3959(03)00065-4.

Shahbaz, M., P. D. Blanc, S. J. Domeracki, and S. Guntur. 2019. Shoulder injury related to vaccine administration (SIRVA): An occupational case report. *Workplace Health & Safety* 67(10):501–505. https://doi.org/10.1177/2165079919875161.

Shaikh, M. F., T. J. Baqai, and H. Tahir. 2012. Acute brachial neuritis following influenza vaccination. *BMJ Case Reports* 2012. https://doi.org/10.1136/bcr-2012-007673.

Shaw, F. E., Jr., H. A. Guess, J. M. Roets, F. E. Mohr, P. J. Coleman, E. J. Mandel, R. R. Roehm, Jr., W. S. Talley, and S. C. Hadler. 1989. Effect of anatomic injection site, age and smoking on the immune response to hepatitis B vaccination. *Vaccine* 7(5):425–430. https://doi.org/10.1016/0264-410x(89)90157-6.

Shields, L. B. E., V. G. Iyer, Y. P. Zhang, J. T. Burger, and C. B. Shields. 2022. Parsonage-Turner syndrome following COVID-19 vaccination: Clinical and electromyographic findings in 6 patients. *Case Reports in Neurology* 14(1):58–67. https://doi.org/10.1159/000521462.

Sinha, A., and S. Gupta. 2017. Poster 266: Parsonage-Turner syndrome following influenza vaccination: A case report. *PM&R* 9:S216.

Slette, E., M. Rohrback, and D. V. Ring. 2022. Persistent shoulder pain after vaccine administration is associated with common incidental pathology: A systematic review. *Clinical Orthopaedics and Related Research* 480(7):1251–1258. https://doi.org/10.1097/Corr.0000000000002191.

Smith, S. S., Y. Lee, and L. Wang. 2020. Adolescent with osteomyelitis after intramuscular administration of a vaccine: A case report. *Journal of the American Pharmacists Association* 60(6):e357–e360. https://doi.org/https://doi.org/10.1016/j.japh.2020.03.015.

Sukhija, S., S. Singh, S. Saxena, S. Ambwani, and P. S. Khera. 2022. Shoulder injury related to vaccine administration (SIRVA) with COVID-19 vaccination—a case report. *Journal of Family Medicine and Primary Care* 11(12):7937–7940. https://doi.org/10.4103/jfmpc.jfmpc_798_22.

Sweet, M. C., G. J. Sheena, S. Liu, F. E. Fisk, J. R. Lynch, and S. J. Muh. 2019. Clinical characteristics and long-term outcomes after septic arthritis of the native glenohumeral joint: A 20-year retrospective review. *Orthopedics* 42(1):e118–e123.

Szari, S., A. Belgard, K. Adams, and J. Freiler. 2019. Shoulder injury related to vaccine administration: A rare reaction. *Federal Practitioner* 36(8):380–384.

Taylor, B. C., and D. Hinke. 2014. Shoulder injury related to vaccine administration (SIRVA). *Applied Radiology* 43(12):30–32.

Tempelhof, S., S. Rupp, and R. Seil. 1999. Age-related prevalence of rotator cuff tears in asymptomatic shoulders. *Journal of Shoulder and Elbow Surgery* 8(4):296–299. https://doi.org/10.1016/s1058-2746(99)90148-9.

Teunis, T., B. Lubberts, B. T. Reilly, and D. Ring. 2014. A systematic review and pooled analysis of the prevalence of rotator cuff disease with increasing age. *Journal of Shoulder and Elbow Surgery* 23(12):1913–1921. https://doi.org/10.1016/j.jse.2014.08.001.

Thompson, A. R., and E. R. Ensrud. 2020. Bilateral adhesive capsulitis following influenza vaccination: A case report. *Clinical Case Reports* 8(11):2155–2157. https://doi.org/10.1002/ccr3.3072.

Uchida, S., A. Sakai, and T. Nakamura. 2012. Subacromial bursitis following human papilloma virus vaccine misinjection. *Vaccine* 31(1):27–30.

van Alfen, N., and B. G. M. van Engelen. 2006. The clinical spectrum of neuralgic amyotrophy in 246 cases. *Brain* 129(Pt 2):438–450. https://doi.org/10.1093/brain/awh722.

van Alfen, N., J. Schuuring, B. G. van Engelen, J. J. Rotteveel, and F. J. Gabreëls. 2000. Idiopathic neuralgic amyotrophy in children. A distinct phenotype compared to the adult form. *Neuropediatrics* 31(6):328–332. https://doi.org/10.1055/s-2000-12954.

van Alfen, N., J. J. van Eijk, T. Ennik, S. O. Flynn, I. E. G. Nobacht, J. T. Groothuis, S. Pillen, and F. A. van de Laar. 2015. Incidence of neuralgic amyotrophy (Parsonage-Turner syndrome) in a primary care setting—a prospective cohort study. *PLoS One* 10(5):e0128361. https://doi.org/10.1371/journal.pone.0128361.

Van Eijk, J.J., J. T. Groothuis, and N. Van Alfen. 2016. Neuralgic amyotrophy: An update on diagnosis, pathophysiology, and treatment. *Muscle and Nerve* 53(3):337–350. https://doi.org/10.1002/mus.25008.

VanLancker, J., and D. Sheth. 2022. Brachial neuritis from the mRNA SARS-COV-2 and influenza vaccines. *Annals of Allergy, Asthma & Immunology* 129(5 Suppl):S96–S97. https://doi.org/10.1016/j.anai.2022.08.773.

Vitturi, B. K., M. Grandis, S. Beltramini, A. Orsi, A. Schenone, G. Icardi, and P. Durando. 2021. Parsonage-Turner syndrome following coronavirus disease 2019 immunization with ChAdOx1-S vaccine: A case report and review of the literature. *Journal of Medical Case Reports* 15(1):589. https://doi.org/10.1186/s13256-021-03176-8.

Wharton, B. R., K. C. Doan, and M. L. Wolcott. 2022. Shoulder injury related to COVID-19 vaccine administration: A case report. *JSES Reviews, Reports & Techniques* 2(2):178–181.

Wong, W., C. Okafor, E. Belay, C. S. Klifto, and O. Anakwenze. 2021. Arthroscopic surgical management of shoulder secondary to shoulder injury related to vaccine administration (SIRVA): A case report. *Journal of Shoulder and Elbow Surgery* 30(6):e334–e337.

Wood, C. T., and A. M. Ilyas. 2022. Shoulder injury related to vaccine administration: Diagnosis and management. *Journal of Hand Surgery Global Online* 4(2):111–117. https://doi.org/10.1016/j.jhsg.2021.12.009.

Wright, A., R. Patel, and D. Motamedi. 2019. Influenza vaccine-related subacromial/subdeltoid bursitis: A case report. *Journal of Radiology Case Reports* 13(6):24.

Wright, J. O., W. Wiggins, M. S. Smith, J. J. King, and T. W. Wright. 2023. Shoulder pain and dysfunction after vaccination: A systematic review. *JBJS Reviews* 11(1). https://doi.org/e22.0013410.2106/JBJS.RVW.22.00134.

Yamamoto, A., K. Takagishi, T. Kobayashi, H. Shitara, and T. Osawa. 2011. Factors involved in the presence of symptoms associated with rotator cuff tears: A comparison of asymptomatic and symptomatic rotator cuff tears in the general population. *Journal of Shoulder and Elbow Surgery* 20(7):1133–1137.

Yuen, W. L. P., Y. J. Loh, and D. B. Wang. 2022. SIRVA (shoulder injury related to vaccine administration) following mRNA COVID-19 vaccination: Case discussion and literature review. *Vaccine* 40(18):2546–2550.

Zeldin, E. R., D. M. Boyette, and J. W. Norbury. 2023. Shoulder pain after influenza vaccine administration: A clinical vignette. *American Journal of Physical Medicine and Rehabilitation* 102(10):e141–e143. https://doi.org/10.1097/PHM.0000000000002242.

Zheng, C., J. Duffy, I. A. Liu, L. S. Sy, R. A. Navarro, S. S. Kim, D. S. Ryan, W. Chen, L. Qian, C. Mercado, and S. J. Jacobsen. 2022. Identifying cases of shoulder injury related to vaccine administration (SIRVA) in the United States: Development and validation of a natural language processing method. *JMIR Public Health Surveillance* 8(5):e30426. https://doi.org/10.2196/30426.

# 11

# Crosscutting Remarks

This chapter summarizes the conclusions made for each of the four COVID-19 vaccines under review and then presents the conclusions, including those about shoulder injuries related to intramuscular administration of any vaccine, by causal category. It offers a summary of information regarding evidence in children. Finally, it identifies methodologic challenges the committee encountered during its review.

The committee makes 85 conclusions about the causal relationship or lack thereof between vaccines and possible harms. Although it lacked evidence to establish, accept, or reject a causal relationship for many possible harms, it identified sufficient evidence for 20 conclusions. It is not surprising that evidence is insufficient for the majority; National Academies of Sciences, Engineering, and Medicine (National Academies) committees conducting similar reviews had similar results. The literature on the relationship between the four COVID-19 vaccines and many of the adverse events in the Statement of Task is sparse, not directly applicable to the question of causality, or conflicting or unconvincing due to study design problems, such as sample size limitations or case ascertainment. Fortunately, important research that sheds light on both the benefit and the potential harms of COVID-19 vaccines is published regularly. As discussed in Chapter 1, the committee incorporated into its definitions of the causal conclusions the understanding that further research may change a conclusion, although the committee thinks it is unlikely for conclusions establishing causality.

Given that this review occurred shortly after vaccines were available, the information in this report is a snapshot in time. New COVID-19 vaccines will be developed, and research will continue on many fronts. Understanding causation is a dynamic process; conclusions are refined as information accumulates. For example, the evidence reviewed in this report does not address real-world use in which many individuals received a "mix and match" sequence (i.e., some with BNT162b2 for their primary series received mRNA-1273 as a booster). Many people vaccinated for COVID-19 received other vaccines (e.g., influenza) simultaneously, and the effect of combined vaccination is not yet well explored. Most of the evidence regarding COVID-19 vaccines was from the primary series. Because children were among the last vaccinees, less evidence exists about them, especially for the youngest age groups (see subsequent section). These areas pose great opportunities for future research.

## COVID-19 VACCINE–SPECIFIC CONCLUSIONS

The committee was not charged to evaluate the benefits of COVID-19 vaccines. All conclusions must be assessed in the context of the established harms of severe acute respiratory syndrome coronavirus-2 (SARS-CoV-2) infection and the well-documented benefits of COVID-19 vaccines in preventing those harms. Most of the evidence the committee reviewed included BNT162b2 (see Box 11-1), which is not surprising, as it was the first vaccine available in the United States and many other countries; mRNA-1273 quickly followed, and many studies addressed it as well (see Box 11-2). The U.S. Food and Drug Administration (FDA) revoked the authorization of Ad26.COV2.S, and the number of studies reflected that short availability (see Box 11-3). NVX-CoV2373 is the most recently available vaccine in the United States—FDA issued an emergency use authorization (EUA) in July 2022 (FDA, 2022)—and the committee identified no epidemiological studies relevant to its review (see Box 11-4).

---

**BOX 11-1**
**Conclusions Regarding BNT162b2**

**Conclusion 3-1: The evidence favors rejection of a causal relationship between the BNT162b2 vaccine and Guillain-Barré syndrome.**

**Conclusion 3-9: The evidence favors rejection of a causal relationship between the BNT162b2 vaccine and Bell's palsy.**

**Conclusion 5-1: The evidence favors rejection of a causal relationship between the BNT162b2 vaccine and thrombosis with thrombocytopenia syndrome.**

**Conclusion 6-1: The evidence favors rejection of a causal relationship between the BNT162b2 vaccine and myocardial infarction.**

**Conclusion 6-5: The evidence favors rejection of a causal relationship between the BNT162b2 vaccine and ischemic stroke.**

**Conclusion 7-1: The evidence establishes a causal relationship between the BNT162b2 vaccine and myocarditis.**

**Conclusion 9-1: The evidence favors rejection of a causal relationship between the BNT162b2 vaccine and female infertility.**

For all other possible harms studied, the conclusion was that the evidence was inadequate to accept or reject a causal relationship with the BNT162b2 vaccine.

---

**BOX 11-2**
**Conclusions Regarding mRNA-1273**

**Conclusion 3-2:** The evidence favors rejection of a causal relationship between the mRNA-1273 vaccine and Guillain-Barré syndrome.

**Conclusion 3-10:** The evidence favors rejection of a causal relationship between the mRNA-1273 vaccine and Bell's palsy.

**Conclusion 5-2:** The evidence favors rejection of a causal relationship between the mRNA-1273 vaccine and thrombosis with thrombocytopenia syndrome.

**Conclusion 6-2:** The evidence favors rejection of a causal relationship between the mRNA-1273 vaccine and myocardial infarction.

**Conclusion 7-2:** The evidence establishes a causal relationship between the mRNA-1273 vaccine and myocarditis.

**Conclusion 9-2:** The evidence favors rejection of a causal relationship between the mRNA-1273 vaccine and female infertility.

For all other possible harms studied, the conclusion was that the evidence was inadequate to accept or reject a causal relationship with the mRNA-1273 vaccine.

---

**BOX 11-3**
**Conclusions Regarding Ad26.COV2.S**

**Conclusion 3-3:** The evidence favors acceptance of a causal relationship between the Ad26.COV2.S vaccine and Guillain-Barré syndrome.

**Conclusion 5-3:** The evidence favors acceptance of a causal relationship between the Ad26.COV2.S vaccine and thrombosis with thrombocytopenia syndrome.

For all other possible harms studied, the conclusion was that the evidence was inadequate to accept or reject a causal relationship with the Ad26.COV2.S vaccine.

---

**BOX 11-4**
**Conclusions Regarding NVX-CoV2373**

For all possible harms studied, the evidence was inadequate to accept or reject a causal relationship with the NVX-CoV2373 vaccine.

The committee made separate conclusions for each vaccine, even if they were of the same platform. However, the conclusions for the two messenger ribonucleic acid (mRNA) vaccines were almost identical:

- Evidence establishing a causal relationship with both vaccines and myocarditis;
- Evidence favoring rejection of a causal relationship between both vaccines and thrombosis with thrombocytopenia syndrome (TTS), infertility, Guillain-Barré syndrome (GBS), Bell's palsy (BP), and myocardial infarction (MI) (numerous studies support the conclusions about GBS, BP, and MI; the evidence for TTS and infertility was more limited but still suggested no effect); and
- Evidence favoring rejection of a causal relationship between BNT162b2 and ischemic stroke, but the evidence was inadequate to accept or reject a causal relationship for mRNA-1273, as the data were more limited.

Despite the limited use of Ad26.COV2.S in the United States and a limited number of published studies, the committee identified sufficient evidence to favor acceptance of a causal relationship with two specific adverse events, TTS and GBS. The evidence bases for these two conclusions were very different. The conclusion about TTS relied heavily on strong mechanistic evidence that vaccination induced anti-PF4 antibody to platelets in people with TTS. Although the mechanistic findings for ChAdOx1-S were strong, it was not used in the United States. The similar, although less striking, mechanistic findings with Ad26.COV2.S, combined with pharmacovigilance data, led the committee to Conclusion 5-3: the evidence favors acceptance of a causal relationship between it and TTS. The data supporting Conclusion 3-1 about GBS were based on strong epidemiological studies and pharmacovigilance data.

## SHOULDER INJURY CONCLUSIONS

The committee concentrated on case reports as the primary source of analysis, evaluating individual cases to arrive at the conclusions (see Box 11-5). Here, the committee was not limited to COVID-19 vaccines. The committee has examined evidence regarding shoulder injuries post-vaccination, exploring three potential mechanisms: direct trauma from improper placement, injury following injection regardless of technique, and vaccine constituents inducing harm, aiming to determine primary causative factors.

---

**BOX 11-5**
**Conclusions Regarding Shoulder Injuries**

**Conclusion 10-1:** The evidence establishes a causal relationship between vaccine administration and subacromial/subdeltoid bursitis caused by direct injection into the bursa.

**Conclusion 10-2:** The evidence establishes a causal relationship between vaccine administration and acute rotator cuff or acute biceps tendinopathy caused by direct injection into or adjacent to the tendon.

**Conclusion 10-3:** The evidence favors rejection of a causal relationship between vaccine administration and chronic rotator cuff disease.

**Conclusion 10-6:** The evidence establishes a causal relationship between vaccine administration and bone injury caused by direct injection into or adjacent to the bone.

**Conclusion 10-7:** The evidence establishes a causal relationship between vaccine administration and axillary or radial nerve injury caused by direct injection into or adjacent to the nerve.

For all other shoulder injuries studied, the conclusion was that the evidence was inadequate to accept or reject a causal relationship.

---

## SUMMARY BY CAUSAL CATEGORY

The committee made six conclusions that the evidence *establishes* a causal relationship with vaccination (see Box 11-6); the evidence fell into two broad categories. The conclusions regarding the mRNA vaccines, BNT162b2 and mRNA-1273, and myocarditis relied on large epidemiological studies that were consistent with well-supported mechanistic evidence. Studies in animal models and ex vivo human samples show a connection between myocarditis and the activation of immune pathways, such as Toll-like receptor 4/inflammasome/interleukin (IL)-1β, triggered by mRNA COVID-19 vaccines. In patients with vaccine-associated myocarditis, the spike protein has been detected in myocardial tissue and is accompanied by elevated blood levels. The conclusions regarding certain shoulder injuries after intramuscular vaccination (independent of type) relied heavily on numerous well-documented case reports and a good mechanistic understanding that injection directly into certain areas of the shoulder could lead to injury.

The committee also made two conclusions that the evidence *favors acceptance* of a causal relationship for Ad26.COV2.S and GBS and TTS (see Box 11-7). As described, the evidence bases for these two conclusions varied.

---

### BOX 11-6
### Conclusions for Which the Evidence Establishes a Causal Relationship

**Conclusion 7-1:** The evidence establishes a causal relationship between the BNT162b2 vaccine and myocarditis.

**Conclusion 7-2:** The evidence establishes a causal relationship between the mRNA-1273 vaccine and myocarditis.

**Conclusion 10-1:** The evidence establishes a causal relationship between vaccine administration and subacromial/subdeltoid bursitis caused by direct injection into the bursa.

**Conclusion 10-2:** The evidence establishes a causal relationship between vaccine administration and acute rotator cuff or acute biceps tendinopathy caused by direct injection into or adjacent to the tendon.

**Conclusion 10-6:** The evidence establishes a causal relationship between vaccine administration and bone injury caused by direct injection into or adjacent to the bone.

**Conclusion 10-7:** The evidence establishes a causal relationship between vaccine administration and axillary or radial nerve injury caused by direct injection into or adjacent to the nerve.

---

### BOX 11-7
### Conclusions for Which the Evidence Favors Acceptance of a Causal Relationship

**Conclusion 3-3:** The evidence favors acceptance of a causal relationship between the Ad26.COV2.S vaccine and Guillain-Barré syndrome.

**Conclusion 5-3:** The evidence favors acceptance of a causal relationship between the Ad26.COV2.S vaccine and thrombosis with thrombocytopenia syndrome.

The committee made conclusions *favoring rejection* of causality for 12 vaccine–adverse event relationships (see Box 11-8). Although the committee concluded that the evidence establishes a causal relationship with Ad26. COV2.S for GBS and TTS, it concluded that the evidence favored rejection with each of the mRNA vaccines. This supports the understanding that vaccine platform distinctly influenced the adverse physiologic and immune response. The committee also favored rejection of a causal relationship for the mRNA vaccines and several other outcomes: female infertility, BP, and MI. The committee favored rejection of a causal relationship between BNT162b2 and ischemic stroke but found that the evidence was inadequate to accept or reject a causal relationship between mRNA-1273 and ischemic stroke. The evidence base varied widely for these conclusions. The committee made one conclusion related to shoulder injuries, favoring rejection of a causal relationship for chronic rotator cuff disease following vaccination with any vaccine.

---

**BOX 11-8**
**Conclusions for Which the Evidence Favors Rejection of a Causal Relationship**

**Conclusion 3-1:** The evidence favors rejection of a causal relationship between the BNT162b2 vaccine and Guillain-Barré syndrome.

**Conclusion 3-2:** The evidence favors rejection of a causal relationship between the mRNA-1273 vaccine and Guillain-Barré syndrome.

**Conclusion 3-9:** The evidence favors rejection of a causal relationship between the BNT162b2 vaccine and Bell's palsy.

**Conclusion 3-10:** The evidence favors rejection of a causal relationship between the mRNA-1273 vaccine and Bell's palsy.

**Conclusion 5-1:** The evidence favors rejection of a causal relationship between the BNT162b2 vaccine and thrombosis with thrombocytopenia syndrome.

**Conclusion 5-2:** The evidence favors rejection of a causal relationship between the mRNA-1273 vaccine and thrombosis with thrombocytopenia syndrome.

**Conclusion 6-1:** The evidence favors rejection of a causal relationship between the BNT162b2 vaccine and myocardial infarction.

**Conclusion 6-2:** The evidence favors rejection of a causal relationship between the mRNA-1273 vaccine and myocardial infarction.

**Conclusion 6-5:** The evidence favors rejection of a causal relationship between the BNT162b2 vaccine and ischemic stroke.

**Conclusion 9-1:** The evidence favors rejection of a causal relationship between the BNT162b2 vaccine and female infertility.

**Conclusion 9-2:** The evidence favors rejection of a causal relationship between the mRNA-1273 vaccine and female infertility.

**Conclusion 10-3:** The evidence favors rejection of a causal relationship between vaccine administration and chronic rotator cuff disease.

For most of the potential harms studied, the evidence was inadequate. Reasons for this include a paucity of studies (e.g., capillary leak syndrome [CLS]), difficulty in diagnostic accuracy (e.g., tinnitus), or methodological flaws, such as difficulty controlling for confounders. For some outcomes, the evidence was inadequate even given a large body of literature because the studies had conflicting results (e.g., pulmonary embolism after mRNA vaccination).

## EVIDENCE IN CHILDREN

As noted in Chapter 1, potential vaccine-associated harms may differ in children and adults. For this reason, the committee conducted an in-depth review of the literature on adverse events to vaccines against SARS-CoV-2 specifically in children (under 18 years of age). At the time of committee review, data were available only for BNT162b2 and mRNA-1273. EUAs were later than for adults, and decreased uptake of vaccines in children, particularly those younger than 11, has led to far less data. Among the potential harms evaluated by the committee, infertility is not relevant to the pediatric population and has not been studied in children.

### Children Younger Than 12

Few data exist for any possible harm other than myocarditis in children younger than 12. For myocarditis, surveillance studies of risk after COVID-19 vaccination have been conducted in children aged 5–11 (Walter et al., 2022), in addition to the original randomized clinical trials (Creech et al., 2022), as noted in the chapter on myocarditis. Multiple studies provide point estimates of risk (e.g., 1.3 cases per million children after the first dose and 1.8 cases per million after the second dose in one systematic review evaluating risk after either BNT162b2 or mRNA-1273 [Simões et al., 2023] or 1–5 cases per million according to the surveillance database used in a study of BNT162b2 [Watanabe et al., 2023]). A Danish surveillance study after BNT162b2 estimated incidence at 4.8 cases per million and used historical background incidence data to calculate a vaccine-associated myocarditis risk ratio of 4.6 (95% confidence interval: 0.1–156.1) (Hause et al., 2022). The absolute increase in risk from BNT162b2 and mRNA-1273 in the 5–11 age group appears to be less than in the 12–17 years and young adult age groups, but because of the epidemiological evidence, the magnitude of risk in this age group is uncertain. Additional research could shed light on the risk in this age group.

Data are sparse on the risk of myocarditis after COVID-19 vaccine in children 6 months to 4 years. The largest surveillance study, using the Vaccine Adverse Event Reporting System data, documented no cases of myocarditis after 599,457 doses of BNT162b2 or 440,773 doses of mRNA-1273 (Hause et al., 2021). Data in children 6 months to 4 years of age are insufficient to evaluate risk of myocarditis after COVID-19 vaccination, since myocarditis is rare in this age group.

Data in children under 12 on the association of COVID-19 vaccines with immune-mediated mechanisms (TTS, immune thrombocytopenic purpura. CLS), neurologic syndromes (GBS, chronic inflammatory demyelinating polyneuropathy, BP, transverse myelitis), postural orthostatic tachycardia syndrome (POTS), sensorineural hearing loss or tinnitus, sudden death, or thromboembolic events (MI, ischemic stroke, hemorrhagic stroke, deep vein thrombosis, pulmonary embolism, venous thromboembolism) are limited to small observational studies, case series, and case reports. In some cases, no data are available at all. The paucity of data on most adverse events in children, particularly children <12 years of age, highlights both the poor immunization rates in children, an equity issue that is important to address with improved access to COVID-19 vaccines for children, and the need for further study of acute and long-term adverse events after COVID-19 vaccination in children.

### Children Older Than 12

More data are available on potential harms in children 12+ than in those younger. As outlined in Chapter 7, substantial data are available on the risk of myocarditis in children 12+ and show an increased risk of myocarditis for boys. Findings are summarized in that chapter; for example, in the systematic review Living Evidence Synthesis conducted by the Canada's Strategy for Patient-Oriented Research, findings from 16 studies of children 12–17 years old provided an estimated range in boys of 13–390 cases per million, all estimates above population norms, but the range for girls was 1–50 cases per million (Su, 2021). The findings in children 12–17 are consistent with findings in adults of increased risk of myocarditis, particularly in boys.

For a number of other potential harms, data in large surveillance studies include children 12+ and adults, but pediatric-specific findings on potential harms were not analyzed. For example, some studies of neurologic outcomes included children 12–17, but none described findings specific to children. Similarly, a large study of multiple immune-mediated, thromboembolic, and neurologic outcomes included children 12–17 but did not include age-specific risk estimates (Hause et al., 2022). For these outcomes, multiple studies included individuals 16+, as outlined in the previous chapters, but made no separate evaluation of them. Data on chronic headache, POTS, or sudden death in association with the COVID-19 vaccine in children 12+ were limited to case reports.

The data reviewed highlight the paucity of information specifically in children on possible harms after COVID-19 vaccination. Because so little data are available for children, particularly those under 12, for most of the harms reviewed, and because of the insufficient time or immunization of younger children to detect infrequent harms, including harms that are infrequent or nonexistent in adults, ongoing and future pharmacovigilance and epidemiology studies will produce more definitive data on the risk and relative incidence of harms.

## Shoulder Injuries in Children

Data on shoulder injury, as summarized in Chapter 10, are largely limited to case reports or small case series. Among specific shoulder injury diagnoses, pediatric case reports of the potential harm after vaccination were not found for subacromial/subdeltoid bursitis, axillary or radial nerve injury, bone injury, acute rotator cuff injury, or septic arthritis, suggesting that these are very rare in children. Pediatric cases or case series were reported for Parsonage-Turner syndrome, adhesive capsulitis, and complex regional pain syndrome after vaccination did not provide sufficient evidence for conclusions regarding risk.

## CONCLUDING REMARKS

The COVID-19 pandemic resulted in voluminous research in many disciplines on many topics by many investigators conducted very quickly. Many factors complicated this research. Vaccines were approved or authorized for use at different times for different populations in different countries. Older people were among the first groups to receive the vaccine; they often have comorbidities that could have put them at risk for health problems simply concurrent with vaccination. The communities being vaccinated had widespread SARS-CoV-2 infection, so that few studies were able to exclude patients with an infection that occurred simultaneously with vaccination. Thus, some of the conditions might reflect harms from infection rather than vaccination. Epidemiological patterns of non-COVID-19 infections changed dramatically during the early days of the pandemic and the vaccination campaigns due to social distancing and other public health interventions. See the discussion on GBS in Chapter 3 as an example. This complicates the use of historical controls in some studies. Many publications report surveillance findings, which do not use comparison populations. Rather, comparisons are made to historical trends, not a true contemporaneous unvaccinated population. Other methodologic limitations in many of the studies include challenges in confirming vaccine receipt and in diagnostic validity.

Many studies reviewed by the committee in this report were not initiated to support causal inference reviews such as this. Thus, although a particular paper might have had limited utility to this committee, it likely has relevance and immense purpose to others. The committee appreciates the work of the researchers and participants involved in these studies often under the very difficult circumstances of an ongoing public health emergency and hopes that the information and conclusions in this report are useful to the vaccine research community at large.

# REFERENCES

Creech, C. B., E. Anderson, V. Berthaud, I. Yildirim, A. M. Atz, I. Melendez Baez, D. Finkelstein, P. Pickrell, J. Kirstein, C. Yut, R. Blair, R. A. Clifford, M. Dunn, J. D. Campbell, D. C. Montefiori, J. E. Tomassini, X. Zhao, W. Deng, H. Zhou, D. Ramirez Schrempp, K. Hautzinger, B. Girard, K. Slobod, R. McPhee, R. Pajon, R. Das, J. M. Miller, and S. Schnyder Ghamloush. 2022. Evaluation of mRNA-1273 COVID-19 vaccine in children 6 to 11 years of age. *New England Journal of Medicine* 386(21):2011–2023. https://doi.org/10.1056/NEJMoa2203315.

FDA (U.S. Food and Drug Administration). 2022. *Coronavirus (COVID-19) update: FDA authorizes emergency use of Novavax COVID-19 vaccine, adjuvanted.* https://www.fda.gov/news-events/press-announcements/coronavirus-covid-19-update-fda-authorizes-emergency-use-novavax-covid-19-vaccine-adjuvanted (accessed December 20, 2023).

Hause, A. M., J. Baggs, P. Marquez, T. R. Myers, J. Gee, J. R. Su, B. Zhang, D. Thompson, T. T. Shimabukuro, and D. K. Shay. 2021. COVID-19 vaccine safety in children aged 5–11 years—United States, November 3—December 19, 2021. *MMWR: Morbidity and Mortality Weekly Report* 70(51–52):1755–1760. https://doi.org/10.15585/mmwr.mm705152a1.

Hause, A. M., D. K. Shay, N. P. Klein, W. E. Abara, J. Baggs, M. M. Cortese, B. Fireman, J. Gee, J. M. Glanz, K. Goddard, K. E. Hanson, B. Hugueley, T. Kenigsberg, E. O. Kharbanda, B. Lewin, N. Lewis, P. Marquez, T. Myers, A. Naleway, J. C. Nelson, J. R. Su, D. Thompson, B. Olubajo, M. E. Oster, E. S. Weintraub, J. T. B. Williams, A. R. Yousaf, O. Zerbo, B. Zhang, and T. T. Shimabukuro. 2022. Safety of COVID-19 vaccination in United States children ages 5 to 11 years. *Pediatrics* 150(2). https://doi.org/10.1542/peds.2022-057313.

Simões, E. A. F., N. P. Klein, C. Sabharwal, A. Gurtman, N. Kitchin, B. Ukkonen, P. Korbal, J. Zou, X. Xie, U. N. Sarwar, X. Xu, S. Lockhart, L. Cunliffe, C. Lu, H. Ma, K. A. Swanson, K. Koury, P. Y. Shi, D. Cooper, Ö. Türeci, K. U. Jansen, U. Şahin, and W. C. Gruber. 2023. Immunogenicity and safety of a third COVID-19 BNT162b2 mRNA vaccine dose in 5- to 11-year-olds. *Journal of the Pediatric Infectious Diseases Society* 12(4):234–238. https://doi.org/10.1093/jpids/piad015.

Su, J. R. 2021. Adverse events among children ages 5–11 years after COVID-19 vaccination: Updates from V-Safe and the Vaccine Adverse Event Reporting System (VAERS). Centers for Disease Control and Prevention.

Walter, E. B., K. R. Talaat, C. Sabharwal, A. Gurtman, S. Lockhart, G. C. Paulsen, E. D. Barnett, F. M. Muñoz, Y. Maldonado, B. A. Pahud, J. B. Domachowske, E. A. F. Simões, U. N. Sarwar, N. Kitchin, L. Cunliffe, P. Rojo, E. Kuchar, M. Rämet, I. Munjal, J. L. Perez, R. W. Frenck, Jr., E. Lagkadinou, K. A. Swanson, H. Ma, X. Xu, K. Koury, S. Mather, T. J. Belanger, D. Cooper, Ö. Türeci, P. R. Dormitzer, U. Şahin, K. U. Jansen, and W. C. Gruber. 2022. Evaluation of the BNT162b2 COVID-19 vaccine in children 5 to 11 years of age. *New England Journal of Medicine* 386(1):35–46. https://doi.org/10.1056/NEJMoa2116298.

Watanabe, A., R. Kani, M. Iwagami, H. Takagi, J. Yasuhara, and T. Kuno. 2023. Assessment of efficacy and safety of mRNA COVID-19 vaccines in children aged 5 to 11 years: A systematic review and meta-analysis. *JAMA Pediatrics* 177(4):384–394. https://doi.org/10.1001/jamapediatrics.2022.6243.

# Appendix A

# Committee Member and Staff Biographies

## COMMITTEE MEMBERS

**George J. Isham, M.D. M.S.** (*Chair*), is a senior fellow at the HealthPartners Institute and a senior advisor for the Alliance of Community Health Plans. He was HealthPartners' medical director and chief health officer, responsible for quality of care and health and health care improvement. He was a member of the Centers for Disease Control and Prevention's Task Force on Community Preventive Services and the Agency for Healthcare Research and Quality's United States Preventive Services Task Force and the founding cochair of the National Committee for Quality Assurance's committee on performance measurement and the National Quality Forum's Measurement Application Partnership. Dr. Isham is a member of the National Academy of Medicine. He has an M.D. from the University of Illinois Chicago and an M.S. in preventive medicine and administrative medicine from the University of Wisconsin–Madison.

**Anne R. Bass, M.D.** (*Vice Chair*), is a professor of clinical medicine at Weill Cornell Medicine and a practicing rheumatologist at the Hospital for Special Surgery and New York Presbyterian Hospital (Cornell). She was the principal investigator for the 2022 American College of Rheumatology (ACR) Guideline for Vaccinations in Patients with Rheumatic and Musculoskeletal Diseases (RMD) and a member of the core group for the ACR Guidance for COVID-19 Vaccination in Patients with RMD. Dr. Bass is currently the treasurer of the ACR and the Rheumatology Research Foundations. Her clinical research focuses on the autoimmune effects of immune checkpoint inhibitor cancer therapy, particularly inflammatory arthritis. She received her undergraduate degree at Harvard and earned her M.D. and was a resident at Columbia, followed by a rheumatology fellowship at New York University.

**Alicia Christy, M.D.,** was the deputy director of reproductive health at the Veterans Health Administration. She served as the chair of the Department of Obstetrics and Gynecology and a consultant to the Army Surgeon General. She was a clinical researcher at the National Institutes of Health (NIH), where her research focused primarily on the areas of contraception, treatment of leiomyoma, and health disparities. She has been involved in evidence review for two U.S. Department of Veterans Affairs (VA) and U.S. Department of Defense clinical practice guidelines. She was the coeditor of *Contraception and Reproductive Medicine*. She held the rank of professor at the Uniformed Services University and adjunct professor at Howard University. Dr. Christy has received the NIH Award of Merit, multiple research awards, the NIH Collaborator Award, a Humanism in Medicine Award, an Excellence in Teaching Award, and a Mentor of the Year Award. She was the chair of the American Society of Reproductive

Medicine Health Disparities Special Interest Group and the VA liaison to an American College of Obstetricians and Gynecologists committee. Dr. Christy received her undergraduate degree from Princeton University, is an Alpha Omega Alpha graduate of Northwestern University School of Medicine, and received an M.A. in health science and clinical research from the Duke University School of Medicine.

**DeLisa Fairweather, Ph.D.,** is a professor of medicine, the director of translational research in the Department of Cardiovascular Medicine, and the codirector of research for the Ehlers-Danlos Syndrome Clinic at the Mayo Clinic in Jacksonville, Florida. In addition to an interest in myocarditis, dilated cardiomyopathy, and heart failure, Dr. Fairweather specializes in how sex differences in inflammation caused by environmental exposures, such as viruses, lead to chronic inflammatory diseases, such as autoimmune diseases, cardiovascular disease, cancer, and lung disease. She was a coinvestigator and leader of the Mayo-led U.S. Food and Drug Administration–funded Expanded Access Program that provided convalescent plasma to patients with COVID-19 during the first year of the pandemic. She was a standing member of the Atherosclerosis and Inflammation of the Cardiovascular System Study Section at the National Institutes of Health for 6 years, and she serves on the Medical Advisory Board for the Myocarditis Foundation. She obtained her Ph.D. at the University of Western Australia in microbiology and immunology and conducted a postdoctoral fellowship at Johns Hopkins University.

**James S. Floyd, M.D., M.S.,** is a physician at the Harborview Medical Center, an associate professor of medicine (general internal medicine) and adjunct associate professor of epidemiology at the University of Washington, and an affiliate investigator at the Kaiser Permanente Washington Health Research Institute. He has expertise in cardiovascular epidemiology and drug safety, including postmarket surveillance using electronic health data, and is an active investigator in several National Heart, Lung, and Blood Institute–funded prospective cohort studies and international research consortia. In 2019 he acted as a consultant for Shionogi.[1] Dr. Floyd earned his M.D. from Duke University. He completed a T32 Fellowship in cardiovascular epidemiology at the University of Washington Cardiovascular Health Research Unit, where he is the codirector.

**Eric J. Hegedus, Ph.D., D.P.T., M.H.Sc.,** is an orthopedic physical therapist and a professor with the Tufts University School of Medicine. He was a professor at High Point University, where he developed its Doctor of Physical Therapy (D.P.T.) program, and an associate professor at Duke University. He has more than 30 years of clinical experience and has taught in the United States and abroad. Dr. Hegedus answers clinical questions in the orthopedic and sports prevention, diagnosis, and rehabilitation realm and translates the findings to clinical practice. He has been a member of the American Physical Therapy Association since 1991 and received its national James A. Gould Teaching Award, given annually to the single most deserving teaching professor of musculoskeletal physical therapy. Dr. Hegedus earned a Ph.D. from the University of Ulster, a D.P.T. from Slippery Rock University, and an M.H.Sc. from Duke University.

**Chandy C. John, M.D., M.S.,** holds the Ryan White Endowed Chair in Pediatric Infectious Diseases and is the director of the Ryan White Center for Pediatric Infectious Diseases and Global Health at Indiana University. He investigates why children develop, survive, or die from malaria and studies ways to prevent malaria and other infections in children with sickle cell disease. Dr. John is a cochair of the Thrasher Research Fund Scientific Advisory Committee and a member of the Fogarty International Center Advisory Board, the American Academy of Pediatrics Committee on Infectious Diseases, and the Centers for Disease Control and Prevention Advisory Committee on Immunization Practices Polio Working Group. Dr. John received the Bailey K. Ashford Medal from the American Society of Tropical Medicine and Hygiene in 2011 and was its president in 2019. He earned his M.D. and was a resident in internal medicine and pediatrics at the University of Michigan and completed fellowship training in pediatric infectious diseases at Case Western Reserve University.

---

[1] Dr. Floyd's biography was updated since the release of the report to disclose his prior relationship with Shionogi.

**John E. (Jed) Kuhn, M.D., M.S.,** is the Kenneth D. Schermerhorn Professor in the Department of Orthopedic Surgery in the Vanderbilt University Medical Center and the director of the Sports Medicine and Shoulder Surgery Division; he joined in 2003 to build that division. Dr. Kuhn is the founder of the Multicenter Orthopedic Outcomes Network Shoulder Group—a multicenter research collaboration designed to study conditions about the shoulder. He is the president elect for the American Shoulder and Elbow Surgeons and the deputy editor in chief for the *Journal of Shoulder and Elbow Surgery*. He earned his M.D. and was a resident in orthopedic surgery at the University of Michigan and then a fellow in sports medicine and shoulder surgery at the Steadman Howking Clinic in Vail, Colorado. He returned as a faculty member at the University of Michigan for 8 years.

**Evan Mayo-Wilson, Ph.D., M.P.A.,** is an associate professor of epidemiology at the University of North Carolina Gillings School of Global Public Health. His research aims to improve public health and to advance methods for conducting health and behavioral research. He focuses on (1) evaluating the effectiveness of pharmacological and behavioral interventions, (2) improving methods for clinical trials and systematic reviews, and (3) developing methods and interventions to increase research transparency and openness. Dr. Mayo-Wilson serves on several editorial boards, including as the associate editor for systematic reviews for the *American Journal of Public Health*. He has contributed to several reporting guidelines and to guidance for increasing transparency and openness. Dr. Mayo-Wilson completed his D.Phil. in the Department of Social Policy and Intervention at University of Oxford. He also has degrees in public administration (M.P.A., University of Pennsylvania) and evidence-based intervention (M.Sc., University of Oxford).

**Thomas Lee Ortel, M.D., Ph.D.,** the chief of hematology and a professor of medicine and pathology at Duke University, is nationally and internationally recognized for his clinical and research expertise in hemostatic and thrombotic disorders. His primary interests focus on rare antibody-mediated thrombotic disorders, including antiphospholipid antibody syndrome and heparin-induced thrombocytopenia, and developing and managing novel antithrombotic therapies. His experience conducting prospective, randomized, multicenter clinical trials and interest in rare thrombotic disorders resulted in becoming the study chair for the National Heart, Lung, and Blood Institute–sponsored Accelerating COVID-19 Therapeutic Interventions and Vaccines Post-Hospital Thrombosis Prevention Study, investigating the use of extended thromboprophylaxis to prevent thromboembolic complications. Dr. Ortel has been the site principal investigator at Duke University for studies funded by Takeda Pharmaceutical Company on the treatment of patients with congenital and acquired thrombotic thrombocytopenic purpura since 2020, and, previously, a study on acquired hemophilia, during which he also received compensation for a steering committee meeting. As of December 2023, he is serving as a consultant to Takeda on the steering committee for the phase 3 study using recombinant ADAMTS13 in patients with acquired thrombotic thrombocytopenic purpura. In 2023 he reviewed the results of a clinical trial for a drug to treat hemophilia, for which he was compensated by Sanofi.[2] During the past year, he collaborated with colleagues at the Centers for Disease Control and Prevention on the Clinical Immunization Safety Assessment Project related to the development of thrombosis with thrombocytopenia syndrome after COVID-19 vaccination. He completed a combined M.D./Ph.D. program at Indiana University in 1985, followed by internship and residency training in internal medicine and fellowship training in hematology and medical oncology, both at Duke University.

**Nicholas S. Reed, Au.D., Ph.D.,** is an assistant professor in the Department of Epidemiology at the Johns Hopkins Bloomberg School of Public Health with a joint appointment in the Department of Otolaryngology—Head and Neck Surgery (Audiology) at the Johns Hopkins University School of Medicine. He is the director of the Audiology Core at the Johns Hopkins Cochlear Center for Hearing and Public Health, where he oversees integrating and managing hearing measures in multiple large epidemiological cohort studies and clinical trials. His research focuses on the association of hearing loss among older adults with healthy aging outcomes, including cognitive

---

[2] Dr. Ortel's biography was updated since the release of this report to disclose his role as a site principal investigator for studies at Duke University funded by Takeda Pharmaceutical Company related to treatment of patients with congenital and acquired thrombotic thrombocytopenic purpura and hemophilia, as well as service on steering committees during the course of the study.

decline and health resource use, the impact of hearing intervention on health outcomes, and novel models of hearing care delivery. He earned the Early Career Research Award in 2021 from the American Auditory Society. Dr. Reed received his Ph.D. in audiology from Towson University and completed his audiology clinical fellowship at Georgetown University Hospital. He sat on the National Academies of Sciences, Engineering, and Medicine's Committee on Evaluating Hearing Loss for Individuals with Cochlear Implants.

**Andy S. Stergachis, Ph.D., B.Pharm.,** is a professor of pharmacy and global health and the director of the Global Medicines Program and the associate dean for research, graduate studies, and new initiatives, School of Pharmacy, University of Washington (UW). He is the director of the UW Biomedical Regulatory Affairs Program and an adjunct in the UW Departments of Health Metrics and Evaluation, Epidemiology, and Health Systems and Population Health. He is an author of publications in areas such as pharmacovigilance, pharmacoepidemiology, pharmaceutical services, and clinical epidemiology. He has developed and evaluated novel approaches for safety surveillance of essential medicines and vaccines. A licensed pharmacist, he served as the editor in chief of the *Journal of the American Pharmacists Association* for 6 years, until 2019. He is a member of the CEPI Maternal Immunization Working Group (formerly via COVAX). Dr. Stergachis is an elected member of the National Academy of Medicine, a fellow of the American Pharmacists Association, and a fellow of the International Society for Pharmacoepidemiology. He received a Ph.D. in social and administrative pharmacy from the University of Minnesota.

**Michel Toledano, M.D.,** is an assistant professor of neurology and the medical director for inpatient neurology services at the Mayo Clinic in Rochester, Minnesota. He completed his neurology residency at the Mayo Clinic, where he pursued a fellowship in multiple sclerosis. He then undertook a fellowship in neuroinfectious diseases at Chelsea and Westminster Hospital in London, United Kingdom. His research interests include improving care delivery models for hospitalized neurology patients and optimizing diagnostic test use, especially for patients presenting with encephalitis and other infectious or neuroinflammatory syndromes. Dr. Toledano earned his M.D. from Ben-Gurion University of the Negev.

**Robert B. Wallace, M.D., M.Sc.,** is an emeritus professor of epidemiology and internal medicine at the University of Iowa (UI) College of Public Health. He was trained in general internal medicine. After his residency, he worked at the Centers for Disease Control and Prevention, where he specialized in the epidemiology and control of several communicable and vaccine-preventable diseases, including measles, mumps and rubella, smallpox, and agents more common in tropical countries, and the infectious causes of chronic illnesses, such as some cancers. During his long career at UI, he researched the prevention and control of several chronic illnesses of older people, such as cardiovascular disease, cancer, and other disabling conditions, including Alzheimer's disease and other neurodegenerative conditions. He received the National Academy of Medicine (NAM) Walsh McDermott Medal in recognition for his distinguished service, having participated in more than 20 National Academies of Sciences, Engineering, and Medicine consensus committees, and is an elected member of the NAM. Dr. Wallace has an M.D. from Northwestern University in Illinois and an M.Sc. from the State University of New York at Buffalo.

**Ousseny Zerbo, Ph.D.,** is a research scientist II at the Vaccine Study Center at Kaiser Permanente Northern California, Division of Research. He is an epidemiologist with expertise in infectious diseases, neurodevelopmental disorders (autism), vaccine safety, and effectiveness. He is the principal investigator on two National Institutes of Health–funded projects to investigate the effectiveness of influenza vaccination, COVID-19 vaccination during pregnancy, and infant risk of influenza and COVID-19. He holds a Ph.D. in epidemiology from the University of California, Davis, and a B.S. in biological sciences from the Université de Ouagadougou.

## NATIONAL ACADEMY OF MEDICINE FELLOW

**Inmaculada (Inma) Hernandez, Ph.D.,** is an associate professor with tenure at the University of California, San Diego, Skaggs School of Pharmacy and Pharmaceutical Sciences. She has authored more than 100 scientific articles, including first-authored papers in *JAMA*, *JAMA Internal Medicine*, and *Annals of Internal Medicine*, among other leading journals. Her research has been covered by media worldwide and featured by main media outlets, including *The New York Times*, *The Washington Post*, NPR, CNN, *Forbes*, and BBC. Dr. Hernandez has studied extensively the underuse of anticoagulation in stroke prevention in patients with cardiac arrhythmias. She is the principal investigator of an R01 award from the National Institutes of Health to study the impact of the COVID-19 pandemic on patients with cardiovascular disease. She has made important contributions to the study of pharmaceutical pricing. In 2020, she was the first to quantify the role of manufacturer discounts in rising drug prices. In 2020–2021, Dr. Hernandez led a group of investigators evaluating geographic access to COVID-19 vaccine administration locations. Their analyses informed the Pennsylvania Department of Health vaccine distribution in medically underserved areas. Dr. Hernandez received her Pharm.D. from the University of Navarra in Spain, her M.S. in health economics and pharmacoeconomics from the Universitat Pompeu Fabra in Spain, and her Ph.D. in health services research and policy from the University of Pittsburgh. She was on the *Forbes* 30 under 30 list in 2018, and in 2021, she became the first pharmacist to be recognized with the Academy Health Alice S. Hersh Emerging Leader Award. She is a fellow of the American College of Cardiology and the American Heart Association.

## STAFF

**Kathleen Stratton, Ph.D.,** began her career at the National Academies of Sciences, Engineering, and Medicine in 1990 in the Institute of Medicine (IOM). She has spent most of her time with the Board on Population Health and Public Health Practice. She has staffed committees addressing vaccine safety and development, pandemic preparedness, environmental and occupational health, drug safety, clinical prevention research, and tobacco control. She was given the IOM Cecil Research Award for sustained contributions to vaccine safety and made a staff scholar in 2005. She received a B.A. in natural sciences from Johns Hopkins University and a Ph.D. in pharmacology and toxicology from the University of Maryland at Baltimore. She conducted postdoctoral research in the Department of Neuroscience at the Johns Hopkins University School of Medicine.

**Ogan K. Kumova, Ph.D.,** is a program officer for vaccine safety at the National Academies of Sciences, Engineering, and Medicine in the Health and Medicine Division. Prior to joining the National Academies, he was a research fellow at the U.S. Food and Drug Administration's (FDA's) Office of Vaccine Research and Review, where he worked on developing vaccines for infectious diseases. During his time at FDA, Dr. Kumova was a coinvestigator on grants evaluating the safety and immunogenicity of vaccine adjuvants and developing vaccines for meningococcal and gonococcal infections. He obtained his Ph.D. in immunology from the Drexel University College of Medicine in Philadelphia, Pennsylvania. In his graduate work, Dr. Kumova studied neonatal immune responses and modifiable risk factors for respiratory viral infections and collaborated with several labs, including Wistar Cancer Institute, to develop a DNA-based HIV vaccine. He holds a B.S. in biochemistry and bioinformatics from the University of the Sciences in Philadelphia and an M.S. in clinical infectious diseases from Drexel University.

**Dara Rosenberg, M.P.H.,** is an associate program officer in the Health and Medicine Division on the Board of Population Health and Public Health Practice. Before joining the National Academies of Sciences, Engineering, and Medicine, Ms. Rosenberg was an epidemiologist at a local health department. She has experience with communicable disease investigations, public health emergency preparedness, and data analysis, specifically with STI/HIV and COVID-19 data. She completed her B.S. in health sciences at the New York Institute of Technology and has an M.P.H. in epidemiology from The George Washington University.

**Olivia Loibner, B.A.,** is a senior program assistant in the Health and Medicine Division on the Board of Population Health and Public Health Practice. While at the National Academies of Sciences, Engineering, and Medicine, she has contributed to the Review of the Department of Veterans Affairs Presumption Decision Process and workshops on health equity. She received her B.A. in international studies from the American University School of International Service.

**Rose Marie Martinez, Sc.D.,** is the senior director of the Board on Population Health and Public Health Practice (1999–present) at the National Academies of Sciences, Engineering, and Medicine. The board conducts evidence-based studies that help shape health policy at the federal, state, and local levels. Dr. Martinez was a senior health researcher at Mathematica Policy Research (1995–1999), where she conducted health policy research. Dr. Martinez is a former assistant director for health financing and policy with the U.S. General Accounting Office, where she directed evaluations and policy analysis in the area of national and public health issues (1988–1995). Her experience also includes 6 years directing research studies for the Regional Health Ministry of Madrid, Spain (1982–1988). Dr. Martinez received a D.Sc. from the Johns Hopkins University School of Hygiene and Public Health.

# Appendix B

# Public Meeting Agenda

**COMMITTEE TO REVIEW RELEVANT LITERATURE REGARDING
ADVERSE EVENTS ASSOCIATED WITH VACCINES**

**The Keck Center, 500 Fifth Street, NW
Washington, DC 20001**

**Thursday, March 30, 2023**

| | |
|---|---|
| 12:00–12:05 ET | Welcome<br>**George J. Isham, M.D., M.S.,** *Committee Chair* |
| 12:05–1:15 | Public comment period for preregistered attendees |
| 1:15 | OPEN SESSION ENDS |